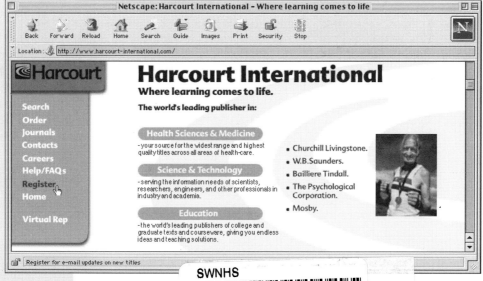

Essential Anatomy and Physiology in Maternity Care

For Churchill Livingstone:

Publishing Manager: Inta Ozols
Project Manager: Derek Robertson
Design Direction: George Ajayi

Essential Anatomy and Physiology in Maternity Care

Linda Wylie BA MN RGN RM RMT

Lecturer, Department of Nursing, Midwifery and Health Care,
University of Paisley, Scotland

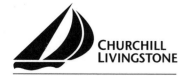

EDINBURGH LONDON NEW YORK PHILADELPHIA ST LOUIS SYDNEY TORONTO 2000

CHURCHILL LIVINGSTONE
An imprint of Harcourt Publishers Limited

© Harcourt Publishers Limited 2000

⬙ is a registered trademark of Harcourt Publishers
Limited

First published 2000

ISBN 0443 05998 5

British Library Cataloguing in Publication Data
A catalogue record for this book is available from the British
Library.

Library of Congress Cataloging in Publication Data
A catalog record for this book is available from the Library
of Congress.

Note
Medical knowledge is constantly changing. As new
information becomes available, changes in treatment,
procedures, equipment and the use of drugs become
necessary. The author and the publishers have taken care to
ensure that the information given in this text is accurate and
up-to-date. However, readers are strongly advised to
confirm that the information, especially with regard to drug
usage, complies with the latest legislation and standards of
practice.

The
publisher's
policy is to use
**paper manufactured
from sustainable forests**

Printed in China

Contents

Preface

With the introduction of 3-year preregistration midwifery programmes in the UK, it has become increasingly evident that student midwives require textbooks directly related to midwifery practice, rather than those relevant to nursing students. Life sciences is a subject that has traditionally been taught to student nurses and then supplemented during subsequent midwifery programmes. The number of life sciences textbooks for nurses reflects this. An obvious need has arisen for a life sciences textbook written specifically for student midwives, which relates the anatomy and physiology of the human body directly to midwifery practice.

This book is intended to meet this need. It covers all aspects of human anatomy and physiology at a fundamental level, and goes on to apply this knowledge to the changing physiology of pregnancy, childbirth and the puerperium. As student midwives frequently ask why they require a knowledge of certain aspects of human anatomy and physiology, boxes are included in each chapter, giving a clear indication of the relevance of each topic to midwifery.

References are included throughout the book, and relate specifically to the sections on pregnancy, labour and the postnatal period. The references have been selected with three purposes in mind:

1. Where possible, they are from recent research documented in journals that are stocked in most British university libraries. These will automatically lead the student to a wider selection of research papers, if these are required.

2. Evidence-based practice is expected to underpin midwifery, and rightly so. Therefore, where research-based evidence is not available, evidence from experts in the particular fields is referred to, cited in standard textbooks readily available.

3. References have been chosen to point the student midwife in the direction of articles which explore the topic more fully, and therefore should be a valuable resource for learning more about any of the topics introduced in this book.

November 1998

Note: For the purposes of this book, the midwife is referred to throughout as 'she', and the baby as 'he'.

Acknowledgements

Writing a book, as I now know, takes considerably more time than expected. I must therefore thank firstly my family – my husband Robert, and my children Sarah, Katie and Andrew – who have given up the dining room and more significantly the computer, for the majority of the evenings and weekends of the past year, to allow me to undertake this project.

Professionally, I thank all my colleagues in the Department of Nursing, Midwifery and Health Care at the University of Paisley, who have offered support and guidance on issues relating to this book. Specifically I would like to thank: members of the Life Science team, and especially Ivan Mills, for their guidance; the members of the midwifery team for listening to my monologues on format and inclusions; and members of the library, particularly Margot Stewart, for help in formatting references.

The human body through the childbearing year

PART CONTENTS

Part 1 begins with a brief introduction to the cells and tissues that make up the human body. It moves on to cover all body systems, except those involved in reproduction, firstly from the non-pregnant perspective and then through pregnancy, labour and the puerperium. The physiology of the neonate is also considered.

The sequence of the chapters does not reflect their order of importance to the student midwife, but represents a natural progression through control and integration, transportation, digestion and excretion.

1

Cells and tissues

Every living organism needs to carry out certain functions in order to survive. These include such activities as respiration, metabolism, excretion and reproduction. For the single-celled organism these can all be carried out via direct contact with the environment, through the cell membrane. For more complex organisms this is not possible, because layers of cells prevent all cells being in contact with the external environment. Cells therefore develop specific roles for the good of the organism as a whole. With increased complexity comes increased specialisation. The human animal is the most complex animal and so is highly specialised.

The human body is made up of the fundamental unit of all living animals: the *cell*. These cells are similar in structure, but differ according to their function. Collections of like cells become concentrated together to carry out their functions in *tissues*. Tissues then build up into a complex *organ* responsible for one or more essential functions. Finally these organs are organised into *systems*, which each have a vital role in the physiology of the body as a whole.

THE CELL

Cells are the smallest functional unit in the body (Fig. 1.1). They are not visible to the naked eye, but when viewed under a microscope they can be seen to contain small structures called *organelles*.

The *cell membrane* is a semipermeable double layer of phospholipids and proteins. The molecules of the double membrane are arranged in

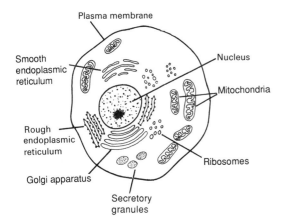

Figure 1.1 Microstructure of a typical animal cell. (Reproduced with permission from Wilson K J W, Waugh A 1996 Ross and Wilson Anatomy and Physiology in Health and Illness. Churchill Livingstone, Edinburgh)

such a way that the interior of the membrane repels water-soluble substances. By this means the membrane can control the substances that enter the cell, a vital factor in maintaining the equilibrium of the cell. Many essential substances can however freely diffuse across the membrane. Others that cannot are transported across by cell membrane proteins which act as carriers. Some proteins also act as receptors for chemical messengers and as markers which identify the cell as belonging to the body.

Inside the cell membrane is a fluid known as cytosol. *Cytosol* can be considered a chemical 'soup' which contains many different substances used in the chemical reactions that are constantly taking place within the cell. These reactions constitute the process known as metabolism. The functioning of the human body is the sum of all these metabolic processes.

Suspended in the cytosol are many organelles which each have specific functions. One such organelle is the cell nucleus. The *nucleus* is the principal player in the cell's metabolic processes. Surrounding the nucleus is a nuclear membrane containing pores, which allows selective movement of substances between the nucleus and the cytosol. The nucleus contains the genetic information that controls the cell's activities. This information is stored on long molecules of *deoxyribonucleic acid* (DNA). DNA is made up

of nucleotides that carry the genetic code of the organism. It contains one hundred thousand genes which can each be translated into the formula for an enzyme. Metabolic processes in the cell are carried out in the presence of enzymes. Specific metabolic processes are controlled therefore by specific genes expressed in the nucleus of the cell.

Each DNA molecule in the nucleus can be seen as a *chromosome* during the process of cell division (Fig. 1.2). There are 46 chromosomes in the human cell. On close examination these can be seen to be arranged in 23 pairs, 22 of which are identical. The 23rd pair of chromosomes is responsible for the sex of the person: a male has one X and one Y chromosome; a female has two X chromosomes. One of each of the chromosomes of the 23 pairs originated from the gamete (reproductive cell) of each parent. These interact, resulting in a person who is a unique individual taking on some of the characteristics of each parent.

When a cell divides, the genetic code is passed on to each subsequent cell. During cell reproduction each molecule of DNA becomes closely wound into the visible chromosome and at the same time makes a copy of itself. So when the cell divides, each new cell receives a copy of every

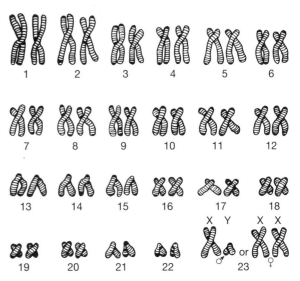

Figure 1.2 Chromosomes visible during cell division.

DNA molecule. This process is called *mitosis*. *Meiosis* is the specialised form of cell division responsible for the formation of gametes. In meiosis only one of each of the pair of chromosomes is passed on to the ovum or spermatozoon, ensuring that the subsequent fertilised ovum will contain the requisite 46 chromosomes.

Other organelles found in the cell include:

- *mitochondria*, involved in the production of energy to fuel the chemical reactions constantly taking place in the cell
- *golgi apparatus*, which packages the products of the cell into easily transported parcels for export through the cell membrane
- *endoplasmic reticulum*, along which substances are produced
- *ribosomes*, the sites of protein synthesis
- *lysosomes* and *peroxisomes*, which contain enzymes required for the breakdown of unwanted particles and microorganisms
- structural proteins such as *filaments* and *tubules* which maintain the shape of the cell and are involved in the functioning of cell membrane projections such as flagella and cilia.

FROM CELLS TO TISSUES

Cells with the same function are collected together as tissues. Tissues require access to all necessary nutrients and this is facilitated by the presence of fluids in the spaces between cells. Chemical substances dissolved or suspended in fluids are more mobile and the presence of fluid prevents dramatic changes in the physical environment.

There are two main types of fluid in the body.

1. intracellular fluid
2. extracellular fluid.

Intracellular fluid is found within cells. Its composition changes very little, ensuring that metabolic processes are not disrupted.

Extracellular fluid includes all other collections of fluid in the body, and can be subdivided into interstitial fluid, surrounding cells, and other fluids such as plasma, cerebrospinal fluid and lymph. The presence of these tissue fluids enables the body as a whole to maintain homeostasis.

Homeostasis is the maintenance of the body's internal environment within certain physiological limits. Body systems are structured to maintain homeostasis by, for example, providing nutrients from the external environment and removing wastes as required. Chemical buffers are also present within all tissue fluids to maintain the correct acid-base balance.

Substances move in and out of cells by both passive and active processes. Passive processes allow substances to move from areas of high concentration to areas of low concentration. This can happen by *diffusion* (e.g. oxygen and carbon dioxide across membranes), and *osmosis*, which moves water. Proteins can speed up these processes by binding with and transporting essential nutrients, such as glucose. Some body organs are structured to move large volumes of substances rapidly. The kidneys, for example, filter blood, due to the increased pressure produced, as blood enters the glomerulus. Similarly in the lungs, gases are moved more rapidly across membranes because of the pressure differences between the alveoli and the capillaries.

Active processes move substances against a gradient, or move larger particles in and out of the cell. These require an input of energy, which is usually provided by the cell itself. Active processes may set up a physiological process, or ensure that essential substances are not lost to the body. Alternatively they may be required as part of the body's defence mechanism against microorganisms.

An example of a physiological process can be found in the cells of the nervous system. An electrical differential between the inside and outside of a neurone is required to enable an action potential to be generated by the movement of ions when the neurone is stimulated. This differential is maintained by active transport.

Glucose is an example of an essential substance which is actively moved across membranes. As much glucose as possible is removed from the intestines – even when the concentration of glucose is higher in the cells than in the gut itself.

There are two main types of active processes:

1. active transport
2. endocytosis.

In *active transport* protein molecules in the cell membranes attach themselves to substances and transport them into the cell up a concentration gradient.

In *endocytosis* the cell membrane can change its configuration and move substances in bulk into the cell. An example of this is phagocytosis. Exocytosis is movement out of the cell.

TISSUES

There are four main types of body tissue:

1. epithelial tissue, which lines cavities and covers organs
2. connective tissue, which maintains structure and provides protection to some organs
3. muscle fibres, which make movement possible
4. nervous tissue, which responds to internal and external changes in the environment.

Muscle and nervous tissue are described in later chapters, in the context of the systems to which they relate. Epithelial and connective tissue are described below.

Epithelial tissue

Epithelial cells are involved in protection, secretion and absorption. These cells are packed closely together to form a membrane. The two main types of epithelial tissue are:

1. simple epithelium
2. stratified epithelium.

Simple epithelium

Simple epithelium is a single layer of identical cells involved in absorption or secretion. Several different types can be identified (Fig. 1.3). *Squamous epithelium* is composed of irregular-shaped flattened cells forming a thin, smooth membrane. Fluids and other substances can

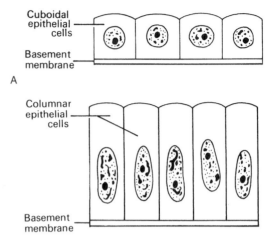

A

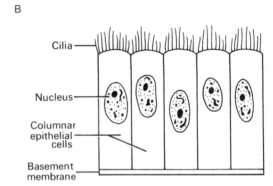

B

C

Figure 1.3 Simple epithelium. A: Cuboidal epithelium. B: Columnar epithelium. C: Ciliated columnar epithelium. (Reproduced with permission from Wilson K J W, Waugh A 1996 Ross and Wilson Anatomy and Physiology in Health and Illness. Churchill Livingstone, Edinburgh)

diffuse easily through these cells, so squamous epithelium forms the linings of structures such as blood and lymph vessels, where it is known as *endothelium*.

Cuboidal and columnar epithelia (named after the shape of their cells) are involved in absorption, secretion and excretion. *Cuboidal epithelium* is found in areas such as the tubules of the kidneys. *Columnar epithelium* is found in the gastrointestinal tract and includes cells which secrete mucus and digestive juices. *Ciliated columnar epithelium* is made up of cells with projections from the cell membrane called *cilia*. These are responsible for moving cells and

particles along tubes, as is the case with the ovum along the uterine tube.

Stratified epithelium

Stratified epithelium is composed of layers of cells of different types (Fig. 1.4). These cells are found in areas where there is a lot of wear and tear, and perform a protective function. The surface cells may contain keratin (e.g. in the skin), to waterproof and add strength to the tissue. As surface cells are damaged, cells in lower levels divide and migrate upwards to replace them. *Transitional epithelium* is a form of stratified epithelium in which the cells can alter shape. This is found in the bladder, where there is need for expansion.

Membranes and glands

Membranes are sheets of epithelial cells. There are three main types of membrane:

1. mucous membranes
2. serous membranes
3. synovial membranes.

Mucous membranes contain goblet cells which secrete mucus and therefore keep the membrane moist. *Serous membranes* consist of a double

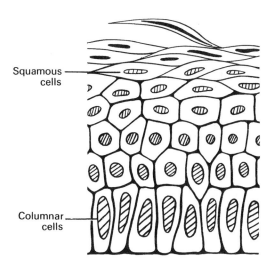

Squamous cells

Columnar cells

Figure 1.4 Stratified epithelium. (Reproduced with permission from Wilson K J W, Waugh A 1996 Ross and Wilson Anatomy and Physiology in Health and Illness. Churchill Livingstone, Edinburgh)

membrane which secretes a watery fluid, allowing the organs they cover to move without friction. The inner membrane is called the visceral layer and covers the organ itself. The outer membrane, the parietal layer, lines the cavity in which the organ lies. Serous fluid collects between the layers allowing free movement. *Synovial membranes* are found in joints, where they secrete synovial fluid to lubricate the joint, allowing free movement of the bones involved.

Epithelial cells can also collect into glands of two types:

1. *exocrine glands*, which secrete substances onto the surface of the membrane
2. *endocrine glands*, which secrete directly into blood or lymph.

Connective tissue

Connective tissue is a supporting material found in all areas of the body. Cells are arranged within a matrix of extracellular material, and as well as supporting, they are involved in transportation, insulation and protection. Five main types of cells are involved in these functions:

1. fibroblasts
2. macrophages
3. mast cells
4. fat cells
5. blood cells.

Fibroblasts are large cells which produce collagen and elastic fibres, the scaffolding of the tissue. *Macrophages* are irregular cells which act as phagocytes, seeking out and engulfing micro-organisms and dead or damaged cell material. *Mast cells* release heparin, serotonin and histamine when cells are damaged, as part of the body's inflammatory response to injury. *Fat cells* are found in many tissues in the body and provide insulation and a source of energy. *Blood cells* provide nutrients for the tissues.

These cells make up a variety of tissues with specific functions:

- *Areolar tissue* supports most organs of the body by providing an array of elastic and collagen fibres (Fig. 1.5).

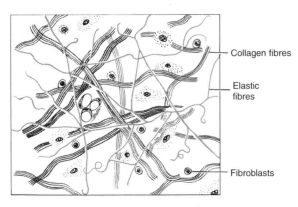

Figure 1.5 Areolar tissue. (Reproduced with permission from Wilson K J W, Waugh A 1996 Ross and Wilson Anatomy and Physiology in Health and Illness. Churchill Livingstone, Edinburgh)

- *Fibrous tissue* is composed principally of collagen fibres and forms ligaments, coverings for muscles, periosteum to cover bones, and an outer layer to protect organs of the body.
- *Elastic tissue* consists principally of elastin which provides flexibility in organs such as blood vessels, so allowing efficient vasodilation and vasoconstriction.
- *Adipose tissue* contains fat cells which provide insulation and support.
- *Cartilage* is composed of specialised cells called chondrocytes, supported by both elastic and collagen fibres.
- *Bone* is composed of osteocytes supported by collagen fibres and strengthened by mineral salts.

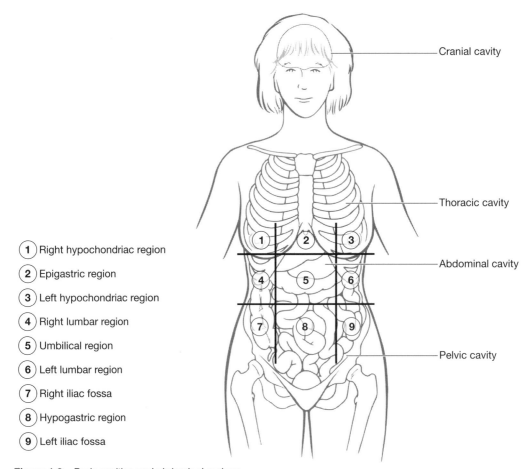

1. Right hypochondriac region
2. Epigastric region
3. Left hypochondriac region
4. Right lumbar region
5. Umbilical region
6. Left lumbar region
7. Right iliac fossa
8. Hypogastric region
9. Left iliac fossa

Figure 1.6 Body cavities and abdominal regions.

BODY CAVITIES

The body is divided into cavities in which specific systems are found. The *cranial cavity* is located in the skull and holds the brain. Within the rib cage is the *thoracic cavity*, which contains the respiratory system and the heart along with other associated structures. The *abdominal cavity* is the largest cavity in the body, and is subdivided into regions (Fig. 1.6), where organs of the gastrointestinal and the renal systems are situated. The *pelvic cavity*, formed by the boundaries of the pelvic girdle, contains the reproductive organs as well as some organs of the renal and gastrointestinal tract.

2

The nervous system

Within the human body, all systems are inter-related and depend on each other to function efficiently. The nervous system, in collaboration with the endocrine system, is responsible for coordinating all of these systems. It is the nervous system that detects any changes in either the internal or external environment and responds to them to maintain homeostasis. It is also the means by which we explore the world we live in: we learn from our surroundings and from other members of our species, and so become unique, individual human beings who are able to reason and explain.

Within the pregnant woman there is very little alteration in the physiological functioning of the nervous system. Coping with the pain of labour, however, is a challenge to both the midwife and the labouring woman. Psychologically, the stress of labour can have a deleterious effect on its progress.

At birth the full-term baby is able to react to both internal and external stimuli, and as the baby grows the nervous system matures to enable the infant to become a fully functional adult.

The nervous system is commonly considered in two parts, the central and the peripheral nervous systems. The central nervous system consists of:

- the brain, which receives, interprets and responds to, stimuli
- the spinal cord, through which nerves are relayed to and from the brain and body.

The peripheral nervous system consists of:

- cranial and spinal nerves, by which stimuli are detected and acted on
- the autonomic nervous system, which controls the functioning of systems without conscious thought.

THE CENTRAL NERVOUS SYSTEM

Macrostructure

The brain

The *brain* is a large organ situated in the cranial cavity in the skull. It is anatomically divided into (Fig. 2.1):

- the forebrain
- the midbrain
- the hindbrain.

The forebrain. The *forebrain* is the largest section of the brain and is divided into the cerebrum and the diencephalon. The *cerebrum* is divided into a right and left *cerebral hemisphere* by a deep longitudinal fissure (Fig. 2.2). This separation is complete superiorly, anteriorly and posteriorly, but deep in the substance of the cerebrum the hemispheres are joined by a broad band of nerve fibres forming the *corpus callosum*.

Each cerebral hemisphere is a 'mirror twin' of the other and each has a complete set of centres for sending, receiving and interpreting information. Each hemisphere is associated with the opposite side of the body but if either cerebral hemisphere is damaged, the corresponding area in the other hemisphere may be able to take over some of the destroyed functions.

The outer layer of the cerebrum is thrown into folds named *gyri* (singular, gyrus) separated by

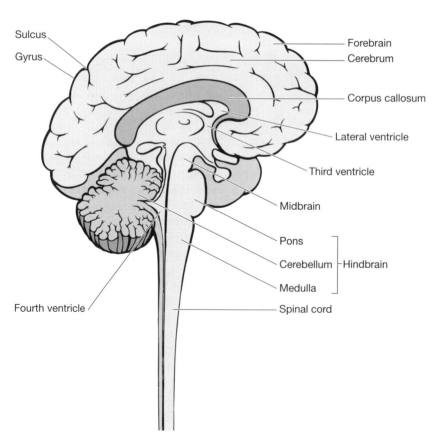

Figure 2.1 Sagittal section to show the macrostructure of the brain and spinal cord.

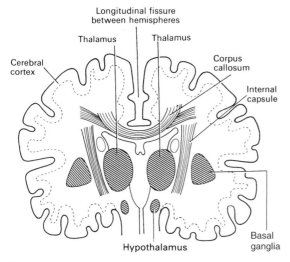

Figure 2.2 Longitudinal section of the cerebral hemispheres. (Reproduced with permission from Wilson K J W, Waugh A 1996 Ross and Wilson Anatomy and Physiology in Health and Illness. Churchill Livingstone, Edinburgh)

fissures known as *sulci* (sulcus). This allows the surface area of the brain to be increased considerably. Three sulci, the central, lateral and parietal-occipital sulci, divide each cerebral hemisphere into four lobes – *frontal, parietal, occipital* and *temporal*, named after the bones that cover them (Fig. 2.3).

A longitudinal section through the hemispheres will expose two distinct types of tissue, grey matter and white matter (Fig. 2.2). *Grey matter* is mainly situated beneath the surface of the cerebrum to a depth of 2–4 mm. A lighter shade of tissue fills the substance of the cerebrum. This is *white matter* through which neurones travel. The layer of grey matter beneath the surface of the cerebrum is the *cerebral cortex,* and contains billions of neuronal cell bodies. Interspersed throughout the white matter are areas of grey matter called nuclei. Several significant groups of these are found within the cerebral hemispheres, one such group being the *basal ganglia.* Also buried deep in the cerebral hemispheres are structures forming the *limbic system* which, together with the hypothalamus, is involved in emotion and motivation.

The second structure of the forebrain, the *diencephalon*, consists of the thalamus and hypothalamus (Fig. 2.2), areas of grey matter situated near the base of the hemispheres with specific responsibilities in the interpretation and regulation of nerve impulses. The *thalamus* is the principal relay station through which most sensory information is passed. Here the sensation is crudely interpreted and passed on to the appropriate region of the cerebral cortex for action. The thalamus is also thought to have a role in knowledge and awareness.

The *hypothalamus* is linked to, and controls, the pituitary gland that is situated immediately beneath it. The hypothalamus controls many body activities, including eating and temperature control, and is thus a major regulator of homeostasis. Control of these activities is influenced not just by nerve activity but also by hormones that are released from the hypothalamus.

The midbrain. The *midbrain* lies between the forebrain and the hindbrain and is approximately 20 mm long (Fig. 2.1). It consists of two stalk-like bands of white matter known as the *superior cerebral peduncles,* and four small prominences called the *quadrigeminal bodies.* The peduncles convey impulses between the brain and spinal cord, whilst the quadrigeminal bodies are associated with sight and hearing reflexes. The pineal gland lies between the two upper quadrigeminal bodies.

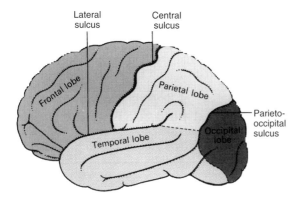

Figure 2.3 Principal lobes of the brain. (Reproduced with permission from Wilson K J W, Waugh A 1996 Ross and Wilson Anatomy and Physiology in Health and Illness. Churchill Livingstone, Edinburgh)

The hindbrain. The *hindbrain* consists of three structures:

1. the pons
2. the medulla oblongata
3. the cerebellum.

The *pons* lies between the midbrain and the medulla oblongata. It forms a bridge between the spinal cord and the cerebrum, and also connects the two hemispheres of the cerebellum. Anatomically, grey matter is found in the centre surrounded by white matter at the surface. Within the pons are nuclei that contain cell bodies of neurones concerned with respiration.

The *medulla oblongata* is situated between the pons and the spinal cord. It is 25 mm long and is shaped like an inverted pyramid. Many vital centres are situated within the medulla, including those that regulate heart and respiratory rate and essential reflex actions. In one area, the *decussation of the pyramids*, many neural pathways cross to the opposite side of the body.

The *cerebellum* projects backwards beneath the occipital lobes of the cerebrum. It is separated into two hemispheres and is thrown into folds. Grey matter is situated on the outside with white matter in the centre. However the deep folds give the impression that much of the cerebellum is composed of grey matter. The cerebellum is concerned with learned patterns of movement, and with posture and balance.

The brain stem. The midbrain, pons and medulla have many similar functions and are collectively known as the *brain stem*.

In the centre of the brain stem lies an area of grey matter that is an extension of the spinal cord. This area, plus small nuclei surrounding it, is the *reticular formation*. This area is responsible for the fine control of muscles and in one specific area, the *reticular activating system*, for consciousness and waking from sleep.

Microstructure

The nervous system is made up of millions of small functional units called *neurones*, supported by a network of specialised connective tissue known as *neuroglia*. Neurones are cells that have been modified to carry out their function of transmitting information between an area of the body and the nervous system, or between one area of the nervous system and another.

A neurone consists of (Fig. 2.4):

- a *cell body* in which the nucleus and other cell organelles are situated
- an *axon* of varying length, which is an extension of the cell body
- *dendrites* which are stimulated by external factors
- *synaptic end bulbs* which pass on an impulse to another neurone or a structure such as a muscle fibre.

There are two main types of neurone: those with myelin surrounding their axon, and those without. *Myelin* is a white fatty substance that insulates the axon from the external environment. It is wrapped around the axon in several

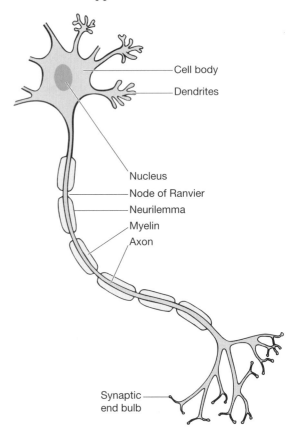

Figure 2.4   Microscopic structure of a neurone.

layers and is enclosed by a layer of cells, the *neurilemma*. At intervals along the length of the axon there are gaps in the myelin sheath where the neurone can come into contact with the surrounding tissues, enabling exchange of materials such as nutrients, water and waste products. These gaps are called *nodes of Ranvier*.

Neurones that are surrounded by a myelin sheath form the white matter of the nervous system. The cell bodies of these neurones do not have a covering of myelin and appear darker in colour to form the grey matter of the nervous system. Myelinated nerve fibres transmit impulses much more rapidly than unmyelinated fibres: myelinated at 120 m/s, compared with unmyelinated at 5–10 m/s.

Neurones are easily damaged by toxins or lack of oxygen and once they die they are not replaced. Their function can occasionally be taken over by other cells. Alternatively, if the cell body is undamaged, the nerve cell may regenerate.

Conduction of impulses

The function of a neurone is to transmit an impulse resulting from a stimulus from one area to another. This is carried out by the generation of an action potential. This action potential is then passed on to another neurone or a structure such as a muscle fibre. Once the action potentials reach the cerebral hemispheres they are interpreted and acted on.

An *action potential* is a change in electrical potential across the cell membrane. This can be measured and is found to alter from −70 mV to +35 mV. Movement of ions across the cell membrane brings about this action potential.

Most cell membranes of the body maintain an electrical imbalance between intracellular and extracellular fluids surrounding the cell. This is the result of an imbalance in the concentration of potassium ions (K^+) and sodium ions (Na^+) and related anions. The inside of the cell has an increased concentration of K^+ and a decreased concentration of Na^+. The outside of the cell has a decreased concentration of K^+ and an increased concentration of Na^+. This imbalance is maintained through active transport across the cell membrane by means of a sodium–potassium pump, and also because of the greater permeability of the membrane to K^+ than to Na^+. Diffusion also occurs down the concentration gradients, but at a much slower rate.

In a neurone this imbalance is also present, and it is used to initiate a rapid change in electrical charge that can be transmitted along the length of the axon. This is the basis of the action potential. Only nerve and muscle cells are capable of changing the electrical charge rapidly across a cell membrane.

A neurone that has not been stimulated has an electrical potential of −70 mV. This is known as its *resting potential*. When a neurone is stimulated, the difference in charge between the inside and the outside of the cell is reduced next to the stimulation. When this difference reaches the threshold level, the sodium channels open, allowing these ions to flood in. This process is called *depolarisation* and it results in the inside of the cell becoming positively charged in relation to the outside of the cell. This is the action potential.

The next region of the neurone will still be maintaining its resting potential – inside negatively charged, outside positively charged. Because unlike charges attract, the positive ions within the cell will be attracted towards the area of negativity. In this way the impulse will be transmitted along the neurone.

Once a section of the cell has become depolarised, K^+ will leak out of the cell and the sodium channels close again, so restoring the resting potential. This is termed *repolarisation*. Until its resting potential has been restored, the neurone cannot respond to another stimulus.

The whole cycle of producing an action potential takes only a millisecond, and when stimulated 200 action potentials per second can be passed along the neurone (Box 2.1).

Because myelinated neurones are only in contact with surrounding fluids at the nodes of Ranvier, impulses cannot pass smoothly along these fibres. Instead, an impulse 'jumps' from one node to the next, a process known as *saltatory conduction*. This enables the impulse to pass

---

dendrite from another neurone or a cell of another organ such as a muscle fibre. Dendrites and cell bodies are often covered in synaptic end bulbs from many different neurones. When an impulse arrives at the synapse, a chemical substance known as a *neurotransmitter* is released from vesicles situated in the synaptic end bulb. This neurotransmitter diffuses across the synaptic gap and causes either an increase or a decrease in the permeability of the membrane of the receiving cell (Fig. 2.5). Accordingly, an action potential will either be initiated or the impulse will be inhibited from spreading along the receiving cell. Once the action potential has been passed on to the next neurone, the neurotransmitter is rapidly broken down by enzymes present in surrounding fluids.

Within synapses several different neurotransmitters may be in use. Acetylcholine, dopamine and noradrenaline are all examples of chemicals that may function as neurotransmitters. Many drugs act at the synapse by binding to the receptors on the dendrites, thus blocking the action of the neurotransmitters. Neurotransmitters are synthesised either in the synaptic end bulb or in the cell bodies, and so some may need to be transported continuously along the length of the axon.

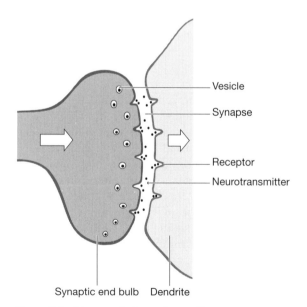

Figure 2.5 Movement of neurotransmitters across a synapse.

much more rapidly along these fibres. Once the impulse arrives at the end of a neurone, it must be passed on to the next nerve cell or muscle cell, across a space known as a synapse.

The synapse

At the terminal end of a neurone, branches of the axon extend to pass the information in several potential directions. At the end of each of these branches is a synaptic end bulb terminating at a *synapse*. Meeting each synaptic end bulb is a

Properties of nerve transmission

Certain fundamental principles govern the transmission of impulses along a neurone. These are outlined below:

- An action potential will either be generated or not – the 'all or nothing' principle. A stimulus received by a dendrite must be sufficient for an action potential to be generated, or else no impulse will result.
- All action potentials for a specific neurone are of the same intensity – it is not possible to stimulate a weak impulse.
- Action potentials can travel in either direction along a neurone, but will only be effective in one direction, i.e. towards synaptic end bulbs where neurotransmitters are available.
- The speed of an action potential along a neurone is related to the diameter of the neurone and to the presence of a myelin sheath, not to the strength of the stimulus (Box 2.2).
- Transmission of an impulse across a synapse may be delayed, because of the time required for the release of the neurotransmitter and its diffusion across the synapse.
- Some synapses are inhibitory – they prevent action potentials being transmitted along all interconnecting neurones.

Box 2.2   Multiple sclerosis

Multiple sclerosis is a degeneration of the myelin sheath that surrounds the axons of most neurones. The myelin sheaths 'sclerose' or become hardened in 'multiple' areas of the body. Action potentials can then spread into surrounding areas and become slowed. This results in early symptoms of double vision, abnormal sensations and muscle weakness. These often improve initially, during periods of remission, but with each recurrence the symptoms become worse.

The cause of this disease is not fully understood but is thought to be the result of a viral attack that results in an inappropriate autoimmune response (Lange 1990). Oligodendrocytes are destroyed and the myelin sheaths cannot be maintained. It is a disease of early adulthood and as it is twice as common in women as in men (Carty 1995) it may have an affect on pregnancy. The risk of inheriting this condition is considered to be 10–15% (Robinson et al 1990).

Once sufficient neurones have been formed to enable the nervous system to function, no new ones are created. Instead, throughout life new connections can be made between existing neurones, along which impulses can pass. Everything the human animal learns is the result of new connections that have been formed between neurones.

Supporting structures

Neurones within the central nervous system are embedded in and supported by a network of specialised tissue known as neuroglia. *Neuroglia* is composed of three principal types of glial cells that carry out different functions: astrocytes, oligodendrocytes and microglia.

Astrocytes form the main supporting tissue of the central nervous system and are found in particularly large numbers around the blood vessels situated within the nervous system. Here they provide an extra layer of cells between the blood and the nervous tissue, forming an important component of the *blood–brain barrier*. This selective barrier protects the nervous tissue from damaging chemicals carried in the blood. Astrocytes are also involved in the metabolic processes relating to the functioning of the neurones.

Oligodendrocytes carry out the function of forming and maintaining the myelin sheath surrounding many neurones.

Microglia are phagocytic cells that are involved in the defence and repair of nerve tissue.

Blood supply

The brain needs a continuous supply of oxygen and nutrients, and mechanisms are in place to ensure this is maintained even when the supply to other systems is inadequate. When the body is in homeostasis the brain consumes 200 times more oxygen than organs of similar size. If this supply is disrupted for just 1 or 2 minutes, brain cells may not be able to function and unconsciousness may result. Complete lack of oxygen for 4 minutes results in permanent damage to brain cells.

To ensure a good supply of blood, the brain

receives arterial blood from the cerebral arterial circle, the *circle of Willis*, situated at the base of the brain. Blood vessels travel over the surface of the brain before branching into smaller vessels to plunge deep into the cortex of the brain. Most essential substances such as oxygen, glucose and water readily and rapidly diffuse out of the blood vessels into the brain cells, along with fat-soluble substances such as alcohol, nicotine and many anaesthetics. Carbon dioxide moves in equally rapidly. However, because of the blood–brain barrier formed by the astrocytes, substances such as electrolytes and urea move more slowly, and proteins and antibiotics cannot pass out of cerebral blood vessels at all.

Venous return from the brain is carried out by venous sinuses situated between two layers of dura mater which are part of the meninges, or coverings, of the brain.

The meninges

Completely covering the brain and the spinal cord are the *meninges* (Fig. 2.6), which are three layers of membrane that give protection to the nervous tissue.

The innermost layer is called the *pia mater* and is a thin connective tissue containing an array of fine blood capillaries. This membrane is in close contact with the surface of the brain, following the contours of the sulci and gyri.

Covering the pia mater is a delicate membrane called the *arachnoid mater*, which follows the principal contours of the brain. Between the pia and arachnoid mater is the *sub-arachnoid space*, which is filled with cerebrospinal fluid (CSF).

The outermost membrane is the tough, fibrous *dura mater*, with two layers. The outer layer lines the inner surface of the skull; the inner layer forms a protective covering for the brain and follows the contours of the brain. Between dura mater and the arachnoid mater is the *subdural space*. Between the layers of the dura mater are the venous sinuses that take the place of a venous drainage system for the brain.

The three meninges are closely associated, and form folds of membranes between the two cerebral hemispheres (the *falx cerebri*), between the

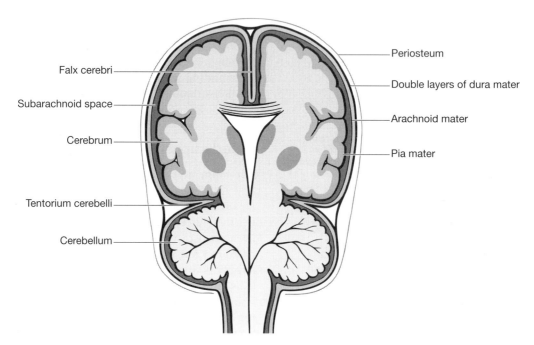

Figure 2.6 Longitudinal section of the cerebral hemispheres showing meninges.

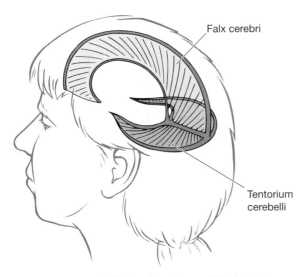

Falx cerebri

Tentorium
cerebelli

Figure 2.7 Principal folds of meninges within the brain.

cerebrum and the cerebellum (the *tentorium cerebelli*), and between the two hemispheres of the cerebellum (the *falx cerebelli*) (Fig. 2.7). The three membranes extend downwards to enclose the spinal cord in a protective sheath and complete the circulation of CSF throughout the nervous system.

The ventricles

Enclosed within the brain are four cavities, or *ventricles*. These ventricles are linked to allow circulation of CSF (Box 2.3).

Two *lateral ventricles* are situated within the cerebral hemispheres on either side of the midline below the corpus callosum. The *third ventricle* is situated beneath the lateral ventricles, between the two portions of the thalamus. This ventricle is connected to the fourth ventricle by a canal, the *cerebral aqueduct*. The *fourth ventricle* is situated between the pons and the cerebellum, and is continuous with the central canal of the spinal cord, so allowing a complete circulation of CSF.

Cerebrospinal fluid (CSF)

Cerebrospinal fluid is a clear, colourless fluid, which fills the sub-arachnoid space and the

Box 2.3 Congenital abnormalities of the nervous system

Box 2.3 Congenital abnormalities of the nervous system

Abnormalities of the central nervous system are responsible for a large number of congenital defects that occur in the fetus, with 3–4 affected per 1000 pregnancies (Brunner & Suddarth 1991). These may take the form of abnormal development of the brain or an anatomical defect which allows the protrusion of part of the nervous system.

Hydrocephalus is a congenital condition in which an abnormality blocks the circulation of CSF. CSF collects in the ventricles of the brain causing an increase in the size of the ventricles. The soft skull bones of the fetus allow the brain to swell, causing damage to brain tissue. Difficulty in delivery may occur. Treatment may be possible by the insertion of a drain from a lateral ventricle to the jugular vein. If damage has not been too severe before treatment, the neonate may develop normally (Brunner & Suddarth 1991).

Anencephaly and microcephaly occur as a result of incorrect development of the brain. The cause of *anencephaly* is unknown, but it is believed that many factors are involved in its development (Holmes 1990). The condition commonly occurs in female fetuses, and is characterised by a complete or partial absence of the cerebral hemispheres and the overlying skull. Anencephaly is incompatible with life. In cases of *microcephaly* the head and brain are smaller than normal, with resulting severe mental retardation. The condition is associated with infections in pregnancy such as rubella or cytomegalovirus (Kelnar et al 1995).

Neural tube defects are commonly associated with dietary deficiency, such as a lack of folic acid in the first trimester of pregnancy (Hibbard 1993). A defect occurs in the vertebral column or skull sometimes allowing the protrusion of the meninges (a *meningocele*), which occasionally includes nervous tissue (a *meningomyelocele*). Both of these conditions can also occur in the lower back, where they are associated with a malformed vertebra, a *spina bifida*. Many of these conditions cannot be successfully treated, and result in serious physical and mental handicap. They carry a risk of inheritance of up to 5% (Tinkle & Sterling 1997). Tests can be carried out during early pregnancy which will pick up many of these conditions. A maternal blood sample can be examined for high levels of *alpha-fetoprotein*, a protein found only in the fetus early in gestation and present in the maternal blood in increased quantity if body fluids are leaking from an abnormally developing fetus (Smith 1995). Termination of pregnancy can then be offered.

ventricles of the brain. It is secreted by the *choroid plexus* found in each ventricle, circulates through the nervous system and is finally reabsorbed into the venous sinuses.

The composition of CSF is very similar to that of blood plasma, but with a smaller amount of protein. Approximately 500 ml of CSF are produced each day. Because it is constantly being recycled by reabsorption, the normal amount of CSF present within the system is 120–150 ml.

The function of CSF is to cushion and support the brain and spinal cord from the bony structures that surround them. It also maintains a constant pressure within the cranial cavity and removes waste and toxic substances from the nervous system. There is free diffusion of substances between intracranial and interstitial tissue, and CSF.

The spinal cord

The *spinal cord* is an extension of the central nervous system. It is responsible for the transmission of nerve impulses from the body to the brain and vice versa. It is protected by the meninges, containing CSF, and by the bony vertebrae of the spinal column.

Structure

The spinal cord is a thin, cylindrical structure composed of nervous tissue. It is approximately 450 mm long and is continuous with the medulla. It leaves the cranial cavity through a hole in the base of the skull, the *foramen magnum*, and terminates at the level of the first lumbar vertebrae. The spinal cord is covered along its whole length by the meninges through which CSF circulates (Fig. 2.8). These membranes and CSF are continuous with those surrounding the brain (Box 2.4).

Nerves leave the spinal cord in pairs along its entire length. Each nerve has two roots, an *anterior* or *motor root*, which leaves from the front of the cord, and a *posterior* or *sensory root*, which leaves at the rear of the cord. Each posterior root has a swelling known as a *ganglion*, containing the cell bodies of the neurones passing through. The anterior and posterior roots join as they leave the spinal cord to form the spinal nerves.

A cross-section of the spinal cord shows an H-shaped arrangement of white and grey matter, with the grey matter centrally positioned

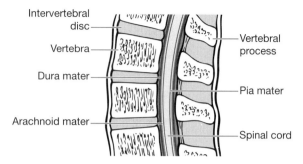

Figure 2.8 Longitudinal structure of the spinal cord showing meninges.

Box 2.4 Epidural and spinal anaesthesia

One very effective method of relieving pain is to administer a long-lasting local anaesthetic into the meninges surrounding the spinal cord, so preventing the transmission of impulses along spinal nerves that run through this area. This is the basis of an *epidural* or *spinal anaesthetic*. A solution of an anaesthetic such as bupivacaine is injected either into the epidural space surrounding the dura mater of the spinal cord (an epidural anaesthetic), or into the sub-arachnoid space containing CSF (a spinal anaesthetic). The anaesthetic acts by preventing the movement of sodium ions across the membrane of the neurones, so maintaining all relevant nerves in their resting state. This includes both sensory and motor neurones, causing loss of mobility as well as relief from pain. The effect of an epidural on the course and duration of labour may be a lengthening of both the first and second stages, and an increase in instrumental delivery (Dickersin 1989). To diminish this effect, more dilute solutions of anaesthetic have been used with the addition of a narcotic such as fentanyl. This gives good analgesia with less effect on nerve function (Youngstrom et al 1996).

Epidurals are successful in the majority of women, but must be used only with 24-hour anaesthetic cover and with midwives experienced in their use (Bevis 1997) as, rarely, complications may occur. Informed consent by the mother is therefore vital (Moore 1997).

(Fig. 2.9). This provides the cell bodies of the neurones passing through the cord with maximum protection from injury. Regeneration may be possible if the axon of a neurone is damaged, but once destroyed, a cell body cannot be repaired.

The grey matter of the spinal cord is divided into regions called *horns*. Within these areas, cell bodies are arranged in layers or *laminae*. White

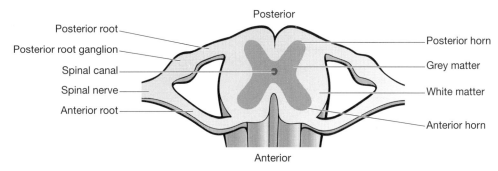

Figure 2.9   Cross-section of the spinal cord.

matter is also arranged in specific columns along which nerve pathways or tracts pass.

THE PERIPHERAL NERVOUS SYSTEM

The peripheral nervous system consists of 12 cranial nerves and 31 spinal nerves. A nerve is composed of many neurones or nerve fibres collected into bundles. A protective covering known as the *endoneurium* surrounds each nerve fibre. Surrounding each bundle is a second protective covering, the *perineurium*, and enclosing the entire nerve is the *epineurium*.

Cranial nerves

Cranial nerves are made up of either sensory or a mixture of sensory and motor nerve fibres. Ten of them originate specifically from the brain stem. They all convey impulses to and from the brain, and have been named according to their function and by roman numerals that indicate the order in which the nerve arises from the brain (Table 2.1).

Spinal nerves

Spinal nerves connect the central nervous system to sensory receptors, muscles and glands. Spinal nerves leave the spinal cord through the spaces in between each vertebra. There are 31 pairs of spinal nerves, named according to the vertebra superior to the site of their exit, i.e.:

- 8 cervical
- 12 thoracic
- 5 lumbar
- 5 sacral
- 1 coccygeal.

Both motor and sensory nerve fibres leave the spinal cord to form the nerve, so each spinal nerve is a mixed nerve. Every spinal nerve also contains a nerve fibre from the autonomic nervous system.

Associated with all spinal nerves (except the thoracic nerves) are an intertwined collection of nerves called a plexus. A *plexus* is made up of spinal nerves from several areas of the spinal cord, which join together and are rearranged before proceeding to the area of the body that they supply. There are five such plexuses:

1. The *cervical plexus*, which is composed of the first four cervical nerves. These regroup to produce nerves associated with the head, muscles of the neck and the diaphragm.

2. The *brachial plexus*, which consists of the four lower cervical nerves. These reform to supply the upper body, arms and part of the chest wall.

3. The *lumbar plexus*, which is formed by the nerves from the first three lumbar nerves and part of the fourth. These become rearranged to supply the lower abdomen, groin and thighs. One branch also joins the sacral plexus.

4. The *sacral plexus*, which consists of the first three sacral nerves, plus the contribution from the lumbar plexus. It reforms to supply the pelvic floor, hip joint and pelvic organs and, with the

Table 2.1 Cranial nerves and their function

Cranial nerve	Function
I (Olfactory)	Smell
II (Optic)	Vision
III (Oculomotor)	Motor function of the eyes
	Sensation of touch around the eyes
IV (Trochlear)	Movement of the eyeballs
	Sensation of touch around the eyes
V (Trigeminal)	Chewing
	Sensation of pain, touch and temperature around and within the face
VI (Abducens)	Movement of the eyeball
	Sensations within the eye
VII (Facial)	Movement of facial muscles
	Sensations from the muscles of the face, scalp and tongue
VIII (Vestibulocochlear)	Hearing and equilibrium
IX (Glossopharyngeal)	Secretion of saliva
	Taste
	Regulation of blood pressure
X (Vagus)	Smooth muscle function
	Sensations from lungs, heart and gut
XI (Accessory)	Movement of head
	Swallowing
	Sensations from oral cavity and throat
XII (Hypoglossal)	Movement of tongue, for speech and swallowing
	Sensations from the tongue

addition from the lumbar plexus, the legs and feet.

5. The *coccygeal plexus*, a small plexus formed by the fourth and fifth sacral nerves and the coccygeal nerves. After reorganisation the nerves from this plexus supply the coccyx, pelvic floor and external anal sphincter.

The thoracic nerves do not form plexuses. Each nerve as it originates from the spinal cord supplies a specific area of the thorax associated with the ribs. The seventh to twelfth thoracic nerves also supply the abdominal walls.

The area of skin that is supplied by one nerve is known as a *dermatome*. Each spinal nerve receives sensory information from this area of the skin as well as control of motor function for a specific segment of the body. There is often considerable overlap between adjacent dermatomes. Knowledge of these dermatomes and the underlying structures served by the same spinal nerves can give an indication of damage to internal organs of the body.

PHYSIOLOGY OF THE NERVOUS SYSTEM

The nervous system functions via two main systems, the sensory and the motor system. The *sensory system* gathers information from both the external environment and internal structures, and sends this information to the brain. The *motor system* uses this information to create actions such as walking and running, or to maintain homeostasis by altering a physiological process. Linking these two main systems are many integrating neurones that allow the modification of sensory and motor information, which produce actions such as writing, speaking and thinking.

Within the cortex of the brain are areas that are concerned with the interpretation of sensory information from specific parts of the body, or relating to specific functions, such as speaking. The sensory area of the cerebrum is situated behind the central sulcus. Sensations are received, interpreted and passed on to the motor area or other regions of the cortex for action. The sensory area is divided into specific regions relating to particular parts of the body. The size of each region depends on the sensitivity of the related body part, rather than its size (Fig. 2.10). The sensory area functions in conjunction with another region of the cortex called the *somato-sensory association area*, situated in the parietal lobes of the cortex. This area enables previous knowledge to aid sensory perception.

There is also a motor area in the frontal lobe, immediately anterior to the central sulcus. Again specific areas of this region are related to the control of motor function for a specific area of the body. The size of each area relates to the complexity of the muscular network of that part, not to its size. An association area, the *premotor area*, is situated in the frontal lobe and acts with the motor area to allow coordination and the learning of skilled movements.

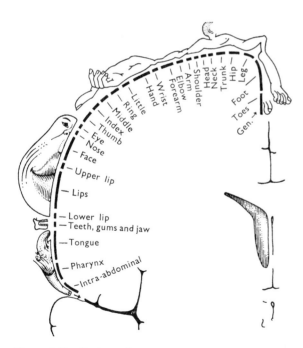

Figure 2.10 Regions of the right sensory cortex associated with body parts. (Reproduced with permission from Wilson K J W, Waugh A 1996 Ross and Wilson Anatomy and Physiology in Health and Illness. Churchill Livingstone, Edinburgh)

There are many other areas which have been identified and defined within the cortex of the brain, but much of their physiology is still poorly understood.

The sensory system

The *sensory system* receives and interprets the impulses that are constantly stimulating it. Many of these stimuli do not reach the level of consciousness because the nervous system deals with them automatically, via the autonomic nervous system. Other sensations which the body needs to act on to protect itself from harm, are transmitted to the cerebral cortex. Impulses are also transmitted to the central nervous system from sensory organs such as the eyes and nose, from receptors in the skin and from deep within the body.

Sensory input is received by sensory receptors of various types. Many have specialised nerve endings feeding into the dendrites of neurones. These respond to a range of different stimuli such as touch, temperature, light, smell, levels of chemicals and change in pressure (including in joints). Three sets of neurones transmit sensory information to the cerebral cortex. The first neurone runs from the site of stimulation, along a specific tract in the spinal cord, to the medulla of the brain (Fig. 2.11). Here it synapses with a second neurone which crosses to the opposite side of the medulla and then travels to the thalamus. In the thalamus the sensation is crudely interpreted and then directed via a synapse along a third neurone to the relevant region of the sensory cortex where it is fully interpreted and acted on.

Many pathways are involved in the transmission of sensations to the cerebral cortex. Most follow a similar route to that described above. Pain and temperature follow a different route, however, synapsing firstly in the posterior horn of the spinal cord, crossing at that level to the opposite side of the body, travelling directly to the thalamus and then to the sensory cortex. Other sensations relating to posture and balance travel to the cerebellum without crossing to the other side of the body.

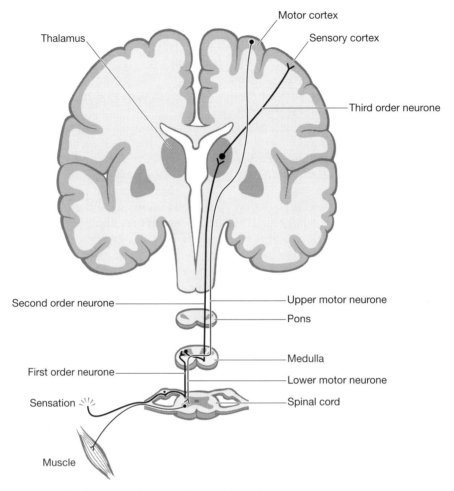

Figure 2.11   Sensory and motor pathways to/from the cortex.

The motor system

The motor system is mostly concerned with muscular activity. Many of the actions it initiates are subconscious and maintain body function. Others are the result of conscious thought, or a response to sensory input. An impulse arises from the motor cortex, then travels down specific pathways in the brain through a white area of the cerebral cortex situated between the thalamus and the basal ganglia. Without synapsing, the impulse continues down through the brain stem to the medulla where it crosses to the opposite side of the body. This first neurone continues down to the spinal column where it synapses at the relevant level with a second neurone in the anterior root of the spinal cord. This neurone then transmits the impulse to the site of required action.

Action is achieved because the synaptic end of the neurone divides into many fine filaments, terminating in minute motor end plates on a muscle fibre. This arrangement ensures that the muscle contracts in a coordinated fashion. To ensure smooth movement, many different neurones will act on the muscles involved in any one action.

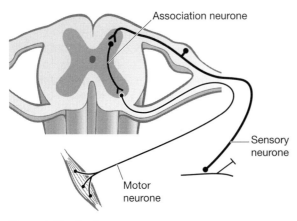

Figure 2.12 A reflex arc.

A reflex action

Reflex actions are ones in which there is no involvement of the cerebral cortex (Fig. 2.12). The pathway involved occurs entirely within the spinal cord. Reflex actions ensure that prompt actions can be rapidly initiated without conscious thought. For example, if the skin detects a sensation such as extreme temperature, this stimulus will initiate an impulse which is passed to the spinal cord, through the posterior root, where it synapses with an association neurone. The impulse is then transmitted along this neurone to the anterior horn where it is passed on to a motor neurone. It then passes back out of the spinal cord through the anterior root to the site of action (in this case muscle fibres), to initiate movement away from the source of danger. This is known as a *reflex arc*.

Although these reflex arcs do not involve the cerebrum, it can be brought consciously into play if there is a need. For example, if the source of extreme heat mentioned above is a valuable plate, then conscious thought can ensure that fingers are burnt whilst the plate is placed on a surface rather than dropped onto the floor.

Reflex actions are found at three levels within the nervous system: at the level of the spine, at the base of the brain, and within the cerebrum.

1. The spinal reflex is involved in simple reactions such as those described above.
2. The reflex initiated at the base of the brain involves the cerebellum. This includes reflexes such as sneezing, coughing and walking.
3. In the cerebrum, association fibres are involved, resulting in reflex actions such as salivating in response to the smell of food, or getting 'goosebumps' in anticipation of an exciting event.

THE AUTONOMIC NERVOUS SYSTEM

The *autonomic nervous system* serves all the internal organs of the body and the blood vessels. As suggested by the name this control is automatic, and not under the conscious will. This means the internal organs can function without any conscious thought – although the effects, such as an increase in respiratory rate, may be noticed.

Sensory receptors for the autonomic nervous system are present in many organs, large blood vessels and many supporting structures of the body. These receptors monitor the levels of chemicals (such as carbon dioxide, hydrogen and sodium ions), blood pressure, degree of stretch in some organs (e.g. the stomach and bladder), and other factors that can disrupt homeostasis. This information is passed on to the autonomic nervous system, which alters the functioning of organs to correct any imbalance.

The autonomic nervous system consists of two parts:

1. the sympathetic nervous system
2. the parasympathetic nervous system.

These two systems usually work in an opposing manner to maintain balance in the functioning of the body systems and therefore maintaining homeostasis.

The sympathetic nervous system

The *sympathetic nervous system* consists of a double chain of ganglia running down the sides of the vertebral column inside the thoracic and abdominal cavities (Fig. 2.13). Nerve fibres run from the spinal cord to the ganglia and then to the organs and blood vessels of the body, often sharing the same nerve as bundles of fibres from the peripheral nervous system.

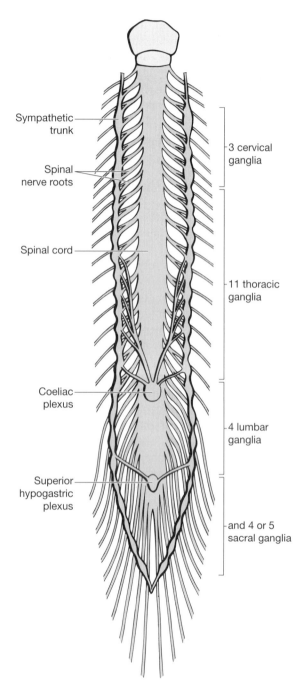

Sympathetic trunk

Spinal nerve roots

Spinal cord

Coeliac plexus

Superior hypogastric plexus

3 cervical ganglia

11 thoracic ganglia

4 lumbar ganglia

and 4 or 5 sacral ganglia

Figure 2.13   Position of the ganglia of the sympathetic nervous system.

The sympathetic nervous system causes the well-known *fight or flight* reaction to external stimuli. It prepares the body for the initiation of a body-wide response to physical danger. All unnecessary procedures, such as digestion, are temporarily halted so that oxygen and nutrients can be rerouted to essential organs such as the muscles, brain and heart.

The parasympathetic nervous system

The *parasympathetic nervous system* has the opposite effect to the sympathetic nervous system: it returns the body to normal functioning. Nerve fibres from the parasympathetic nervous system run from the brain or spinal cord directly to the organ concerned – although the fibres associated with organs in the head synapse in ganglia first.

PHYSIOLOGICAL CHANGES THROUGH THE CHILDBEARING YEAR

Pregnancy

Along with many other systems, the nervous system is affected by the hormones produced in abundance during pregnancy. Although many women experience *mood swings* and *headaches* during this time, little is known about any specific changes in neural function (Davis 1996). Short periods of *depression* are common and many women *lack confidence*. Many women also experience *changes in sleep patterns* especially during the third trimester (Blackburn & Loper 1992). Whether these are due to neurological changes or to discomforts associated with other systems, such as heartburn or frequency of micturition, is not known.

In the later months of pregnancy, women may experience *numbness* and *tingling of the fingers and hands* at the beginning of the day. This is the result of oedema causing pressure on the median nerve in the wrists, a condition known as *carpel tunnel syndrome* (Symonds & Symonds 1998). Diuretics, and splinting and raising the affected limb at night may improve this condition.

Labour

During labour, as well as at times during pregnancy and the puerperium, *discomfort* and *pain sensations* are transmitted to the brain by nerve fibres. Two types of pain are felt during labour:

1. visceral pain from the contracting uterus
2. somatic pain from the pressure exerted on the birth canal and surrounding structures.

Visceral pain is transmitted via the spinal nerves at levels T10–L1 during the first stage of labour and this is often felt as referred pain in the lower abdominal wall and sacrum. During the second stage somatic pain is transmitted through spinal nerves at levels S2–S4 and referred to the abdomen, lower back and upper thighs (Yerby 1996).

Pain perception varies considerably between women (Box 2.5) and is greatly influenced by psychological, social and cultural factors (Lowe 1996, Weber 1996). The pain of labour and how labouring women perceive this pain may affect the *progress of labour*. It has been shown that one way of reducing the need for analgesia at this time is to provide good antenatal information regarding the process of birth (Simkin & Enkin 1989).

The midwife can apply her knowledge of the physiology of pain when advising a woman on pain relieving techniques. By recognising the factors which moderate and amplify pain, the midwife is in a better position to advise about both pharmacological methods, e.g. narcotics or epidural, and non-pharmacological ones, such as massage and aromatherapy.

Postnatal

Headaches are common during the first week of the puerperium (MacArthur et al 1991) and are thought to be due to alterations in fluid and electrolyte balance (Blackburn & Loper 1992). *Sleep* is frequently disturbed, but this tends to be as a result of feeding and caring for the neonate, and the discomforts and pain of birth trauma. However, other diagnoses such as pregnancy induced hypertension (PIH) or stress must be considered by the midwife.

Box 2.5   Gate Control theory

For many years physiologists have attempted to explain the differences in pain perception in terms of basic pain pathways to the brain and subsequent interpretation. Early theories have not been able to explain how the emotional state of the person in pain can affect the pain felt, or how various physical factors such as warmth or massage diminish the pain. The most popular theory at present is the *Gate Control theory* devised by Melzack and Wall in 1965. This theory explains pain perception in terms of physiological, psychological and sociological factors.

Nerve fibres vary in diameter and the Gate Control theory identifies three main fibres that have an affect on pain transmission (Melzack & Wall 1988). A β fibres are large-diameter fibres that carry sensations of pressure and temperature, whereas A δ fibres and C fibres are small-diameter fibres which transmit pain sensation. These fibres synapse within the spinal cord in an area known as the substantia gelatinosa. This theory suggests that the *substantia gelatinosa* acts as a gate, allowing only so many impulses to be passed up to the cortex of the brain. If, therefore, A β fibres can be encouraged to transmit sensations in sufficient bulk, the pain impulses will be blocked. Massage or warmth in the form of hot pads or baths can achieve this. Another factor involved in pain transmission according to this theory is the production of natural endorphins, the body's own analgesics. This will also influence transmission of pain across synapses.

Psychological moderation or enhancement of pain is explained by the suggestion that nerve pathways descend from specific areas of the brain to the spinal cord and, depending on the emotional state of the person in pain, either encourage or depress endorphin production. Again this can be demonstrated by the use of Transcutaneous Electrical Nerve Stimulation (TENS). A TENS device can be placed over the lower back where it will administer small electrical shocks, which both stimulate A β fibres and encourage the production of endorphins (Johnson 1997).

A knowledge of the Gate Control theory and the physiology which underpins its physiology enables those caring for people in pain to make appropriate and full use of any of the pain control methods described here (Davis 1993).

Pain as a consequence of delivery can be severe and must be treated adequately. Analgesics can be used, as can local agents such as heat and ultrasound. *Afterpains* are common (Niven & Gijsbers 1996), particularly in women having had their second or subsequent delivery. These are the result of the continued contraction of uterine muscle as it returns to its prepregnant state.

Many women experience transitory periods of *minor depression* for a few days after birth, commonly known as *postnatal* or *baby blues* (Romito 1989). The symptoms vary but tend to be associated with mood swings, anxiety, tearfulness and fatigue. This is an accepted normal physiological process, although the cause is not known. Occasionally a true depression occurs and, rarely, a puerperal psychosis is diagnosed (Box 2.6).

The neonate

At birth the nervous system of the full-term neonate is not fully developed, but it has a range of reflexes to enable him to carry out basic functions such as rooting for the breast, sucking, swallowing and blinking. The neonatal brain has to deal rapidly with the greater changes in temperature, light and other environmental variations not present in the uterus. Additionally the autonomic nervous system has to regulate systems not fully functioning up until birth, such as the respiratory and digestive systems. At term, the blood–brain barrier is not fully developed, leaving the neonatal brain more vulnerable to toxic substances present in the blood stream.

In the preterm infant many reflexes are lacking and the neonate requires extra help with feeding and temperature control, as well as with many other physiological functions.

Box 2.6 Postnatal depression

Postnatal 'blues' commonly occurs in mothers around the third or fourth day of the puerperium and describes an abrupt change of mood (Gregoire 1995). It is thought to be due to changing hormonal levels and is aggravated by the physical discomforts of the postnatal period.

Postnatal depression however is a more serious condition affecting approximately 10% of women to some degree (Llewellyn-Jones 1994). Again the cause is not known and diagnosis may be difficult as the mother and her family may not recognise the problem. Common symptoms are depression, sleep disturbances unrelated to childcare, a feeling of inability to cope or fear of harming the baby, and extreme anxiety (Lambert 1994). Treatment may be by support if not severe, or else by antidepressants possibly with admission to a specialist unit with the baby (Vincenti 1996).

Rarely a true *puerperal psychosis* may occur. The incidence of this condition is 1–2 in every 1000 births (Ball 1993). Within a few days of delivery the mother will show an abrupt change of behaviour with agitation, loss of memory, hallucinations and possibly suicidal thoughts. She may deny the baby is hers or believe that he is dead (Riley 1995). Admission to the care of a psychiatrist is vital. Recurrence in later pregnancies is between 10% and 25%, with up to 33% developing a psychosis outside pregnancy later in life (Sweet 1997).

Rapid neurological development continues throughout childhood and into adulthood, with increasing myelination of neurones enabling more efficient functioning, and the development and connecting of nerve pathways.

REFERENCES

Alden K R, Durham C F 1995 Endocrine, cardiovascular and medical-surgical problems during pregnancy. In: Bobak I M, Lowdermilk D L, Jenson M D (eds) Maternity nursing, 4th edn. Mosby, St Louis, p 654

Ball J 1993 Complications of the puerperium. In: Bennett V R, Brown L K (eds) Myles textbook for midwives, 12th edn. Churchill Livingstone, Edinburgh, p 487

Bevis R 1997 Regional anaesthesia: epidural and spinal block. In: Moore S (ed) Understanding pain and its relief in labour. Churchill Livingstone, New York, p 174

Blackburn S T, Loper D L 1992 Maternal, fetal and neonatal physiology. W B Saunders, Philadelphia, p 522–580

Brunner L S, Suddarth D S 1991 The Lippincott manual of paediatric nursing, 3rd edn. Harper Collins Nursing, London, p 494–506

Carty E 1995 Disability, pregnancy and parenting. In: Alexander J, Levy V, Roch S (eds) Aspects of midwifery practice. Macmillan, Basingstoke, p 57

Crawford P 1997 Epilepsy and pregnancy: good management reduces the risks. Avoiding fetal malformation. Professional Care of the Mother and Child 7(1):17–18

Davis D C 1996 The discomforts of pregnancy. Journal of Obstetric, Gynecologic and Neonatal Nursing 25(1):73–81

Davis P 1993 Opening up the Gate Control theory. Nursing Standard 7(45):25–27

Dickersin K 1989 Pharmacological control of pain during labour. In: Chalmers I, Enkin E, Keirse M J N C (eds) Effective care in pregnancy and childbirth. Oxford University Press, Oxford, p 944

Gregoire A 1995 Hormones and postnatal depression. British Journal of Midwifery 3(2):99–104

Hibbard B M 1993 Folates and fetal development. British Journal of Obstetrics and Gynaecology 100(4):307–309

Holmes L B 1990 Congenital malformations. In: Oski F A, DeAngelis C D, Feigin R D, Warshaw J B (eds) Principles and practice of paediatrics. J B Lippincott, Philadelphia, p 259

Johnson M I 1997 Transcutaneous electrical nerve stimulation in pain management. British Journal of Midwifery 5(7):400–405

Kelnar C J H, Harvey D, Simpson C 1995 The sick newborn baby, 3rd edn. Baillière Tindall, London, p 322

Lambert C 1994 Depression: aetiology and features. Part 1. Nursing Standard 8(4):49–56

Lange L S 1990 Multiple sclerosis: neurology. In: De Souza L Multiple sclerosis. Approaches to management. Chapman and Hall, London, p 16–17

Llewellyn-Jones D 1994 Fundamentals of obstetrics and gynaecology. Mosby, London, p 91

Lowe N K 1996 The pain and discomfort of labour and birth. Journal of Obstetric, Gynecologic and Neonatal Nursing 25(1):82–92

MacArthur C, Lewis M, Knox E G 1991 Health after childbirth. HMSO, London, p 85

Melzack R, Wall P D 1988 The challenge of pain, 2nd edn. Penguin, Harmondsworth, p 83

Moore S (ed) 1997 Understanding pain and its relief in labour. Churchill Livingstone, New York, p 170

Niven C, Gijsbers K 1996 Perinatal pain. In: Niven C A, Walker A (eds) Conception, pregnancy and birth. Butterworth Heinemann, Oxford, p 131

Reynolds F 1991 Pharmacokinetics. In: Hytten F, Chamberlain G (eds) Clinical physiology in obstetrics, 2nd edn. Blackwell Scientific Publications, London, p 226

Riley D 1995 Perinatal mental health. Radcliffe Medical Press, Oxford, p 106–128

Robinson I, Jones R, Segal J 1990 Patients, their families and multiple sclerosis. In: De Souza L Multiple sclerosis.

Approaches to management. Chapman and Hall, London, p 159–160

Romito P 1989 Unhappiness after childbirth. In: Chalmers I, Enkin E, Keirse M J N C (eds) Effective care in pregnancy and childbirth. Oxford University Press, Oxford, p 1433

Sawle G 1995 Epilepsy and anticonvulsant drugs. In: Rubin P (ed) Prescribing in pregnancy, 2nd edn. BMJ Publishing Group, London, p 126

Silverton L 1993 The art and science of midwifery. Prentice Hall, New York, p 197

Simkin P, Enkin M 1989 Antenatal classes. In: Chalmers I, Enkin E, Keirse M J N C (eds) Effective care in pregnancy and childbirth. Oxford University Press, Oxford, p 318–334

Smith L 1995 Antenatal screening for neural tube defects. Modern Midwife 5(7):27–29

Sweet B R (ed) 1997 Mayes' midwifery. A textbook for midwives. 12th edn. Baillière Tindall, London, p 735

Symonds E M, Symonds I M 1998 Essential obstetrics and gynaecology, 3rd edn. Churchill Livingstone, New York, p 45

Tinkle M B, Sterling B S 1997 Neural tube defects. A primary prevention role for nurses. Journal of Obstetric, Gynecologic and Neonatal Nursing 26(5):503–512

Vincenti G 1996 Treating postnatal and other depressions. Professional Care of the Mother and Child 6(4):86–87

Weber S E 1996 Cultural aspects of pain in childbearing women. Journal of Obstetric, Gynecologic and Neonatal Nursing 25(1):67–72

Yerby M 1996 Managing pain in labour. Part 1. Perceptions of pain. Modern Midwife 6(3):22–24

Youngstrom P C, Baker S W, Miller J L 1996 Epidurals redefined in analgesia and anaesthesia: a distinction with a difference. Journal of Obstetric, Gynecologic and Neonatal Nursing 25(4):350–354

3

The endocrine system

No body system functions in isolation: they all influence and respond to one another. To maintain homeostasis, there needs to be some form of central control. Providing this is one of the roles of the endocrine system. Information from all the systems of the body is relayed swiftly to the nervous system, which either influences function through nerve impulses or stimulates endocrine glands to secrete chemicals to alter function. As endocrine adjustment involves the production of hormones and their transmission via the blood stream, it is a slower process than nervous control.

The reproductive system is continuously affected by hormones after puberty. In women, a cyclical alteration in the levels of certain essential hormones results in the release of an ovum ready for fertilisation and prepares the uterus for its supporting role throughout pregnancy.

During pregnancy there is a dramatic increase in many of the hormones. Most systems of the body are affected by the pregnancy and these will require adjustment to cope with the changes pregnancy brings. Labour itself, it is thought, is largely initiated by hormonal triggers, and so is controlled by the endocrine system.

Postnatally the endocrine system, like most other body systems, rapidly returns to normal functioning. However the initiation of lactation and the subsequent production of milk are both fully dependent on the endocrine system. The neonate, both throughout the pregnancy and after birth, is influenced by maternal endocrine function and has its own functional endocrine system at birth.

The endocrine system produces hormones in many ductless, or *endocrine, glands* scattered around the body, and in *endocrine cells* situated in tissues of the body (Fig. 3.1). These hormones diffuse into the blood stream and are transported to target organs where they alter function.

Hormones are involved in the *control and regulation of tissues and organs*. These include the regulation and chemical composition of body fluids, the regulation of metabolic processes and muscle function, and the maintenance of homeostasis.

The glands and tissues that make up the endocrine system are:

- the hypothalamus, which controls most endocrine functioning through the pituitary gland
- the pituitary gland, which secretes hormones responsible for the homeostasis of many organs of the body
- the pineal gland, which is involved in body biorhythms
- the thyroid gland, which influences metabolic activities
- four parathyroid glands, involved in the homeostasis of blood calcium and phosphate levels

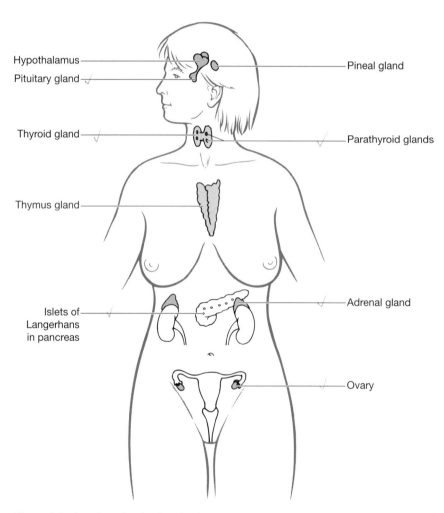

Figure 3.1 Location of endocrine glands.

- the thymus gland, which releases hormones related to the immune system
- two adrenal glands, involved in autonomic nervous system responses and renal function
- endocrine cells, situated in organs such as the ovaries and testes, placenta, pancreas and digestive system.

THE HYPOTHALAMUS

The *hypothalamus* is a small area of the brain situated beneath the two lobes of the thalamus. It is a major integrating link between the brain and endocrine function. The hypothalamus receives information from many areas of the brain and from body organs and structures. In response to this information it alters function either by nerve impulses or by releasing its own hormones. In this way the hypothalamus functions both as a part of the nervous system and as an endocrine gland in its own right.

The hypothalamus produces hormones that act on the pituitary gland to which it is physically linked (Fig. 3.2). These hormones act by increasing or decreasing the hormonal secretion of the pituitary gland. The hypothalamus produces its own hormones in specialised nerves, *neuro-endocrine cells*, which are transported rapidly to the anterior lobe of the pituitary by a network of blood vessels, called the pituitary portal system.

THE PITUITARY GLAND

The *pituitary gland* is situated at the base of the brain in the hypophyseal fossa of the sphenoid bone, and consists of an anterior and a posterior lobe. It is a very small structure, weighing only 4 g yet, with the hypothalamus, it has a vital role in the maintenance of homeostasis. The hypothalamus and pituitary gland are physically connected by the pituitary stalk through which many nerve fibres run.

The anterior lobe

The *anterior lobe* of the pituitary gland, the adeno-hypophysis, produces hormones that have a variety of functions. They can stimulate or inhibit the release of other hormones produced by many of the endocrine glands and cells of the body. They can also have a direct effect on tissues of the body. Anterior pituitary hormones are released

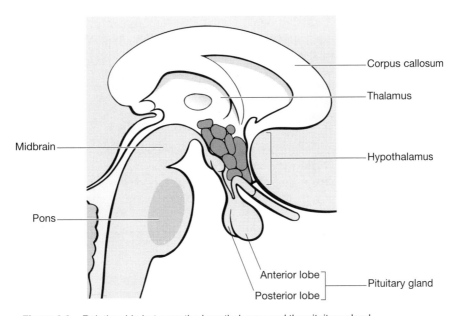

Figure 3.2   Relationship between the hypothalamus and the pituitary gland.

in response to the action of the hypothalamus. The hypothalamus monitors the levels of many chemicals in the body. If any of these levels become inappropriately low, it releases hormones which act on the pituitary gland. The pituitary gland then produces the hormones necessary to stimulate the target gland to increase its production. If body chemical levels become too high, the hypothalamus reduces the amount of hormone produced, resulting in a reduction of hormones from the pituitary gland and therefore from the target organs or tissues. This is an example of a negative feedback system.

There are six different types of hormone secreted by the anterior pituitary gland in response to hypothalamic hormones. These are:

1. *Gonadotrophins*, released in response to gonadotrophin-releasing hormone (GRNH) from the hypothalamus. Follicle-stimulating hormone (FSH) is a gonadotrophin which is released from the pituitary in the female after puberty to stimulate the ovary to produce a Graafian follicle containing a mature ovum. Later a second gonadotrophin, luteinising hormone (LH), is produced to trigger ovulation and to maintain the corpus luteum in the ovary. In the male, FSH stimulates the production of spermatozoa in the testes, and LH stimulates Leydig (interstitial) cells also in the testes to produce testosterone.

2. *Prolactin*, produced during the puerperium to initiate and maintain the production of breast milk, in response to the release of prolactin-releasing hormone from the hypothalamus.

3. *Growth hormone*, produced in response to growth hormone releasing hormone (GHRH) from the hypothalamus. Growth hormone stimulates the growth of many tissues and organs in the body such as bones, muscles, the kidneys and the liver. An inhibiting hormone from the hypothalamus related to GHRH is growth hormone release inhibiting hormone (GHRIH). This affects the production of many other hormones including those of the thyroid and the digestive system.

4. *Thyroid-stimulating hormone* (TSH), which affects the development and production of hormones by the thyroid gland. It is released in response to thyrotrophin releasing hormone.

5. *Adrenocorticotrophic hormone* (ACTH) is released in response to corticotrophin-releasing hormone from the hypothalamus. It stimulates blood flow to the adrenal glands and the production, by them, of steroids.

6. *Melanocyte-stimulating hormone* (MSH) affects skin pigmentation.

Both ACTH and MSH are released in response to corticotrophin-releasing hormone from the hypothalamus.

The posterior lobe

The *posterior lobe* of the pituitary gland, the neurohypophysis, is composed of specialised secretory cells, and nerve fibres from the hypothalamus and other regions of the brain. Two hormones are secreted in the posterior lobe: oxytocin and antidiuretic hormone. Neither of these is produced by the pituitary gland, but rather by the hypothalamus. They are then passed along nerve fibres to the pituitary, where they are stored, and released when required.

Oxytocin is involved in uterine contraction and in the contraction of the myoepithelial cells surrounding the alveoli of the breasts during lactation. *Antidiuretic hormone* is released when a decrease in fluid volume in the blood is detected by the hypothalamus. It acts on the nephrons of the kidney to reabsorb water, resulting in less being lost in urine. It is also a powerful vasoconstrictor and plays an important role in the maintenance of blood pressure.

Blood supply

Arterial blood to the pituitary gland is supplied by branches of the internal carotid artery, and venous blood drains into the venous sinuses between the dura mater of the brain.

THE PINEAL GLAND

The *pineal gland* is very small – only 10 mm in size – and is attached to the roof of the third ventricle of the brain. Many sympathetic nerve pathways terminate in the pineal gland. The exact physiological function of this gland is not fully understood.

The main hormone that is secreted by the pineal gland is *melatonin*, which is associated with biorhythms and possibly, by inhibiting gonadotrophins, with the timing of puberty.

THE THYROID GLAND

The *thyroid gland* is situated in the neck in front of the larynx and trachea (Fig. 3.3). It consists of two conical lobes measuring 50×30 mm joined by a narrow band, the isthmus. The thyroid gland is surrounded by a capsule and is extremely vascular. The gland is composed of follicular cells containing the protein colloid, a thickened fluid in which thyroid hormones are produced and stored, and parafollicular cells scattered around the follicular cells that secrete calcitonin.

Three principal hormones are secreted by the thyroid gland:

1. thyroxine
2. triiodothyronine
3. calcitonin.

Thyroxine (T_4) and *triiodothyronine* (T_3) require iodine from the diet for their manufacture. Once formed these hormones are stored in combination with colloid in the follicular cells. When stimulated by TSH from the pituitary gland, T_4 and T_3 are secreted.

T_4 and T_3 are essential for metabolic processes, and for physical and mental growth. They have an effect on the regulation of the basal metabolic rate, the metabolism of carbohydrates, fats and proteins, and on the normal functioning of the cardiac, nervous and reproductive systems (Box 3.1).

Calcitonin is secreted by the parafollicular cells in response to high levels of calcium and phosphate in the blood. Together with the parathyroid

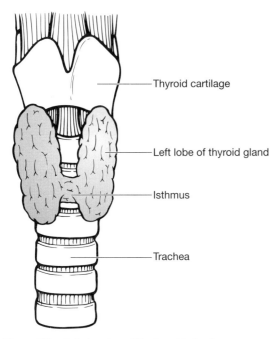

Figure 3.3 Anterior view of the thyroid gland.

- Thyroid cartilage
- Left lobe of thyroid gland
- Isthmus
- Trachea

Box 3.1 Hypo- and hyperthyroidism

Disorders of the thyroid gland are present in many pregnancies. However both hypothyroidism and hyperthyroidism can be associated with infertility (Ramsey 1991), so women with thyroid disorders in pregnancy generally have only mild manifestations. Increased rates of spontaneous abortion are associated with disorders of the thyroid gland (Sweet 1997).

Hypothyroidism is the more common of these disorders (Ramsey 1991). It may be caused by the disease process or be a consequence of treatment for hyperthyroidism. Iodine deficiency also results in hypothyroidism, particularly in third-world countries. In pregnancy, existing medication for hypothyroidism may need to be altered, in line with the increasing demands on the body (Mooney et al 1998). Maternal hypothyroidism can result in *congenital hypothyroidism* (cretinism) in the fetus, which causes deafness, mental retardation, spasticity, and a typical coarse facial appearance (Daker & Bobrow 1989). Congenital hypothyroidism can occur spontaneously, as well as in babies of mothers with hypothyroidism. It affects 1 in 4000 babies (Popovich & Moore 1993), and is screened for in the UK using a blood test (the Guthrie test).

Hyperthyroidism occurs less commonly and is associated with increased congenital abnormalities, pregnancy-induced hypertension and preterm labour (Smith 1990). As drug therapy for thyrotoxicosis crosses the placenta, the condition should, ideally, be remedied surgically before pregnancy. However, if hyperthyroidism is present, the fetus will also develop the condition, but it should return to normal 2–3 weeks after delivery. Drugs for hyperthyroidism are excreted in breast milk, so breast-feeding is contraindicated.

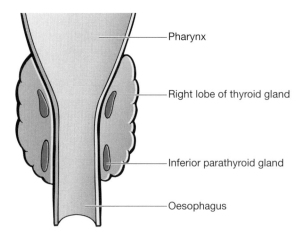

Figure 3.4 Posterior view of the thyroid gland showing location of the parathyroid glands.

glands, it controls the levels of these minerals. Calcitonin causes a reduction in the amount of calcium and phosphate released by bone and an increase in the amount of calcium and phosphate secreted by the renal tubules.

Blood supply

Blood supply to the thyroid glands is through the superior and inferior thyroid arteries, which branch from the external carotid and subclavian arteries respectively. Venous blood drains into the internal jugular veins through the thyroid veins.

THE PARATHYROID GLANDS

The four tiny *parathyroid glands* lie on the posterior surface of the thyroid gland (Fig. 3.4). They secrete *parathyroid hormone* which, with calcitonin from the thyroid gland, maintains the homeostasis of calcium and phosphate. Parathyroid hormone functions as an antagonist to calcitonin: it releases calcium and phosphate from bone and decreases secretion from the kidneys when blood levels of these minerals are low. Parathyroid hormone also promotes the formation in the kidneys of calcitriol, a hormone which is the active form of vitamin D. *Calcitriol* is involved in the absorption of calcium, phosphate and magnesium from the gastrointestinal tract.

Blood supply

Blood supply to parathyroid glands is by the same routes as the thyroid gland.

THE THYMUS GLAND

The principal function of the *thymus gland* is to activate lymphocytes (Fig. 3.5). It does this by

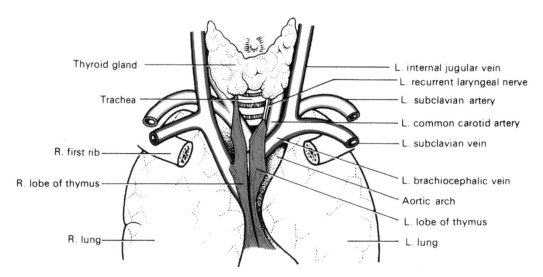

Figure 3.5 Location of the thymus gland. (Reproduced with permission from Wilson K J W, Waugh A 1996 Ross and Wilson Anatomy and Physiology in Health and Illness. Churchill Livingstone, Edinburgh)

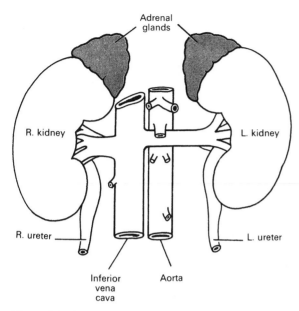

Adrenal
glands

R. kidney

L. kidney

R. ureter

L. ureter

Inferior
vena
cava

Aorta

Figure 3.6 Location of the adrenal glands. (Reproduced with permission from Wilson K J W, Waugh A 1996 Ross and Wilson Anatomy and Physiology in Health and Illness. Churchill Livingstone, Edinburgh)

secreting the hormones *thymopoietin* and the *thymosins*. This is described in detail in Chapter 7.

THE ADRENAL GLANDS

The *adrenal glands* are situated on the superior pole of each kidney (Fig. 3.6). They measure approximately 40 × 30 mm and consist of an outer cortex and an inner medulla, which differ both in structure and function.

The adrenal cortex

The *adrenal cortex* secretes adrenocorticosteroids, or steroid hormones, of three main types:

1. glucocorticoids
2. mineralocorticoids
3. gonadocorticoids.

Glucocorticoids

The *glucocorticoids* include *cortisol* (hydrocortisone) and *corticosterone*, hormones that are essential for life. The release of glucocorticoids is stimulated by ACTH from the anterior pituitary gland, or through the hypothalamus by stress. Glucocorticoids have wide-ranging effects on the body, all resulting in the formation of ATP, the energy-producing molecule required by all body cells. Glucocorticoids are therefore involved in the metabolism of glucose and carbohydrates, and also in sodium and water reabsorption from the renal tubules. They also cause blood vessels to be sensitive to chemicals which cause vasoconstriction, and so contribute to the maintenance of blood pressure. Additionally, glucocorticoids can function as anti-inflammatories, and can suppress the immune response when necessary.

Mineralocorticoids

Mineralocorticoids include the hormone *aldosterone*. This hormone is involved in the reabsorption of sodium in the distal convoluted tubule of the kidney and in the removal of hydrogen ions into urine. It is also involved in the renin–angiotensin control of blood pressure.

Gonadocorticoids

Gonadocorticoids include the sex hormones *oestrogen* and *androgen*. These are involved in the changes in body shape in males at puberty, and in female sexual behaviour. These hormones are normally secreted in very low levels compared with those released by the gonads, and so have a minor role to play in reproductive function.

The adrenal medulla

The adrenal medulla is enclosed by the cortex, and is a component of the sympathetic nervous system. Two hormones are produced by the medulla:

1. adrenaline
2. noradrenaline.

Adrenaline and *noradrenaline* are secreted when there is an expectation of instant action – the 'fight or flight' response. These hormones therefore work in a similar way to the sympathetic nervous system (see Ch. 2, p. 25). They help

---

Box 3.2 Stress

Stress is any undue strain exerted on the mind or body. A *stressor* can be any agent or stimulus that produces stress. A woman entering hospital to give birth can be overwhelmed by stressors such as lack of knowledge, lack of control, the unfamiliar environment, severe pain, or extreme excitement. Each individual's reaction to this will be different.

During childbirth, the physical and psychological stressors on both mother and baby are considerable (Niven 1992). When faced with the challenge of labour, a woman may react positively or negatively. Many women find this a time of great anxiety and tension, leading to physiological and psychological imbalance. This results in *stress*. Midwives are invaluable in reducing stress by giving support and increasing women's confidence in their ability to cope (Too 1997).

Any stressful situation initiates the release of corticotrophin-releasing hormone from the hypothalamus. This raises the amount of ACTH released by the anterior lobe of the pituitary gland. ACTH acts on the adrenal cortex to secrete much larger amounts of cortisol with an increase in aldosterone. These hormones initiate the '*fight or flight*' response: the heartbeat is increased in rate and strength, blood pressure rises, glucose is released into the bloodstream, and peripheral blood supply is decreased to enable more blood to reach essential organs such as the heart, brain and muscles.

For the woman in labour, being anxious increases stress. This can affect the normal functioning of the uterus. Adaptation, *eustress*, will enable labour to be seen as a challenge, an attitude which helps lead to a positive labour experience and normal progress (Ginesi & Niescierowicz 1998). If however labour proves to be much worse than expected, *distress* sets in. This indicates a failure to adapt, and the resulting physiological and psychological imbalance can disrupt the progress of labour (Annie & Groer 1991). Prolonged labour causes greater anxiety and stress.

The midwife's role must be to educate the woman about the process of labour and so minimise her anxiety (Raphael-Leff 1991). This should allow the normal physiological processes to proceed as efficiently as possible.

---

the body to deal with stressful conditions by increasing metabolic processes, muscular contraction and cardiovascular and respiratory function, while decreasing digestion (Box 3.2).

OTHER SITES OF ENDOCRINE ACTIVITY

Endocrine cells are present in many organs of the body. The *pancreas*, for example, though principally made up of exocrine glands, also contains endocrine tissue. The endocrine cells are situated in the islets of Langerhans and consist of alpha, beta, delta and F cells, each secreting a different hormone.

Alpha cells secrete *glucagon* when blood glucose levels are below normal. Glucagon converts glycogen, stored in the liver and skeletal muscles, into glucose.

Beta cells secrete *insulin* when blood glucose and nutrient levels are high. Insulin converts glucose into glycogen for storage, so increasing protein and fatty acid synthesis, the uptake of glucose by cell membranes (particularly in muscle cells), and the storage of fats in adipose tissue (Box 3.3).

Box 3.3 Diabetes mellitus

Diabetes mellitus is a condition in which a deficit or complete absence of insulin, or a resistance of cell membranes to insulin, prevents glucose being used by cells to fuel metabolism. Cells break down fats and proteins for fuel instead. The absence of insulin for whatever reason prevents glucose being converted to glycogen for storage in the liver and muscle cells when blood sugar levels are high. High blood sugar levels (*hyperglycaemia*) result, which can be detected in urine, because the renal threshold for glucose is exceeded.

Hyperglycaemia causes damage to many body systems (Lewis 1992). Water is lost in the urine along with glucose, and so the patient passes excessive amounts of urine (*polyuria*) and becomes excessively thirsty in consequence (*polydipsia*). Because proteins and fats are being broken down, the patient becomes excessively hungry (*polyphagia*). Weight loss occurs too.

There are two types of diabetes mellitus: *insulin dependent diabetes mellitus* (IDDM), and *non-insulin dependent diabetes mellitus* (NIDDM). In IDDM, insulin is required by injection to enable cells to use glucose circulating in the blood. In NIDDM, dietary control and possibly hypoglycaemic drugs maintain blood sugar at the correct level.

The presence of IDDM during pregnancy (NIDDM diabetes tends to occur in later life), increases the risk of *stillbirth* or *congenital abnormality* (Steel et al 1990). Both maternal and fetal mortality and morbidity are increased (Brudenell 1991). A woman who does not have diabetes before becoming pregnant may develop it in pregnancy. This is called *gestational diabetes*. A pregnant woman with either type of diabetes will need to be cared for throughout pregnancy by both a diabetologist and an obstetrician, to minimise complications.

Delta cells secrete several hormones including *GHRIH*, which inhibits the secretion of both glucagon and insulin. *F cells* secrete *pancreatic polypeptide* that regulates the release of pancreatic digestive enzymes.

Endocrine cells are also found:

- In the *ovaries* of the female, where *oestrogen* and *progesterone* are responsible for the reproductive cycle, the development and maintenance of female characteristics, the continuation of a pregnancy and the preparation of the breasts for lactation. The ovaries also secrete *inhibin*, which inhibits secretion of FSH and LH, and *relaxin*, which relaxes pelvic ligaments during pregnancy and plays a role in cervical dilation.
- In the male *testes*, where *testosterone* is synthesised, which is responsible for the development and maintenance of male characteristics and the production of spermatozoa.
- In the *placenta* during pregnancy, releasing *human chorionic gonadotrophin* initially to maintain the corpus luteum until the placenta is fully functional, and then *oestrogen, progesterone, human placental lactogen, corticosteroids, ACTH and TSH* for the remainder of the pregnancy.
- In the *digestive tract*, where hormones are secreted which regulate the release of digestive enzymes.
- In the *atria* of the heart, where *atrial natriuretic peptide* is secreted to help regulate blood volume.
- In the *kidneys*, where *erythropoietin* is synthesised, which increases the production of red blood cells.
- In *blood* and *mast cells*, which secrete *histamine*. This plays a role in the inflammatory response, digestive processes and the contraction of smooth muscle in the bronchi.
- In *platelets*, the *brain* and the *gastrointestinal tract*, where *serotonin* is produced. This plays a role in digestive processes and in smooth muscle contraction.

Prostaglandins are present in most tissues and have a varied role. These are thought, for example, to influence the female reproductive tract, pituitary function, body temperature in response to the inflammatory response and the transmission of pain stimuli.

HORMONAL ACTION

There are thought to be about 50 different hormones in the human body, each responsible for altering the function of just a few types of cell. A hormone identifies its *target cells* by the presence of specific receptors on the cell membrane or within cytosol. The hormone binds to these receptors and chemically alters the metabolic processes of the target cells.

Hormones are transported round the body in the blood. Endocrine glands are very vascular, making it easy for hormones to diffuse into the bloodstream. Some hormones are transported unattached in the plasma, whereas others rely on the presence of transport proteins which they bind to for transportation. Binding with proteins has two main advantages:

1. hormones are readily available to all their target cells as required
2. small hormones are not lost by filtration when they pass through the kidneys.

PHYSIOLOGICAL CHANGES THROUGH THE CHILDBEARING YEAR

Pregnancy

The majority of *hormonal changes* in pregnancy are related to the activity of the placenta. The role of the endocrine system in the placenta, the reproductive cycle, fertilisation and pregnancy is discussed in Part 2.

Many of the alterations in endocrine activity during pregnancy match changing body needs. The resulting physiological changes in organs and tissues lead to the common *discomforts of pregnancy*. These are described in later chapters, in the context of the systems to which they relate.

Some symptoms however, are directly linked to relative hormone levels, rather than to any alterations in function. Early in pregnancy, for example, many women complain of *changes in appetite, sleep patterns* and *food tolerance*. This type of symptom is a result of the increased level of human chorionic gonadotrophin (hCG) (McNabb 1997). Once the amount of hCG lessens the symptoms generally resolve. Altered patterns of sleep are thought to be related to the sedative effect of progesterone (Coutts 1998).

During pregnancy the secretion of *FSH* and *LH* from the pituitary gland is minimal, as a cyclical reproductive cycle is not required. *Prolactin* levels rise from early in pregnancy in preparation for lactation. Other pituitary hormones also increase, specifically *ACTH, TSH* and *MSH* (Llewellyn-Jones 1994).

Largely as a result of these changes in hormone secretion by the pituitary gland, the amounts of hormones in specific endocrine glands are significantly altered. For example, *cortisol* levels from the adrenal glands increase from the second trimester of pregnancy (Klein 1995). Cortisol is involved in many metabolic processes, and is required in greater quantities to meet the body's extra workload during pregnancy. *Corticosteroid* levels overall are increased in pregnancy and are thought to be implicated in the development of *striae gravidarum* (stretch marks), the presence of *glucose in the urine* and in *raised blood pressure* (Llewellyn-Jones 1994).

Hormones released by the thyroid gland play an important role in reproduction. Metabolism is largely controlled by thyroid hormones, so it is not surprising that thyroid function alters during pregnancy. Levels of both T_3 and T_4 increase (Mooney et al 1998), and peak at around 10–15 weeks' gestation. The basal metabolic rate also increases (Lewis & Chamberlain 1990). *Nausea and vomiting* in early pregnancy have been associated with the raised levels of T_4 and hCG, and also with the correspondingly higher amounts of TSH (Blackburn & Loper 1992).

Labour

Both fetal and maternal endocrine systems are thought to be involved in the *initiation of labour* (Box 3.4). The fetus is considered to control this event (Symonds & Symonds 1998). *Cortisol* levels

---

Box 3.4 Induction of labour

Normal human gestation is considered to be 37–42 completed weeks (Cardozo 1993). However, some pregnancies go past 42 weeks with no sign that delivery is imminent. If there is concern regarding the health of the mother or the fetus in utero, it may be considered best to deliver the fetus, rather than continue the pregnancy. Provided dates have been accurately predicted (usually by ultrasound), intervention by induction of labour is thought to reduce both the perinatal mortality rate and the number of caesarian sections (Gardosi et al 1997). However there is some evidence to suggest that induction results in longer labour, increased instrumental delivery and a lower Apgar score (Goer 1995).

Onset of labour can be induced in several ways. Firstly, vaginal examination will determine whether there has been any effacement of the cervix, commonly referred to as ripening of the cervix. Should the cervix not be effaced then prostaglandin gel can be inserted into the posterior fornix to initiate the process (Keirse & van Oppen 1989).

Once the cervix has effaced, uterine contractions can be initiated with a synthetic oxytocin infusion called syntocinon, accompanied by amniotomy. However, the midwife must take care that the uterus is not overstimulated. Too frequent contractions with insufficient rest between them may cause physical distress of both the fetus and the labouring woman (Keirse & Chalmers 1989).

---

from the fetal adrenal gland rise towards term. This is thought to reduce the amount of *progesterone* released by the placenta and increase production of *oestrogen* (Bobak 1995). Progesterone inhibits uterine muscle activity; oestrogens increase it. Late in pregnancy, more oxytocin receptors appear on uterine muscle cell membranes in response to the high levels of oestrogens. *Oxytocin* is then released in greater quantities by the posterior lobe of the maternal pituitary gland, and the uterus is stimulated to contract.

Postnatal

With the expulsion of the placenta, many hormone levels fall dramatically (Cashion 1995). The drop in *oestrogen* levels allows prolactin to act on the alveoli of the breast to begin milk production. *Prolactin* and *oxytocin* levels remain high to maintain breast-feeding. Oxytocin also maintains the contraction of uterine muscle, so minimising blood loss during the puerperium. In women who choose not to breast-feed, prolactin levels gradually fall due to lack of stimulus by the baby at the breast, resulting in the resumption of the reproduction cycle within 14–21 days of delivery (Ball 1993). In women who do breast-feed, this return to normal reproductive functioning generally takes longer.

The endocrine system as a whole generally returns to normal soon after delivery. Changes in *thyroid* levels occur more slowly, returning to prepregnancy levels by 6 weeks postpartum (Popovich & Moore 1993).

The neonate

The endocrine system is largely functional by term in the neonate. However, hormones related to reproduction are not produced until puberty.

During the second half of pregnancy, the fetal adrenal gland begins to produce *cortisol*. This results in the maturation of many fetal organs, in preparation for extrauterine life. The liver increases *glycogen* synthesis and produces many enzymes required for digestion. The storage of glycogen prevents hypoglycaemia for the first days of life whilst feeding is established (Box 3.5). The production of *surfactant*, which enables the lungs to function, is under the control of many hormones, particularly cortisol, oestrogen, adrenaline and thyroid hormones.

Box 3.5 Hypoglycaemia

The stress of labour and delivery into the extrauterine world uses up much of the glycogen stored in the neonate towards the end of pregnancy. Feeding often takes a few hours or even days to establish, particularly if breast-feeding. One concern of those who care for a newborn infant uninterested in feeding, is that he will become *hypoglycaemic*, i.e. have too low a level of glucose in the blood (Hawden et al 1993). However in the full-term infant, glycogen stores normally provide the infant with sufficient energy until feeding is established (Smith 1995). The full-term fetus will also have adequate fat stores for use if required (Dodds 1996).

The preterm infant however may not have had sufficient time in the uterus to produce adequate stores of glycogen or adipose tissue, and so must be closely observed for signs of hypoglycaemia (Henschel & Inch 1996). These include lethargy, irregular respiration and jitteriness of the limbs. Other babies at risk of hypoglycaemia are those who are growth-retarded, and those with diabetic mothers. In all these cases, early feeding and close observation is essential (National Childbirth Trust 1997). If a newborn baby shows signs of hypoglycaemia, blood will be taken to test for glucose levels. Low blood glucose levels can be associated with long-term neurological damage (Kane et al 1997).

Thyroid hormones and noradrenaline are required for the metabolism of brown fat in thermoregulation (see Ch. 5). The full-term neonate can respond to cold by increasing its metabolic rate by up to 100%. The preterm infant responds less rapidly to cold stress and is therefore at greater risk of hypothermia.

REFERENCES

Annie C L, Groer M 1991 Childbirth stress: an immunologic study. Journal of Obstetric, Gynecologic and Neonatal Nursing 20(5):391–397

Ball J A 1993 Physiology, psychology and management of the puerperium. In: Bennett V R, Brown L K (eds) Myles textbook for midwives, 12th edn. Churchill Livingstone, Edinburgh, p 234

Blackburn S T, Loper D L 1992 Maternal, fetal and neonatal physiology. W B Saunders, Philadelphia, p 660–663

Bobak I M 1995 Genetics, conception and fetal development. In: Bobak I M, Lowdermilk D L, Jenson M D (eds) Maternity nursing, 4th edn. Mosby, St Louis, p 82

Brudenell M 1991 Diabetes in pregnancy. Maternal and Child Health 16(6):174–182

Cardozo L 1993 Is routine induction of labour at term ever justified? British Medical Journal 306(6881):840–841

Cashion K 1995 Maternal physiology during the postpartum period. In: Bobak I M, Lowdermilk D L, Jenson M D Maternity nursing, 4th edn. Mosby, St Louis, p 442–443

Coutts A 1998 The 'minor problems' of pregnancy: a review. Professional Care of the Mother and Child 8(4):95–97

Daker M, Bobrow M 1989 Biochemical screening for disease in the newborn infant. In: Chalmers I, Enkin E, Keirse M J N C (eds) Effective care in pregnancy and childbirth. Oxford University Press, Oxford, p 1419–1420

Dodds R 1996 When policies collide: breast feeding and hypoglycaemia. MIDIRS Midwifery Digest 6(4):382–386

Gardosi J, Vanner T, Francis A 1997 Gestational age and induction of labour for prolonged pregnancy. British Journal of Obstetrics and Gynaecology 104(7):792–797

Ginesi L, Niescierowicz R 1998 Neuroendocrinology and birth 1: stress. British Journal of Midwifery 6(10):659–663

Goer H 1995 Obstetric myths versus research realities. Bergin and Garvey, Connecticut, p 179–202

Hawden J M, Ward Platt M P, Ainsley Green A 1993 Neonatal hypoglycaemia: blood glucose monitoring and baby feeding. Midwifery 9(1):3–6

Henschel D, Inch S 1996 Breast feeding: a guide for midwives. Books for Midwives Press, Cheshire, p 90–93

Kane R M, Bennett V R, Crafter H 1997 Management of neonatal hypoglycaemia: a wide disparity in midwives' practice. MIDIRS Midwifery Digest 7(1):100–103

Keirse M J N C, Chalmers I 1989 Methods of inducing labour. In: Chalmers I, Enkin E, Keirse M J N C (eds) Effective care in pregnancy and childbirth. Oxford University Press, Oxford, p 1065–1066

Keirse M J N C, van Oppen A C C 1989 Preparing the cervix for induction of labour. In: Chalmers I, Enkin E, Keirse M J N C (eds) Effective care in pregnancy and childbirth. Oxford University Press, Oxford, p 1051–1052

Klein P M 1995 Anatomy and physiology of pregnancy. In: Bobak I M, Lowdermilk D L, Jenson M D (eds) Maternity nursing, 4th edn. Mosby, St Louis, p 91–108

Lewis P 1992 Diabetes in pregnancy. Modern Midwife 1(6):14–18

Lewis T L T, Chamberlain G V P (eds) 1990 Obstetrics by ten teachers, 15th edn. Edward Arnold, London, p 26

Llewellyn-Jones D 1994 Fundamentals of obstetrics and gynaecology, 6th edn. Mosby, London, p 29

McNabb M 1997 Maternal and fetal physiological responses to pregnancy. In: Sweet B R (ed) Mayes' midwifery. A textbook for midwives. Baillière Tindall, London, p 124

Mooney C J, James D A, Kessenich C R 1998 Diagnosis and management of hypothyroidism in pregnancy. Journal of Obstetric, Gynecologic and Neonatal Nursing 27(4):374–380

National Childbirth Trust 1997 Hypoglycaemia of the newborn. Midwives 110(1317):248–249

Niven C A 1992 Psychological care for families. Butterworth Heinemann, Oxford, p 40–44

Popovich D, Moore L 1993 Pregnancy in women with thyroid disease: a delicate balance. Journal of Perinatal and Neonatal Nursing 7(3):29–38

Raphael-Leff J 1991 Psychological processes of childbearing. Chapman and Hall, London, p 242–251

Ramsey I D 1991 The thyroid gland. In: Hytten F, Chamberlain G (eds) Clinical physiology in obstetrics, 2nd edn. Blackwell Scientific, Oxford, p 361

Smith J 1990 Pregnancy complicated by thyroid disease. Journal of Nurse-Midwifery 35(3):143–149

Smith S L 1995 Hypoglycemia in the neonate. In: Alexander J, Levy V, Roch S (eds) Aspects of midwifery practice. A research-based approach. Macmillan, Basingstoke, p 154–176

Steel J M, Johnstone F D, Hepburn D A, Smith A F 1990 Can prepregnancy care of diabetic women reduce the risk of abnormal babies? British Medical Journal 301(6760):1070–1074

Sweet B R (ed) 1997 Mayes' midwifery. A textbook for midwives. Baillière Tindall, London, p 555

Symonds E M, Symonds I M 1998 Essential obstetrics and gynaecology, 3rd edn. Churchill Livingstone, New York, p 129

Too S 1997 Clinical: stress, social support and reproductive health. Modern Midwife 7(12):15–19

4

The special senses

The body's sense organs detect and transmit information about the external environment to the nervous system so that the body can alter its actions as required to maintain normal functioning. The special senses are responsible for alerting the body to its position relative to other objects, through vision, and for monitoring posture and balance, via the fluid levels in the inner ear. The ear also detects sounds in the environment, by the process of hearing. Pleasure resulting from the taste of ingested foodstuffs (detected by the taste buds) can encourage the process of taking in nutrients. This pleasure may be enhanced by the smell of the food, detected by the sense organs in the nasal cavity. Finally the fifth sense, touch, enables us to explore and learn from the environment in which we live, gathering further information for the nervous system.

During pregnancy many of the senses are enhanced under the influence of the increased levels of hormones. This may aggravate some of the minor disorders commonly associated with pregnancy such as morning sickness or altered taste. The special senses play no direct role in labour, but contribute to the nervous system's overall interpretation of events. Postnatally the functioning of the special senses quickly returns to its prepregnancy state.

In the newborn infant at term all the special senses are functioning sufficiently to enable him to react to the environment. The transition from the muted stimuli of the uterine environment to the outside world may constitute a shock to the neonate, and this factor must be considered when preparing the area where delivery is to take place.

The following organs are responsible for the special senses:

- two eyes, which detect light
- two ears, which detect sound and control balance
- taste buds, situated in the tongue and oral cavity, that detect the presence of chemicals
- olfactory cells in the nasal cavity, which detect the odour caused by chemicals
- touch receptors situated in the skin, which give further information about the external environment.

THE EYES

Vision is the result of the detection of light by the eyes, their transmission to the brain and subsequent interpretation by the cerebral cortex. Accessory structures protect the eyes from damage.

The *eye* is a spherical object, which is largely enclosed within a bony indentation in the skull, called the *orbit*. Fatty tissue forms a protective layer between the eye and the bone of the orbit. The eye is composed of three layers (Fig. 4.1):

1. an outer fibrous layer forming the sclera and cornea
2. a middle vascular layer containing the central iris surrounded by the ciliary body and choroid, behind which the lens is suspended
3. an inner layer of nervous tissue, the retina.

The *sclera* is the white of the eye that forms the posterior and lateral walls and is continuous with the cornea at the front. It consists of fibrous tissue that maintains the eye's rounded shape. It also forms an attachment for the extrinsic muscles required for focusing.

The *cornea* is a transparent membrane of epithelial tissue which allows light to enter the eye. It is involved in bending light rays to focus them on the internal retina.

The circular *iris* is situated beneath the cornea and is formed from the middle vascular layer of the eye. The iris divides the interior of the eye into anterior and posterior chambers. It is com-

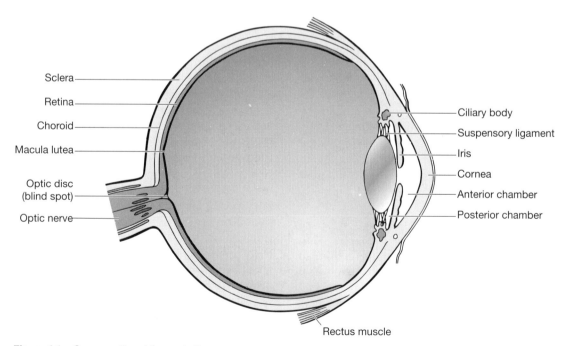

Figure 4.1   Cross-section of the eyeball.

posed of pigment cells, which give the familiar colour to the eye, and two layers of smooth muscle. Centrally there is an aperture, the *pupil* of the eye, which can be increased and decreased in diameter by these layers of smooth muscle, according to the intensity of light entering the eye. The autonomic nervous system is responsible for the action of these muscles.

Surrounding the iris is the *ciliary body*, composed of smooth muscle and secretory epithelial cells. The ciliary body acts as an attachment for the *suspensory ligaments*, which supports the lens. The muscle of the ciliary body is responsible for changing the shape of the lens to focus light on the retina. Again this action is effected by the autonomic nervous system. The secretory epithelium forms the aqueous humor – a specialised fluid that fills the chambers of the eye. The remainder of the middle layer of the eye is composed of the highly vascular *choroid* that lines the sclera and provides nutrients for the retina. It is also responsible for absorbing light after the image has been formed on the retina.

Immediately behind the pupil is the *lens*. This is a transparent circular biconvex structure formed from elastic tissue. It is attached to the ciliary body by the suspensory ligaments, and its thickness can be altered by the action of the ciliary muscle through the suspensory ligament, enabling light entering the eye to be focused on the retina.

The inner layer contains one structure, the *retina*, which is an extremely delicate membrane consisting of several layers of nerve fibres that react to light (Box 4.1). These lie on a pigmented layer of cells attaching it to the choroid. The retina lines most of the eye, and is thickest at the rear becoming thinner towards the anterior. A specialised area of the retina is the *macula lutea*, which is seen as a yellow area towards the centre of the rear of the retina. All the nerve fibres of the retina converge on an area towards the inner aspect of the eye, where they form the optic nerve. At this point there are no light sensitive nerve cells. This area is called the *optic disc* or blind spot, and is where the optic nerve leaves the eye.

The retina is responsible for reacting to the

Box 4.1   Retinopathy of prematurity

Preterm infants require prolonged oxygen therapy at high arterial pO_2 levels to provide sufficient oxygen to the cells of the body. However, when exposed to high oxygen levels for long periods of time, preterm infants run the risk of damage to the eyes (Thomson & Torley 1993). Arterioles in the retina of the eye constrict when exposed to these levels of oxygen, and when prolonged these changes are irreversible (Llewellyn-Jones 1994). Once the infant is able to obtain sufficient oxygen at normal levels, retinal arterioles proliferate, causing the retina to detach and fibrous tissue to form (Sweet 1997). Blindness can be the result. This condition is named retrolental fibroplasia or *retinopathy of prematurity*. The problem for the neonatologist is to balance the amount of oxygen required for respiration to prevent brain damage, against the possible occurrence of retinopathy.

light entering the eye and relaying this information to the cerebral cortex for interpretation.

Between the cornea and the lens of the eye are two chambers divided incompletely by the iris. These are the *anterior* and *posterior chambers*, containing aqueous fluid or humor. *Aqueous fluid* is secreted from the ciliary processes, and flows throughout the eye to the scleral venous sinus, where it is discharged into the circulatory system. Aqueous fluid is maintained at a constant pressure and provides a constant supply of nutrients as well as removing waste products.

Behind the lens, filling most of the eye, is a jelly-like substance called the *vitreous body*. This is mainly composed of water, with the addition of protein and salts. Its function is to give support to the eye as a whole and to maintain the position of the retina against the choroid.

Accessory structures

The accessory structures of the eye are:

• the eyelids
• the lacrimal glands.

Two *eyelids*, the upper and lower, enclose each eyeball. They are made up of connective tissue and muscle into which eyelashes are inserted. A fine transparent membrane, the *conjunctiva*, covers the inner surface of the eyelids and continues over the surface of the eye. The eyelids

---

Box 4.2 Ophthalmia neonatorum

Newborn babies commonly develop sticky eyes. The fluid that bathes the eyes usually drains down the lacrimal ducts, but these can be easily blocked in the early days after delivery. Tears are not generally shed until the baby is a month old, which aggravates the situation. Cleaning the eyes with a saline solution will usually clear the problem. Occasionally an infection will be present and the infant will need treating with the appropriate antibiotic eyedrops. The usual causative organisms for this condition, known as *ophthalmia neonatorum*, are E. coli and staphylococcus (Kelnar et al 1995).

Rarely the neonate may be delivered with an infection obtained from the vagina such as gonococcus or chlamydia. These latter infections must be treated rigorously as they are highly infectious and may cause permanent damage to the eyes (Silverton 1993).

---

protect the eye, inhibiting external stimuli during sleep, and lubricate the surface of the eye with the mucous membrane that lines the eyelids. Additionally, a watery solution called lacrimal fluid containing antibacterial substances such as lysozyme is constantly produced by the *lacrimal glands* and swept over the surface of the eye by the eyelids to moisten and protect (Box 4.2). This fluid drains into two ducts on the inner aspect of the eyelids, the lacrimal ducts, and eventually into the nasal cavity. Any foreign bodies will stimulate the lacrimal glands to increase production to wash the object away from the surface of the eye. Parasympathetic stimulation in the form of strong emotion may also result in increased lacrimal fluid production, i.e. in crying.

Three pairs of *extrinsic muscles* are inserted into the surface of the eye, which enable the eyeball to make precise and rapid movements. The brain stem and cerebellum are involved in the coordination of the two eyes.

Blood supply

Branches of the internal carotid artery, the ciliary arteries and a central retinal artery supply arterial blood to the eye. Venous drainage is down several routes.

Physiology of sight

The retina contains light-sensitive nerve cells known, because of their shapes, as rods and cones. When light from the visible spectrum hits these nerve cells, chemical changes stimulate nerve impulses, which are passed along the optic nerve to the visual cortex of the brain situated in the occipital lobe.

Cones are sensitive to bright light and colour. Colour is identified by the presence of specific pigments. There are three types of cone each containing one type of photosensitive pigment. Each pigment can only be stimulated by one colour. Thus colour is determined in the visual cortex according to which cones are transmitting nerve impulses.

Rods are stimulated by low-intensity light and wave lengths associated with blue/green light. Rods contain a light-sensitive pigment, *rhodopsin*, which changes shape in the presence of light. Regeneration of rhodopsin takes a short period of time, during which the rods cannot be stimulated by light. In the presence of bright light many rods are degraded, and this explains why it takes time for the eyes to adapt when moving from an area of bright light to one of darkness. Because rods are sensitive to dim light and detect only green/blue wavelengths, there is a subdued perception of colour in a darkened area. Not enough light enters the eyes to stimulate the cones to determine specific colour. There is no time lag in adaptation, when moving from dark to light, however, because cones are immediately receptive to light.

Rods and cones are distributed unevenly throughout the retina. In the macula lutea there are only cones, mostly of the type sensitive to red or green. From this point outwards the number of cones decreases and the number of rods increases, until at the periphery there are considerably more rods than cones.

Light is reflected from objects in the field of vision. *Colour* is determined by the wavelength of this light. White light is a combination of all the colours of the visual spectrum. Each colour has a specific wavelength. Objects absorb light of certain wavelengths, and reflect a small range of wavelengths, giving the impression that an object is of the colour of the light reflected.

Rods and cones are responsible for sending information to the brain for interpretation. The eye is designed to enable a clear picture to be focused on the retina. This picture is actually inverted, but the brain interprets it so the world is seen the right way up. This process occurs by: refraction of light onto the retina, by alterations to the aperture of the pupil of the eye, and by accommodation of the eyes.

Refraction is the bending of light, and it occurs at the junction between structures of different density. To enter the eye light must pass through the conjunctiva, cornea, aqueous fluid, lens and vitreous humour. All these structures are denser than air and so refract the incoming light. The lens is the only structure that can alter the degree to which light is refracted. This is essential to focus light clearly on the retina, as light from far distances needs less refraction than light from closer to the eye. The degree of contraction of the ciliary muscle will affect the curvature of the lens and hence its refractive power (Box 4.3).

To enable a clear picture to reach the retina, the amount of light entering the eye must be controlled. Too much light would cause the cones to be excessively stimulated, making interpretation by the brain difficult. The pupil of the eye constricts therefore in the presence of bright light, and dilates when light is diminished. This is carried out by the muscles present in the iris, under the control of the autonomic nervous system.

Box 4.3   Myopia

The normal eye can focus objects up to 6 m away onto the retina by altering the curvature of the lens so that light waves are refracted, as they pass through it. Not all people have this ability. In some, the length of the eyeball prevents correct refraction. Those who suffer myopia – near-sightedness – either have a longer than normal eyeball or a thickened lens. Light is therefore focused in front of the retina. People who are far-sighted have a shortened eyeball, and so the image is focused behind the retina. Astigmatism is a condition where the lens or cornea has an irregular shape, which prevents the image being focused. This results in blurred vision. Contact lenses or glasses can easily correct all of these conditions.

Accommodation of the eyes is achieved by both the above processes, along with movement of the eyes themselves. To enable light to reach the retina centrally, not only must the pupil constrict to allow the correct amount of light to enter, but the eye must also move to a position where the light passes through the pupil centrally. The same is true for the lens. The main factor influencing how good an image is formed on the retina for transmission to the brain is the position of the two eyes: they should be positioned such that the image is formed on the same part of the retina in both eyes. This is called *convergence of the eyes* and is achieved by the use of the eyes' extrinsic muscles. Part of this is a voluntary act – the head and the muscles of the eyes move to look directly at an interesting object. Constant readjustment is required to fine-tune this, carried out by the autonomic nervous system.

There are distinct advantages to having two eyes. Each eye sees a scene slightly differently: the left eye detects light waves from further to the left, and the right eye from further to the right of the body. This creates a larger picture, and so a better interpretation of height, width and distance is possible.

The visual pathways involved in the interpretation of light are shown in Figure 4.2. Nerve fibres from the retina converge at the blind spot where they join to form the optic nerve. The two branches of the optic nerve, one from each eye, meet at the *optic chiasma*, which is situated in front of and slightly above the pituitary gland. At this point fibres from the inner aspect of the retina cross to the opposite side. Those from the outer aspect continue on the same side. All nerve fibres then synapse in the thalamus, continuing on to the visual cortex. Some nerve fibres originate in the thalamus and, stimulated by optic nerve fibres, pass information from the eyes, ears, muscles and joints to the cerebellum, to contribute to the maintenance of balance.

THE EARS

Hearing is the result of the detection by the ears of sound waves, which are transmitted to the

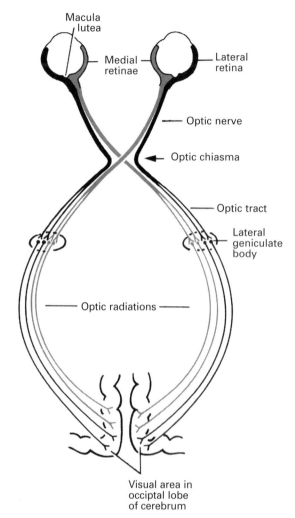

Figure 4.2 Visual pathways. (Reproduced with permission from Wilson K J W, Waugh A 1996 Ross and Wilson Anatomy and Physiology in Health and Illness. Churchill Livingstone, Edinburgh)

auditory cortex in the temporal lobe and interpreted by the brain.

The ear is divided into (Fig. 4.3):

1. the outer ear
2. the middle ear
3. the inner ear.

Except for the pinna of the outer ear, all the structures of the ear are enclosed in temporal bone.

The outer ear

The outer ear consists of the pinna or auricle, and the external auditory meatus. The *pinna* is a trumpet-shaped enlarged portion of cartilage that projects out from the side of the head. Its outer aspect is ridged and is called the helix. At the lower aspect is a highly vascular more pliable structure, the ear lobe. The function of the pinna is to funnel sound waves into the meatus of the ear.

The *external auditory meatus* is a curved tube along which sound waves travel to stimulate the middle ear. This tube is approximately 25 mm long and extends from the pinna to the eardrum. It is formed partly of cartilage and partly by the temporal bone. The external auditory meatus is lined with hair and secretory glands. These glands include wax-producing glands containing lysozyme and immunoglobulins. The presence of hair and glands, plus the curvature of the meatus, prevent foreign materials reaching the eardrum. These become entangled in the wax, which is expelled from the ear by the action of the mandible during eating and talking.

The middle ear

The middle ear consists of the eardrum and the tympanic cavity, which contains three tiny bones. The eardrum, or *tympanic membrane*, separates the external auditory meatus from the sensitive middle ear. It is formed from fibrous tissue, covered externally with skin and internally by a mucous membrane continuous with that of the middle ear.

The *tympanic cavity* is an irregular-shaped cavity within the temporal bone. It is filled with air that enters through the auditory (also called eustachian) tube. The *auditory tube* is 40 mm long, lined with ciliated epithelium, and extends from the pharynx into the tympanic cavity. The function of the auditory tube is to equalise the air pressure on each side of the tympanic membrane so that sound waves will cause the membrane to vibrate.

Within the *tympanic cavity* lie three tiny bones, or ossicles (Fig. 4.4):

1. the malleus

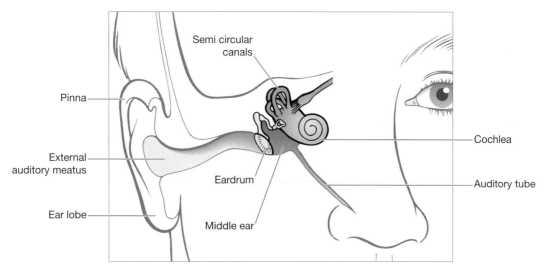

Figure 4.3   Macrostructure of the ear.

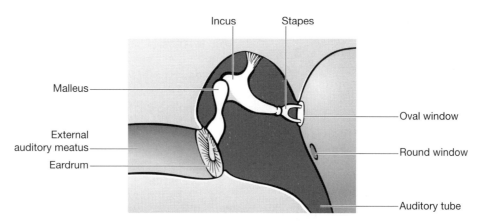

Figure 4.4   Ossicles of the middle ear.

2. the incus
3. the stapes.

These bones stretch from the tympanic membrane to a bony partition that separates the middle ear from the inner ear. The *malleus* is a hammer-shaped bone lying with its handle to the tympanic membrane and head to the incus. The *incus* forms a moveable joint with the malleus and is shaped like an anvil. The body of the incus connects with the malleus: one extremity links with the stapes, the other is anchored on the posterior wall of the tympanic cavity. The *stapes*

is a stirrup-shaped bone, the head meeting the incus at a moveable joint, and the footplate situated on the oval window. The *oval window* is an aperture into the inner ear through the temporal bone. One other aperture is found in the middle ear: the *round window*, which also leads to the inner ear.

The malleus, incus and stapes transmit sound waves from the tympanic membrane to the inner ear by vibrating. Muscles anchoring these tiny bones to the walls of the tympanic cavity limit movement and protect these delicate structures and the inner ear from excessive sound.

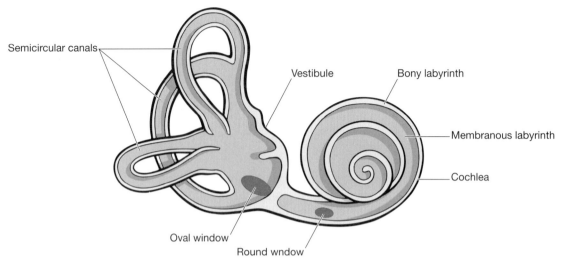

Figure 4.5   Structures of the inner ear.

The inner ear

The inner ear consists of the bony and membranous labyrinths and is responsible for the transmission of information from the ear to the brain where it is interpreted (Fig. 4.5). The *bony labyrinth* is a cavity in the temporal bone, within which the membranous labyrinth lies. The bony labyrinth consists of a vestibule, cochlea and semicircular canals. The *vestibule* is an expanded portion of the cavity, which lies close to the middle ear and contains the oval and round windows. The *cochlea* has the shape of a snail's shell, with a broad base continuous with the vestibule, and spirals around a central bony column. The *semicircular canals* are three tubes continuous with the vestibule, each one lying in one of the three planes of space.

Between the bony and membranous labyrinths there is a layer of fluid called *perilymph*. Contained in the membranous labyrinth is a fluid called *endolymph*. Both of these fluids serve to transmit sound waves.

The *membranous labyrinth* has the same general shape as the bony labyrinth. It is also divided into a vestibule, cochlea and semicircular ducts. Neuroepithelial cells, consisting of hair cells and supporting cells, line the length of the cochlea of the membranous labyrinth and form the sense organ of the ear, the *spiral organ of Corti*. Hair cells are in contact with a membrane, the tectorial membrane. The semicircular ducts and vestibule contain receptors for equilibrium.

Physiology of hearing and balance

Sound is a physical sensation received by the ear. It is caused by a vibrating source and is transmitted through the air as sound waves. High-pitched sound creates short frequency waves; low-pitched sound produces long wavelengths. Sound waves from outside the human body are directed into the external auditory meatus by the trumpet-shaped pinna of the external ear. The sound waves set up vibrations in the tympanic membrane and the bony ossicles of the middle ear. The stapes vibrates against the oval window producing waves in the perilymph and subsequently in the endolymph. These waves are detected by the neuroepithelial cells in the spiral organ along the length of the cochlea. Short wavelengths produce frequent waves and longer wavelengths less frequent waves. The waves stimulate hair cells at specific intervals along the cochlea to bend against the tectorial membrane, initiating nerve impulses. These are transmitted along the eighth cranial nerve – the *vestibulocochlear nerve* – to the medulla where many pathways cross, then to the thalamus and on to the auditory centre in the temporal lobe of the cerebrum for interpretation.

The semicircular ducts provide the body with information about the position of the head in space and contribute to the maintenance of balance and equilibrium. Movement of the head creates movement of the perilymph and endolymph, which stimulates nerve endings and hair cells in the semicircular ducts and the vestibule of the membranous labyrinth. This results in the transmission of nerve impulses – also along the vestibulocochlear nerve – to the cerebellum. The cerebellum sends continuous information to the motor cortex to enable the brain to initiate muscle and joint adjustments to maintain balance and equilibrium.

TASTE AND TASTE BUDS

Chemicals have distinct tastes when dissolved in fluid. Taste buds capable of detecting these chemicals are widely distributed throughout the epithelium of the tongue, soft palate, epiglottis and pharynx (Fig. 4.6). The presence of a pleasant taste enhances the acts of eating and drinking.

Taste buds consist of small collections of cell bodies and nerve endings of the seventh, ninth and tenth cranial nerves – the facial, glosso-pharyngeal and vagus nerves. Chemical activation causes these nerve cells to depolarise and transmit impulses to the thalamus and then to the taste area of the cerebral cortex.

Four types of taste can be distinguished by taste buds found on different parts of the tongue. The tip of the tongue can detect sweet and salty tastes, the lateral aspects of the tongue sour tastes, and the rear of the tongue bitter tastes. The taste of the food ingested also depends on its temperature and texture (detected by other receptors in the mouth), and is also influenced by its smell.

OLFACTORY CELLS AND SMELL

Chemicals release smells which are detected by specialised receptors situated in the epithelium of the superior aspect of the nasal cavity. These *olfactory receptors* enhance the taste of food and drink. Olfactory receptors are nerve cells with ciliated ends that are stimulated by the presence of a chemical. Many receptors join one axon and transmit information along the olfactory nerve – the first cranial nerve – to *olfactory bulbs* situated in the base of the brain. From here the impulses are transmitted along the olfactory tract to the thalamus and from there to the relevant area of the cortex, in the frontal lobes of the brain. Some nerve impulses are transmitted to the limbic system allowing emotional memories to affect the interpretation of the smell.

Olfactory glands are also situated in the nasal

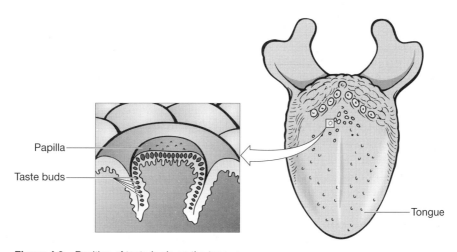

Papilla

Taste buds

Tongue

Figure 4.6   Position of taste buds on the tongue.

epithelium and constantly secrete mucus which moistens the epithelium and dissolves the surface film of fluid, along with any odorous gases, enabling fresh smells to be perceived.

The sensation of smell is poorly understood. Many attempts have been made to distinguish between and classify smells. Recent thinking suggests than that there are hundreds of different smells distinguishable by the olfactory nerve cells. A key characteristic of the sensation of smell is its speed of adaptation. Our perception of smells – even strong smells – quickly decreases and soon ceases altogether. This is thought to be due to adaptation of the olfactory nerves and of the cerebral cortex itself.

TOUCH AND TOUCH RECEPTORS

Receptors for touch, or tactile, sensations are situated in many of the coverings of the body, including the skin and mucous membranes such as those lining the mouth and anus. Touch receptors are not evenly distributed throughout the body, but are more densely situated in areas where exploration of the environment is more likely. For example, they are spread thinly in the skin of the back, which is not commonly used for tactile exploration, whereas they are present in abundance in the lips and fingers.

The sensation of touch has two main components, touch and pressure, each detected by a different type of dendrite. Dendrites make up part of the sensory component of the nervous system (see Ch. 2).

Meissner's corpuscles are an egg-shaped collection of dendrites that enable discriminative touch. They are situated in the papillae of the skin and are therefore stimulated very readily when brought into contact with external stimuli. Meissner's corpuscles are particularly abundant in the tips of fingers, soles of the feet and palms of the hands. They are also found in areas where touch sensation enhances sexual reproduction such as the nipples, clitoris and tip of the penis.

Pressure sensation gives information to the nervous system about the intensity of touch. *Pacinian corpuscles* are found deep in the tissues

of the skin. These are oval structures enclosing a dendrite.

PHYSIOLOGICAL CHANGES THROUGH THE CHILDBEARING YEAR
Pregnancy

Women can develop sight problems during pregnancy. A mild *corneal oedema* is not uncommon, particularly during the third trimester. This could result in minor vision problems, because refraction is altered. Women who wear contact lenses may find that these cause discomfort, due to the change in shape of the eyeball (Imafidon & Imafidon 1992). They should be reassured that this will correct spontaneously after delivery.

If a woman complains of *visual disturbances*, the midwife must be aware that these could be caused by a complication of pregnancy such as diabetes or pregnancy-induced hypertension (Kelly 1993).

Many women experience changes in their sense of taste during pregnancy. The extent of these changes varies, and often leads to the pregnant woman wanting to eat different foods from normal.

The sense of smell may also be affected as a result of the mild vascular congestion in the nose commonly found in pregnant women. Strong smells may aggravate morning sickness.

Hearing and touch do not appear to alter during pregnancy.

Labour

Labour is enhanced by the sensations detected by the special senses. However there is little further change to the physiology of these senses during labour.

Postnatal

Any changes in the functioning of the sense organs during pregnancy quickly returns to normal after delivery.

The neonate

The external environment is dramatically different from that experienced by the fetus in the uterus. Although sounds are present in the womb, they are muffled and rhythmical. The fetus lies in darkness, within amniotic fluid that minimises temperature differences, and keeps taste and smells constant.

With delivery everything changes. The fetus is squeezed firstly by uterine contractions and then during its passage through the birth canal. The neonate's sense of hearing and then sight are bombarded by the noises and lights of the delivery room – where the temperature is considerably lower, and varies continuously. The exploration of the senses of taste and smell begin with the introduction of milk.

The special senses are all functional in the term infant (MacLaren 1994). They are stimulated by sensations, which provide input to the maturing brain. As the brain matures, so do the special senses. Input from the mother, in particular in terms of sights and sounds, smells and tastes, will encourage these developments. Tactile stimulation in the form of cuddles and massage produces pleasure for both the infant and the mother, and encourages bonding. This is especially important for the neonate who is separated from his mother at birth.

REFERENCES

Imafidon C O, Imafidon J E 1992 Contact lenses in pregnancy. British Journal of Obstetrics and Gynaecology 99(11):865–867

Kelly S 1993 Disorders caused by pregnancy. In: Bennett V R, Brown L K (eds) Myles textbook for midwives, 12th edn. Churchill Livingstone, Edinburgh, p 595

Kelnar C J H, Harvey D, Simpson C 1995 The sick newborn baby, 3rd edn. Baillière Tindall, London, p 173

Llewellyn-Jones D 1994 Fundamentals of obstetrics and gynaecology, 6th edn. Mosby, London, p 207

MacLaren A 1994 Maternal-neonatal nursing. Springhouse, Pennsylvania, p 282–283

Silverton L 1993 The art and science of midwifery. Prentice Hall, New York, p 586

Sweet B (ed) 1997 Mayes' midwifery. A textbook for midwives, 12th edn. Baillière Tindall, London, p 867

Thomson E, Torley E 1993 Intensive care of the newborn. In: Bennett V R, Brown L K (eds) Myles textbook for midwives, 12th edn. Churchill Livingstone, Edinburgh, p 595

5

The integumentary system

The integumentary system consists of the skin, the largest organ of the body, and its derivatives. It performs a number of essential functions. It forms protection against external invaders such as microorganisms, and shields internal structures from injury. It contains sense receptors that provide information about the external environment for the nervous system, and is also involved in the process of thermoregulation. The skin becomes easily damaged through contact with the external environment, and so the outer surfaces are continually replenished.

During pregnancy, the surface area of the skin increases in many areas – on the abdomen and breasts in particular. The elasticity of the skin enables this to occur, although some women may develop stretch marks. Under the influence of the hormones produced in pregnancy, skin pigmentation may become visible in many parts of the body.

The process of delivery will be detected by the skin and its underlying structures, adding to the sensory information being transmitted to the brain. Damage to the skin may occur during delivery. Postnatally, the skin may never totally return to its prepregnancy condition.

For the newborn baby, a fully functional integumentary system is essential to life. All the new sensations of extrauterine life will be enhanced by the stimuli detected by the receptors in the skin, which are transmitted to the brain. Although fully functional, the skin will be vulnerable to damage, and until it becomes toughened by exposure to the external world the neonate will require gentle handling.

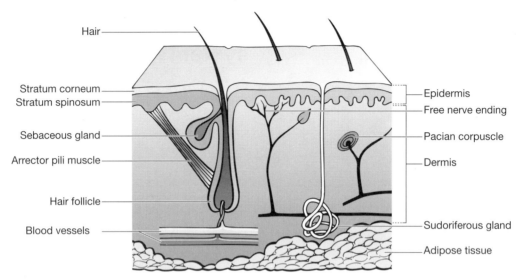

Figure 5.1 Macrostructure of the skin and integral structures.

The integumentary system is composed of (Fig. 5.1):

- the epidermis, which contains keratin to protect the body from damage
- the dermis, which maintains shape
- integral structures such as hair, glands, nails and nerve endings.

THE EPIDERMIS

The *epidermis* is the most superficial layer of the skin, composed of stratified squamous epithelium. The epidermis varies in thickness in different areas of the body, depending on the degree of wear and tear. Four main types of cell make up the epidermis:

1. *keratinocytes*, which produce keratin to toughen and waterproof the skin, and make up 90% of epidermal cells
2. *melanocytes*, which produce the pigment melanin, and transports it to the keratinocytes where it gives the skin colour (Box 5.1) and protects the nucleus (and hence DNA) from ultraviolet light
3. *Langerhans cells*, which are produced in bone marrow and migrate to the skin where they aid the immune response

4. *Merkel cells*, involved in the sensation of touch.

The epidermis consists of four principal layers that contain cells undergoing successive stages of development (Fig. 5.2). Keratinocytes formed in these layers mature as they are pushed to the surface: they gradually accumulate keratin, and lose their cytoplasm, nucleus and remaining organelles, at which point they die. Once dead, these surface cells are shed and replaced by other keratinised cells from lower levels. This cycle takes 3–4 weeks.

THE DERMIS

The *dermis* is made up of connective tissue containing collagen and elastic fibres. Like the epidermis, its thickness varies throughout the body. Embedded within the dermis are hair follicles, nerves, glands and blood vessels. *Collagen fibres* provide strength to the skin, whilst the presence of *elastic fibres* allows a considerable degree of stretch in the skin, including the ability to regain shape once stretch has ceased. *Papillae* in the dermis create projections through the epidermis, which result in natural surface ridges such as fingerprints. The function of these ridges is to increase friction and so improve grip.

The skin gets its colour from three pigments:

1. melanin
2. carotene
3. haemoglobin.

Melanin creates the degree of black and yellow in the skin. The addition of *carotene* creates the shades of brown seen in many races, and the 'suntan' in those of pale skin when exposed to ultraviolet light. A lack of melanin with extra carotene gives the skin a yellowish hue. As only small amounts of melanin are present in the cells of pale skin, *haemoglobin* present in capillaries beneath the surface gives it a pink appearance (Tortora & Grabowski 1993).

Discoloration of the skin may assist in the diagnosis of some pathological conditions. If there is insufficient oxyhaemoglobin in the capillaries, for instance, pale skin will lose its pink hue and appear bluish. This may be an indicator of *cyanosis*. In very pale membranes, such as the mucous membranes inside the eyelids, *anaemia* may be indicated if the membranes appear particularly pale. *Jaundice* is apparent from the yellowish tinge created by bilirubin in the fatty subcutaneous layer under the skin and in the whites of the eyes.

The pigment melanin, in tandem with proteins in the skin, *protects the body from radiation* (Lookingbill & Marks 1993). Melanin absorbs some of the ultraviolet radiation from the sun, whilst proteins scatter it, so that it does not penetrate into the deeper layers of the skin. The more melanin is present in the skin, the more radiation is absorbed. With exposure to the sun, the production of melanin increases to protect the body from the damaging radiation. However excessive exposure to sunlight increases the risk of developing skin cancer (Payling 1995). Ultraviolet radiation damages the skin by altering the structure of DNA, leading to mutation and cancer when the cells subsequently divide.

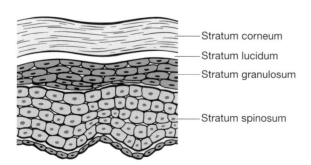

Figure 5.2   Layers of the epidermis.

Stratum corneum

Stratum lucidum

Stratum granulosum

Stratum spinosum

Integral structures

Hairs

Hairs are formed in hair follicles produced by a down growth of the epidermis into the dermis. These are distributed throughout the body. Hair is composed of dead, keratinised cells bonded closely together. The primary function of hair is one of protection.

Sebaceous glands are commonly associated with hair follicles. They produce sebum that keeps the skin and hair soft and pliable, prevents evaporation of water and inhibits some bacterial growth.

Attached to each hair is a bundle of smooth muscle, which can act to pull the hair from its normal position at an acute angle to the skin, to a more upright position. This traps warm air between the hairs and so is an aid in the maintenance of body temperature. This is visible as goose pimples, produced by the elevation of the skin around the hair shaft.

Glands

The skin contains several types of gland, including the mammary glands or breasts, which will be discussed in Chapter 19. Sebaceous glands are usually associated with hair follicles; *sweat glands* are found in most areas of the body. There are several types of sweat glands, the two most common being eccrine and apocrine glands.

Eccrine glands produce a watery secretion, dilute perspiration, which has two functions:

1. it assists in temperature control, by cooling the body as it evaporates
2. it removes waste products, to a limited degree.

The eccrine glands are found in many areas of the skin and are the most abundant form of sweat gland. They are particularly numerous on the palms of the hands and the soles of the feet, which accounts for the 'sweaty' hands associated with high environmental temperatures or moments of stress.

Apocrine glands are present mainly in the axilla, the pubic area and the areola of the breasts. These produce a more viscous solution commonly associated with emotional stress and sexual excitement.

Specially modified sweat glands are found in the ears, where they produce a waxy secretion. These are *ceruminous glands*, and they create a sticky barrier to foreign particles entering the ear.

Nails

Nails are formed from closely packed cells containing keratin. They continuously grow to replace worn down end portions. They make it easier for the fingers to grasp small objects, and they protect the extremities of both fingers and toes.

Blood, nerves and lymph

Nerve endings which are sensitive to touch, temperature, pressure and pain are widely distributed in the dermis. Blood and lymph vessels are also present. These provide nutrients and remove waste products, and also play an important role in temperature regulation.

PHYSIOLOGY OF THE SKIN

The skin is involved in many functions, which it carries out in conjunction with other systems of the body. The principal functions are listed below.

- *Protection*: the skin is a physical barrier to different sorts of trauma, including damaging light waves, microorganisms and loss of body fluids.
- *Sensing*: the skin contains many types of nerve endings which transmit information regarding the external environment to the nervous system.
- *Thermoregulation*: the skin contains sweat glands, which increase their production when core temperature rises, or during physical exertion. This is because muscular activity releases heat as a by-product, and so prolonged physical exertion can upset internal homeostasis. As surface sweat evaporates, the skin is cooled. In this way the temperature of the

body is regulated. If the external temperature decreases, less sweat is produced. Changes in blood flow to the skin contributes to the thermoregulatory process.

- *Excretion*: sweat contains small amounts of salts and organic compounds such as urea. These substances therefore are also lost through evaporation.
- *Immunity*: skin cells contain components of the immune system, so assist in the process of defence against microorganisms.
- *Synthesis of vitamin D*: the process of vitamin D synthesis is initiated in the skin by ultraviolet light from the sun.

PHYSIOLOGICAL CHANGES THROUGH THE CHILDBEARING YEAR

Pregnancy

Many features of the skin are altered markedly by pregnancy. Although rarely of pathological origin, they frequently cause great anxiety to the pregnant woman, as they can alter her *cosmetic appearance* (Blackburn & Loper 1992). As a consequence many creams and lotions have been developed – but they appear to have little or no effect on the changes (Silverton 1993).

Increased *pigmentation* of certain areas of the skin occurs in the majority of women. The cause of this is unknown, but it is widely considered to be of hormonal origin (Lewis & Chamberlain 1990). Pigmentation varies between individuals and is particularly pronounced in women with dark hair or complexions. The nipples and areolae of the breasts become darker, and during the second half of pregnancy a *secondary areola* will develop. The external genitalia also become darker. In the woman experiencing her first pregnancy, the linea alba will darken from the umbilicus down the midline to the pubic area. This becomes the *linea nigra*. The linea nigra may fade between pregnancies but becomes darker again during each subsequent pregnancy. Freckles, birth marks and recent scars may also darken.

In some women a pregnancy mask, *chloasma*, may develop on the face. This is made up of areas of pigmentation, often resembling a butterfly shape around the nose and cheeks. Chloasma is caused by increased production of the hormone melanocyte-stimulating hormone from the anterior pituitary gland (Klein 1995). There appears to be a familial tendency to some of these changes.

The skin contains an abundance of elastic fibres, but in some women the skin appears to 'tear' as it stretches to accommodate pregnancy. This results in 'stretch marks' or *striae gravidarum*, which commonly occur on the abdominal wall, upper thighs, buttocks or breasts. Their number varies considerably between women. During the pregnancy in which they appear, the striae appear an unsightly purple pink in colour. However, after pregnancy colour fades to leave a white mark. The cause of striae is thought to be the increased levels of hormones produced during pregnancy, rather than actual damage from stretching (Symonds & Symonds 1998).

Some women complain of increased itchiness during pregnancy – *pruritis gravidarum* – which is either generalised or felt only over the abdomen. The cause of pruritis gravidarum is unknown (Coutts 1998) but it usually disappears spontaneously after delivery (Stephens & Black 1990). However, the midwife must be alert to the fact that the itchiness may be a sign of a skin infection or infestation, or of other pathological conditions (Box 5.2).

Many pregnant women complain of a general feeling of *greasiness* of the skin. This is the result of increased activity of the sebaceous glands, due to the elevated hormone levels in pregnancy (Bayliss & Tunbridge 1990). Sweat glands, particularly the eccrine glands, also become more active because of changes in thyroid activity resulting from the increased metabolic demands of the body. A consequence of increased sweating is increased *heat loss*. This is useful as heat is being produced not only by the pregnant woman, but by the fetus too.

Labour

With its abundance of nerve endings the integumentary system will add to the *experience of labour*

Box 5.2 Obstetric cholestasis

Itching of the skin is common in pregnancy and is thought to be related to elevated hormone levels and stretching of the skin. However, in rare instances, itching is associated with liver disease. This may be *obstetric cholestasis*. This condition can be distinguished from pruritis gravidarum by the sites of itching which, in obstetric cholestasis, tend to be in areas where little skin stretching is occurring, such as on the arms, legs, hands and soles of the feet. The itch can be severe and is particularly bad at night, leading to constant fatigue (British Liver Trust 1997). Other symptoms of this disorder may be *loss of appetite, malaise* and occasionally *jaundice*.

The cause of obstetric cholestasis is unknown. However one theory is that it is caused by the high levels of oestrogen of pregnancy causing a reduction in the production of bile (Fagan 1994). Excessive bile salts are released into the blood. The condition is of little pathological significance to the mother, because it is a temporary liver disorder, although the effect of the itching can be unbearable. For the fetus, however, there is a high risk of *stillbirth*, possibly due to a biochemical side effect, after 37 weeks of pregnancy (Waine 1995).

If obstetric cholestasis is suspected, liver function tests and blood bile salt levels can confirm the diagnosis. Absorption of fats and *vitamin K* levels may be affected by the condition, so vitamin K may be required to minimise the blood loss associated with delivery (Fagan 1994). The pregnancy must be closely monitored and labour may need to be induced before term to avoid intrauterine death. Once the mother has delivered, the condition quickly resolves with little, if any, effect on her health. However, obstetric cholestasis may recur in 60–70% of subsequent pregnancies (Price 1995).

---

by giving information about external factors such as personal contact with partner and the newborn baby at delivery (Raphael-Leff 1991). Massage and warmth may be applied to the skin to help diminish the discomfort of labour. During the process of labour, the skin may become *damaged* and require subsequent care or repair (Box 5.3).

Postnatal

Many of the changes to the skin's structure will revert to normal during the postnatal period. However the increase in pigmentation may never disappear completely (Stephens & Black 1990). Increased *hair loss* is noticed by many women and is the result of a change in its growth pattern

---

Box 5.3   Wound healing

Any tissue damage that is sustained during the delivery of the fetus will go through several stages of repair. During this time, the way in which the wound is cared for may influence the speed at which it heals, and the amount of permanent damage it leaves.

The physiological stages of wound healing are:

1. the inflammatory stage
2. the destructive stage
3. the proliferative stage
4. the maturation stage.

The *inflammatory* stage begins within minutes and lasts for 4–5 days. During this stage of wound healing, the body is applying 'first aid' to the area. Blood coagulates and blood vessels constrict to prevent further blood loss. Capillaries locally become more permeable allowing leucocytes and antibodies to reach the wound. Neutrophils bring necessary repair materials to the wound and macrophages begin phagocytosis. These changes produce the classic signs of inflammation: *redness, swelling, heat* and *pain*.

The *destructive* stage lasts 1–6 days. During this stage, macrophages phagocytose dead tissue and any invading microorganisms to clean up the site and enable effective repair to take place. They also stimulate the formation of fibroblasts, which lay down an array of collagen fibres to act as scaffolding for repair. The

synthesis of collagen depends on the presence of the slightly acid environment associated with tissue damage. The wound should therefore be left untouched to maintain these conditions. A good diet including *vitamin C* is also required (Guest & Pearson 1997) to provide adequate nutrients to the repairing cells.

During the *proliferative* stage, which lasts 3–24 days, increasing numbers of fibroblasts lay down fibres of collagen. New tissue is formed around the collagen and is organised into the necessary layers of tissue for the area. Blood capillaries increase in number (vascularisation) to supply the necessary nutrients for the intense building programme. Granulation tissue may form. This is fibrous tissue that fills the space between the two edges of the wound. If large, this may cause a permanent *scar*. The presence of infection or retained dead material or a foreign body, will make granulation more extensive.

During the *maturation* stage, which may last 24–365 days, fibroblasts leave the area and collagen fibres become organised into correctly configured supporting structures of normal tissue. Over time this results in a flattening and softening of the wound. Vascularisation also decreases. The wound changes its appearance to pale white, familiar as a scar. This may fade to a large extent, but where granulation tissue has been laid down the area will be *non-functioning* as a tissue.

---

during pregnancy, caused by the high levels of oestrogen (Burton 1990).

The neonate

At term the epidermis of the neonatal skin is well developed and keratinised. Water loss is therefore minimal. Sweat glands are present but initially not very active. However, the neonate is prone to increased heat loss due to the high surface to body mass ratio. The more premature the infant, the thinner and more vulnerable to damage is its skin (Isaacs & Moxon 1991). The postmature infant, on the other hand, has very dry skin, liable to peeling due to its prolonged immersion in amniotic fluid without protection (Berger 1989). Two temporary structures have given the skin protection during intrauterine life:

1. vernix caseosa
2. lanugo.

Vernix caseosa is a fatty film that develops over the skin from the 5th month of pregnancy. It

provides the fetus with protection from the drying effect of constant immersion in amniotic fluid (Michie 1993). Vernix also prevents fluid and electrolyte loss from the fetus. As the fetus nears term, the skin becomes sufficiently mature to become waterproof, so vernix is increasingly absorbed into the body. The neonate born at term will therefore have little vernix, with any remaining layers usually in the creases of the body such as the neck and groin.

Lanugo is a fine covering of hair the fetus develops from the 20th week of pregnancy until it is shed from the 36th week. Little remains on the full-term neonate at birth.

Adequate functioning of the skin is essential for the health and wellbeing of the neonate. At delivery the newborn enters an environment very different to the one it has experienced in the uterus. The gentle cushioning of the amniotic fluid is replaced by clothing and bedlinen that irritates the skin surface. Room temperature is at best several degrees less than inside the uterus, and microorganisms abound.

The skin of the neonate at term is thin and *easily damaged* (Michie 1996). This increases the risks to the body of invasion by microorganisms. Although sterile during fetal life, the skin becomes rapidly *colonised by commensals* within the first few days of birth (Johnston 1994). These commensals will usually prevent invasion by pathogens. Sebaceous and sweat glands are present but are relatively inactive during the first days of life. *Milia* may be seen on the nose and cheeks. These are enlarged sebaceous glands. Nails are formed and hair is present to varying degrees.

Thermoregulation

Thermoregulation is a vital function required by the neonate immediately from birth. As the surface area of the newborn baby is large in proportion to its body mass, it loses heat quickly. The skin is unable to conserve heat as efficiently as an adult's, and the neonate cannot generate heat by shivering (Box 5.4).

Heat is lost from the newborn by four main routes (Fig. 5.3):

1. By *evaporation*. The large surface area of skin when damp, such as immediately after birth

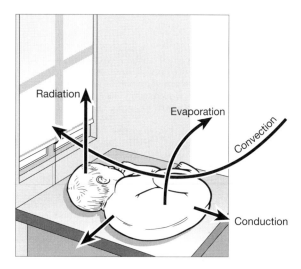

Figure 5.3 Types of heat loss in the newborn.

or subsequently during bathing, will cause rapid heat loss through evaporation, especially if the surrounding environment is cool.
2. By *convection*. Any cool currents of air passing over a partly dressed neonate will remove the warm air close to the skin surface.
3. By *radiation*. If the neonate is placed close to cold objects in his environment, such as a window, heat will radiate from the exposed areas of the baby to the window.
4. By *conduction*. Contact with cold surfaces such as cot sheets and weighing scales will result in direct loss of heat to this surface.

The midwife therefore must ensure that minimal heat is lost both during delivery and during the early days of neonatal life (Kelnar et al 1995). The delivery room must be kept warm, with windows closed to prevent draughts. Cloths and bedding should be warmed before use, and the baby dried and wrapped up either with the mother or in warm coverings as soon after birth as possible (Michie 1996). The midwife must then educate the mother to be alert for ways in which her newborn baby can become cold during the first few weeks of life. In a cold environment, care must be taken to prevent heat loss through the proportionately large head of the neonate. Conversely, it is also important to guard against overheating the baby, as this has been implicated in cot death (Ponsonby et al 1992).

Box 5.4   Non-shivering thermogenesis

To maintain temperature, the neonate has to rely entirely on the heat produced through metabolism, as he is unable to shiver. Provided the neonate has adequate stores of or access to glucose and oxygen, his required body temperature can be maintained (Tyson et al 1989). The fetus lays down a specialised form of adipose tissue called *brown fat* from the 28th week of gestation. Metabolism of brown fat produces heat rapidly when required. Lipolysis, the breakdown of fat, is stimulated by the release of thyroid hormones and noradrenaline (Sweet 1997). This mechanism is termed *non-shivering thermogenesis*.

Brown fat is thought to make up 2–7% of the neonate's weight (Sweet 1997). It is situated in the mediastinum, between the scapulae, next to the spinal column and around the kidneys. It has an increased blood and nerve supply, to enable lipolysis and the rapid production of heat. However, the supply of brown fat is limited, and will be used up rapidly if the neonate is exposed to cold for long periods of time. He will then use up all other sources of glucose in the body, and produce further supplies by anaerobic respiration, producing a metabolic acidosis.

REFERENCES

Bayliss R I S, Tunbridge W M G 1990 Thyroid disease, the facts. Oxford University Press, Oxford, p 99

Berger H 1989 Clinical examination of the newborn infant. In: Chalmers I, Enkin E, Keirse M J N C (eds) Effective care in pregnancy and childbirth. Oxford University Press, Oxford, p 1403–1416

Blackburn S T, Loper D L 1992 Maternal, fetal and neonatal physiology. W B Saunders, Philadelphia, p 491

British Liver Trust 1997 Obstetric cholestasis. http://www.britishlivertrust.org.uk/blt.html

Burton J L 1990 Essentials of dermatology, 3rd edn. Churchill Livingstone, Edinburgh, p 40

Coutts A 1998 The 'minor' problems of pregnancy: a review. Professional Care of the Mother and Child 8(4):95–97

Fagan E A 1994 Intrahepatic cholestasis of pregnancy. British Medical Journal 319(6964):1243–1244

Guest C, Pearson S 1997 Wound care. Recovery on a plate. Nursing Times 93(46):84–86

Isaacs D, Moxon E R 1991 Neonatal infections. Butterworth Heinemann, Oxford, p 6–7

Johnston P G B 1994 Vulliamy's the newborn child, 7th edn. Churchill Livingstone, Edinburgh, p 120

Kelnar C J H, Harvey D, Simpson C 1995 The sick newborn baby, 3rd edn. Baillière Tindall, London, p 115

Klein P M 1995 Anatomy and physiology of pregnancy. In: Bobak I M, Lowdermilk D L, Jenson M D (eds) Maternity nursing, 4th edn. Mosby, St Louis, p 103

Lewis T L, Chamberlain G (eds) 1990 Obstetrics by ten teachers, 15th edn. Edward Arnold, London, p 210

Lookingbill D P, Marks J G 1993 Principles of dermatology, 2nd edn. W B Saunders, Philadelphia, p 6

Michie M M 1993 The normal baby. In: Bennett V R, Brown L K (eds) Myles textbook for midwives, 12th edn. Churchill Livingstone, Edinburgh, p 506

Michie M M 1996 A delicate concern; caring for neonatal skin. British Journal of Midwifery 4(3):159–163

Payling K J 1995 Skin cancer. Professional Nurse 11(3):175–176

Ponsonby A L, Dwyer T, Gibbons L E, Cochrane J A, Jones M E, McCall M J 1992 Thermal environment and sudden infant death syndrome: case-control study. British Medical Journal 304:277–282

Price S 1995 Obstetric cholestasis. Nursing Times 91(48):57–58

Raphael-Leff J 1991 Psychological processes of childbearing. Chapman and Hall, London, p 286–292

Silverton L 1993 The art and science of midwifery. Prentice Hall, New York, p 90

Stephens C J M, Black M M 1990 The skin changes of pregnancy. Maternal and Child Health 15(12):378–381

Sweet B (ed) 1997 Mayes' midwifery. A textbook for midwives, 12th edn. Baillière Tindall, London, p 824

Symonds E M, Symonds I M 1998 Essential obstetrics and gynaecology, 3rd edn. Churchill Livingstone, Edinburgh, p 26

Tortora G J, Grabowski S R 1993 Principles of anatomy and physiology, 7th edn. Harper Collins, New York, p 131

Tyson J, Silverman W, Reisch J 1989 Immediate care of the newborn infant. In: Chalmers I, Enkin E, Keirse M J N C (eds) Effective care in pregnancy and childbirth. Oxford University Press, Oxford, p 1294–1295

Waine C 1995 Beware of itching during late pregnancy. The Practitioner 239(1547):97–100

6

The cardiovascular system

The cells of a multicellular organism such as the human require an efficient transport system to bring them necessary nutrients and to pass on the products of metabolism. The cardiovascular system carries out this function. With the lymphatic system, the cardiovascular system also provides protection against adverse changes in the cells' environment and invasion by microbes.

During pregnancy the cardiovascular system alters considerably to cope with the extra demands of a growing uterus, fetus and other maternal organs. Labour is a time of increased physical effort and the requirements for this are supplied by the cardiovascular system. As the body returns to its prepregnancy state postnatally, the system also returns to normal.

In the fetus, the cardiovascular system is anatomically altered to adapt to a situation in which the placenta is responsible for respiration, absorption of nutrients and disposal of waste. Temporary structures are in place to divert blood flow from the lungs and to pass through the placenta. Labour places increased demands on the fetus, and as soon as the neonate is delivered he must breathe and take over the functions of the placenta in order to survive.

The cardiovascular system consists of:

- the heart, which pumps blood to every cell of the body
- blood vessels, which transport the blood
- blood, which consists of a fluid portion called plasma, in which specialised cells, blood cells, are suspended.

THE HEART

The *heart* is a cone-shaped, muscular, hollow organ situated in the *mediastinum*, the space between the lungs (Fig. 6.1). About two-thirds of the heart lies to the left of the midline and it extends down to the diaphragm. An adult heart weighs 250–350 g and is considered to be approximately the same size and shape as that adult's fist. The lower margin of the heart is known as the *apex*, and the broad upper portion is the *base*.

Structure

The heart wall is composed of three layers:

1. an outer serous layer, the epicardium
2. the middle muscular myocardium
3. an inner endothelial endocardium.

The epicardium

The outermost layer, the *epicardium*, is part of the *pericardium*, which is a double supportive layer which protects the heart. The outermost layer of the pericardium is composed of tough connective tissue, which attaches the heart to the diaphragm and is closely associated with the pleura of the lungs. The inner layer, the serous pericardium, is a thinner double membrane, the outer portion of which is attached to the fibrous pericardium and the inner layer forming the epicardium of the heart. Between the two layers is a potential space containing a thin layer of serous fluid which allows the two membranes to slide over one another as the heart contracts and expands. This space is known as the *pericardial cavity*.

The myocardium

The middle layer of the heart wall consists of muscle, the *myocardium*, which is the thickest layer. It varies in thickness according to the function of the underlying space or chamber. The myocardium is composed of *cardiac muscle* which is found only in the heart (Fig. 6.2). The cells of this muscle are branched and striated, and in close contact with adjacent muscle cells via small channels called *intercalated discs*. These muscles form sheets in two separate networks each of which supplies either the atrial or ventricular chambers of the heart. Because the two separate networks lie in such close proximity, they are stimulated to contract in coordination with one another.

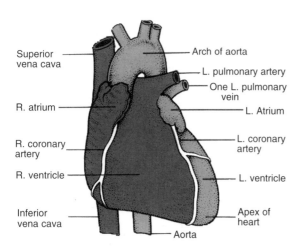

Figure 6.1 External structure of the heart. (Reproduced with permission from Wilson K J W, Waugh A 1996 Ross and Wilson Anatomy and Physiology in Health and Illness. Churchill Livingstone, Edinburgh)

Labels on Figure 6.1:
- Superior vena cava
- R. atrium
- R. coronary artery
- R. ventricle
- Inferior vena cava
- Arch of aorta
- L. pulmonary artery
- One L. pulmonary vein
- L. Atrium
- L. coronary artery
- L. ventricle
- Apex of heart
- Aorta

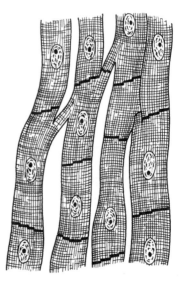

Figure 6.2 Microstructure of cardiac muscle fibres. (Reproduced with permission from Wilson K J W, Waugh A 1996 Ross and Wilson Anatomy and Physiology in Health and Illness. Churchill Livingstone, Edinburgh)

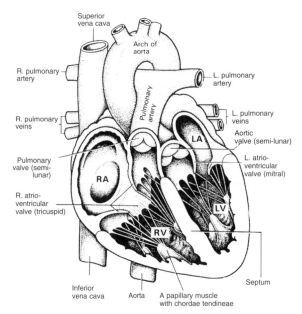

Figure 6.3   Internal structure of the heart. (Reproduced with permission from Wilson K J W, Waugh A 1996 Ross and Wilson Anatomy and Physiology in Health and Illness. Churchill Livingstone, Edinburgh)

Box 6.1   Atrial and ventricular septal defects

An abnormality of the cardiovascular system occurs in 4–8 live births in every 1000 (Thomas 1992). One third of these are insignificant, one third will affect the neonate to some extent, and the remaining third will be life-threatening.

One of the most common defects is an opening in the septum between two chambers of the heart. This may be due to an incomplete closure of the *foramen ovale* (Forfar & Arneil 1984), the temporary opening that exists in the fetus to divert blood from the pulmonary circulation. This defect can be detected on examination by a murmur in the heart sounds. The opening will usually close spontaneously over a few weeks.

However, the opening could be due to a defect in the atrial septum. This is known as an *atrial septal defect*, and it rarely shows any symptoms until adulthood. Even if surgery is required in infancy, it is usually a low-risk procedure.

The most common of all congenital defects is a *ventricular septal defect*, which is an opening between the two ventricles. Again this may not be a life-threatening problem: 80% close spontaneously in the first 8 years of life (Kelnar et al 1995). However, if the condition is severe it may lead to life-threatening complications requiring urgent surgery.

The endocardium

The innermost layer of the heart wall is a thin layer of endothelium, the *endocardium*, which lines the heart, the valves between the chambers and the blood vessels leaving the heart.

Chambers

The three layers of the heart wall enclose four chambers: two *atria* (singular, atrium) and two *ventricles* (Fig. 6.3). The two atria are situated at the base of the heart, the ventricles at the apex.

Externally grooves, or *sulci*, separate the muscles of each chamber, enabling them to function independently. Internally, the chambers of the heart are separated into the right and left atria and ventricles by a septum (Box 6.1). The atrium and ventricle on each side of the heart are separated by valves, with further valves situated at the exits of the heart from the ventricles.

Valves

There are four valves in the heart composed of connective tissue covered by endocardium. Their function is to prevent backflow into the chambers. With each contraction of the heart, the relevant valves open to allow blood to pass through, and close as the heart relaxes. There are four valves in the heart (Fig. 6.3):

- The *tricuspid valve* is situated between the right atrium and ventricle. It is composed of three flaps or cusps.
- The *mitral valve* is situated between the left atrium and ventricle. It is also known as the *bicuspid valve*, because it is composed of two cusps (Box 6.2).
- two *semilunar valves* are situated in the pulmonary artery and aorta as they leave the heart. These valves consist of three semicircular cusps which are attached to the inner surface of the heart.

The mitral and tricuspid valves are opened and closed according to the pressure differences in the atria and ventricles. They are prevented from opening into the atria by the presence of fibres, the *chordae tendinae*, joined to muscles attached to the walls of the ventricles.

Pre-existing heart disease can seriously complicate pregnancy, resulting in a high mortality or morbidity rate for both mother and baby. Cardiac disease in pregnancy accounts for 30% of maternal deaths and occurs in 1% of pregnancies (Kennedy 1995).

Cardiac disease may be congenital or acquired, for example as a result of previous rheumatic fever. The latter is rare nowadays in developed countries, but when it does occur, it damages the heart valves, particularly the mitral valve. Congenital heart defects are more common. These tend to be uncorrected atrial or ventricular septal defects. However, even where surgical repair has been carried out, the fact that there has been a defect may mean that cardiac function is still compromised.

Often women with defects tolerate pregnancy well, but they are checked very carefully throughout the pregnancy by a specialist team of medical staff. The pregnant woman is advised to rest, eat a well-balanced diet, control weight gain and seek medical help for any sign of infection. Labour is monitored carefully and minimal effort allowed in the second stage, the amount allowed depending on the woman's condition. The first 48 hours after delivery will be a time of particular care and observation, while circulatory volume increases due to the shift of fluid from body tissues. On delivery, the baby will be carefully examined because he will be at increased risk of inheriting the condition (Comport & Seng 1997).

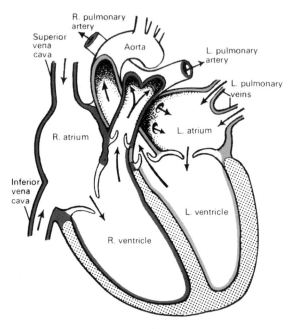

Figure 6.4   Direction of blood flow through the heart. (Reproduced with permission from Wilson K J W, Waugh A 1996 Ross and Wilson Anatomy and Physiology in Health and Illness. Churchill Livingstone, Edinburgh)

Movement of blood through the heart

The right atrium receives blood from the largest veins in the body, the venae cavae (Fig. 6.4). Blood is then passed through the right ventricle and out of the heart via the pulmonary arteries to the lungs. Here it is oxygenated and returns through the pulmonary veins to the left atrium of the heart. Finally the blood exits the heart through the left ventricle into the largest artery of the body, the aorta.

The varying thickness of the myocardium reflects the work required by the underlying chamber of the heart. It is thinnest surrounding the atria, which move blood into the ventricles. The right ventricle moves blood into the lungs and so the myocardium is thicker around this ventricle. The left ventricle, however, must produce sufficient pressure to move the blood to all areas of the body. It is surrounding this ventricle that the myocardium is at its thickest.

Physiology

The heart muscle contracts in order to move blood through the chambers of the heart and into the blood vessels which deliver it to the relevant parts of the body. The heart acts, therefore, as a pump, supplying the pressure required to deliver the blood to all the cells in the body.

In order to carry out this process efficiently, the heart must contract in an organised fashion, maximising the pumping effect. Heart muscle is stimulated to contract in such a way that first the atria contract to move blood into the ventricles, then the ventricles contract to move blood into the general circulation. This is achieved by the rhythmical electrical activity of the heart muscle, which is independent of nervous control – although the rate and force of the contraction are controlled by the autonomic nervous system.

Within the myocardium are groups of specialised muscle cells which initiate action potentials, resulting in muscle contractions. The impulses are then conveyed through the myocardium via specific muscle cells.

The *sinoatrial node* is one such collection of muscle cells situated in the wall of the right

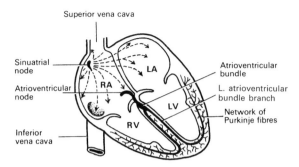

Figure 6.5 Electrical conduction through the heart muscle. (Reproduced with permission from Wilson K J W, Waugh A 1996 Ross and Wilson Anatomy and Physiology in Health and Illness. Churchill Livingstone, Edinburgh)

atrium just below the opening from the superior vena cava (Fig. 6.5). This node is often referred to as the heart's *'pacemaker'* because it is here that the majority of impulses – between 60 and 100 every minute – are initiated. Each of these impulses spreads through the atria of the heart resulting in their contraction. The impulse then arrives at a second group of specialised muscle cells, the *atrioventricular node*, which is situated in the septum between the atria and ventricles. This node is also capable of initiating impulses, but at a slower rate than the sinoatrial node. From the atrioventricular node, the impulse passes down the septum dividing the ventricles via a group of cells known as the *atrioventricular bundle* or *bundle of His*. From here the impulse passes along a series of fibres, the *Purkinje fibres*, that travel through the walls of the ventricles, causing the ventricles to contract.

The majority of heart contractions follow the pathway through the heart described above. However, the atrioventricular node is also capable of initiating impulses. An impulse spreading from this point results in an ectopic beat. In healthy people these are occasionally triggered by substances such as high levels of nicotine and caffeine.

The cycle of muscular activity resulting in one contraction of the heart, followed by relaxation, is known as the *cardiac cycle*. A period of contraction is called *systole* and that of relaxation, *diastole*. An average of 72 cardiac cycles occur every minute in an adult.

Movement of blood through the heart and into the circulation can be described by examination of one cardiac cycle. The cardiac cycle can be divided into three phases: relaxation, ventricular filling and ventricular contraction.

1. *Relaxation*. On completion of each cardiac cycle all heart muscle is in a state of relaxation, in diastole. The semilunar valves close, because the pressure in the pulmonary arteries and aorta is greater than in the ventricles. This prevents back flow of blood. Blood from the pulmonary veins and the vena cava floods into the atria. When the pressure in the ventricles drops to less than that in the atria, the tricuspid and mitral valves open. This phase takes 0.4 s.

2. *Ventricular filling*. Once the valves open between the atria and ventricles, blood rushes into the ventricles. The flow is assisted by the contraction of the atria (atrial systole), initiated by an impulse from the sinoatrial node. This phase lasts 0.1 s.

3. *Ventricular contraction*. Finally the impulse arrives at the Purkinje fibres, initiating contraction of the ventricles (ventricular systole), which moves the blood into the general circulation. This phase takes 0.3 s.

The entire cardiac cycle therefore lasts approximately 0.8 s.

The electrical activity of the heart can be picked up by external monitors, which produce a visual record called an electrocardiogram.

Cardiac output

The specialised cells of the myocardium initiate action potentials that create the rhythm of the heart's contractions. These contractions occur independently of the functioning of the body as a whole. When the body is stressed by exercise or psychological events, the cells require a greater amount of oxygen and nutrients, so the heart has to increase the amount of blood getting to them. It can do this either by speeding up its contraction rate, or by increasing its output, i.e. the amount of blood expelled with each cardiac cycle.

The *cardiac output* is defined as the amount of

blood ejected from the heart each minute, usually from the left ventricle into the aorta. In the average adult at rest, the cardiac output (CO) is determined by the amount of blood pumped out of the left ventricle – the stroke volume – multiplied by the number of contractions or heart beats per minute.

$$CO = \text{stroke volume (70 ml)} \times \text{heart rate}$$
$$(72 \text{ beats})$$
$$= 5040 \text{ ml/min} \triangleq 5 \text{ L/min}$$

The total amount of blood in the average adult is 5 L. When the body is at rest, the heart pumps the equivalent of the entire blood volume around the body every minute. When blood flow needs to be increased due to, for example, exercise, cardiac output can increase to as much as 30 L/min in the well trained athlete.

Cardiac output is regulated by both the autonomic nervous system and by hormones and other chemicals.

Nervous control is initiated by the cardiovascular centre in the medulla of the brain. When the body is involved in exercise, signals are received there from the moving limbs. At the same time chemoreceptors and baroreceptors present in the cardiovascular system monitor the levels of chemicals in the blood and blood pressure respectively, and this information is also sent to the medulla. In response to all these signals, the sinoatrial node, which is innervated by the sympathetic nervous system, is stimulated to increase the heart rate by initiating and increasing the numbers of action potentials. Also the myocardial muscle cells are stimulated to contract more effectively, so raising the stroke volume.

Hormonal regulation of cardiac output involves the adrenal glands. Exercise stimulates them to increase their production of adrenaline. This hormone acts on cardiac muscle to raise both the heart rate and stroke volume. Changes in levels of ions in the blood also affect the rate and volume of the heart's contractions.

Other factors such as age, gender, physical fitness and temperature also influence cardiac output. The heart of a person who undertakes regular exercise works more efficiently and will show less of an increase in heart rate on exercise, because the heart muscle is able to contract more strongly and raise stroke volume more effectively. Any significant increase in body temperature causes the sinoatrial node to initiate impulses more rapidly.

Blood supply

The heart is well supplied with blood to enable it to work effectively (Fig. 6.1). Right and left *coronary arteries* leave the aorta soon after it leaves the left ventricle. These arteries then divide to supply all parts of the heart with necessary oxygen and nutrients. Many *anastomoses* (collateral vessels) are present in the coronary circulation. These are connections between arteries that supply blood to an area through an alternative route. So if one artery is blocked, an anastomosis may still be able to supply that portion of the myocardium.

Venous return is through small veins that empty into the coronary sinus on the posterior surface of the heart, or into the chambers of the heart.

BLOOD VESSELS

From the heart, a series of blood vessels transports blood to all areas of the body, eventually returning it to the heart. Every cell in the body is reached by circulating blood, which means gases, nutrients and chemicals can diffuse between the blood, the interstitial fluid surrounding the cells and intracellular fluid.

There are two main types of blood vessel:

1. arteries and arterioles, which carry oxygenated blood to the cells
2. veins and venules transporting deoxygenated blood away from the cells.

An elaborate array of capillaries connects these two systems.

Arteries

Arteries are large vessels that transport oxygenated blood in bulk. The walls of the arteries are therefore substantial, and are made up of three distinct layers:

1. the tunica interna
2. the tunica media
3. the tunica externa.

The inner *tunica interna* surrounds the lumen of the artery, and is composed of endothelium covering a basement membrane and a layer of elastic tissue. The middle layer, the *tunica media*, is usually the thickest and is composed of smooth muscle interspersed by elastic fibres. The outermost layer, the *tunica externa*, consists of a tough layer of fibrous tissue.

The presence of muscle and elastic fibres gives the arteries two important properties: elasticity and contractility. When the ventricles of the heart contract, they eject blood into the large arteries. The *elasticity* of these arteries allows them to expand to accommodate the extra blood. As the ventricles relax, the elastic recoil of the arteries forces the blood onwards.

The property of *contractility* originates in the middle muscle layer of the walls, in which smooth muscle is arranged longitudinally and in rings. This muscle receives its nerve supply from sympathetic branches of the autonomic nervous system. When stimulated, the walls contract, narrowing the lumen. This process is called *vasoconstriction*. When the stimulation ceases, the muscle wall relaxes and the arterial lumen increases. This is *vasodilation*.

Contractility is important both in maintaining homeostasis and in instances of arterial haemorrhage: the artery can contract, so helping to limit blood loss.

Three main types of arteries are present in the cardiovascular system:

1. elastic or conducting arteries
2. muscular or distributing arteries
3. anastomoses.

Elastic arteries have thin walls in proportion to their overall diameter. Their tunica media is composed mostly of elastic tissue, so they have considerable elasticity, which is necessary as these arteries conduct large quantities of blood from the heart to muscular arteries.

Muscular arteries have thicker walls in proportion to their overall diameter than elastic arteries, and their tunica media contains more muscle cells than elastic fibres. This means these arteries are able to dilate or constrict the lumen diameter to adjust and distribute the quantity of blood supply to the organs required.

Anastomoses occur where two or more arteries join together to supply one area of the body, providing an alternative source of blood should one artery become blocked.

This alternative route is called a *collateral circulation*. Not all tissues are supplied with a collateral circulation. Arteries supplying those that are not are called *end arteries*. If an end artery becomes blocked, the tissue it serves quickly dies.

Arterioles

Arterioles are small arteries that connect the arterial network to the capillary network. The structure of the arterioles reflects that of the vessel joining it, i.e. arteriole walls close to arteries have a similar three-layered structure, with an inner tunica interna, a middle tunica media of mostly muscle cells, and an outer layer, the tunica externa, of elastic and connective tissue. Arterioles closest to the capillary network by contrast have very thin walls consisting of tunica interna enclosed in a few muscle cells.

Those arterioles with a tunica media play a vital role in vasodilation and vasoconstriction, because they contain so much muscle. They therefore control the amount of blood arriving in the capillary bed.

Veins

Veins are made up of the same three layers as arteries (Fig. 6.6). However there is a difference in the thickness of the walls of arteries and veins. In veins the layers of tunica interna and tunica media are very thin, whereas the tunica externa is much thicker than arteries of a similar diameter. Veins are still able to expand to accommodate the quantity of blood passing through. In addition

Box 6.3   Varicose veins

Varicose veins commonly occur in pregnancy, due to the action of progesterone on the smooth muscle of the veins. The muscle tone is diminished and the increased venous pressure from the effects of pregnancy allows pooling of blood in the superficial veins of the legs (Silverton 1993). This condition is hereditary, and in many cases the varicose veins may already be present but are aggravated by each pregnancy.

Occasionally the presence of varicose veins may result in the complication *thrombophlebitis*, in which a clot (a *thrombus*) forms in an inflammed superficial vein. Rarely, the clot forms in a deep vein, giving rise to severe calf pain. An embolus may break away and, if it becomes lodged in the lungs, it creates a life-threatening situation.

Varicose veins can also occur around the anal sphincter as *haemorrhoids*, or in the vulva as *vulval varicosities*. Haemorrhoids often appear for the first time in pregnancy (Sinclair 1995). Haemorrhoids that occur in these circumstances tend to disappear quickly.

many veins contain *valves* to prevent back flow of blood, which is under much less pressure to move forward than in arteries (Box 6.3).

Venous sinuses are specialised types of vein found in the brain and heart. The walls of these veins consist simply of tunica interna with no surrounding muscle cells. Connective tissue surrounds the sinus to give support.

Venules

The structure of *venules*, like that of arterioles, depends on the structure of the vessel adjacent to them. So, the walls at the venous end of the venule are composed of all three layers, whereas at the capillary end, the middle layer of tunica media is absent.

Capillaries

Capillaries supply almost every cell in the body. They are composed of a single layer of tunica interna. This thin wall allows capillaries to carry out their primary function, which is to allow the diffusion of gases, nutrients and wastes between the blood and surrounding tissues. The walls of some capillaries contain pores or *fenestrations* which aid the movement of substances from blood to tissue fluids. These capillaries are called *fenestrated capillaries*. Two other types of capillaries are *continuous capillaries* and sinusoids. In continuous capillaries the cells of the tunica interna form a continuous ring around the lumen. *Sinusoids* consist of walls without a basement membrane containing large gaps rather than pores.

Capillaries form the connections between the arterial and venous system. The numbers of capillaries present in any tissue depends on its function, with an abundance of capillaries in areas where the cells have a high metabolic rate and require greater exchange of gases and nutrients.

In the capillary bed there is constant movement of fluid between plasma and tissues, distributing the chemicals dissolved in the plasma. At the arteriole end of capillaries, fluid is forced out by blood pressure into the surrounding interstitial spaces. At the venous end, blood pressure is very low and the presence of plasma proteins attracts fluid back into the capillaries. Any fluid that escapes this process is returned to the circulatory system via lymphatic vessels.

MOVEMENT OF BLOOD THROUGH BLOOD VESSELS

Blood moves through the circulatory system largely as a result of the pressure created by the contraction of the heart. This means that blood pressure in arteries is high, but it decreases as the blood moves through the arterioles, capillaries, venules and veins until, on return to the heart, it is negligible.

Blood pressure

Blood pressure can be defined as the pressure exerted on the interior walls of blood vessels. The average adult blood pressure during systole – contraction of the ventricles of the heart – is 120 mmHg. During diastole – relaxation of the heart – the blood pressure averages 70 mmHg. Blood pressure depends on physical factors, such as the strength of the ventricular contraction, and on physiological factors such as vasoconstriction in response to body function (Box 6.4).

Box 6.4 Hypertensive disorders of pregnancy

Hypertension, high blood pressure, in pregnancy is associated with high maternal and fetal mortality and morbidity rates (Kwast 1991). It is usually a symptom of a disease process involving many systems of the body, and can either predate the pregnancy, or occur as a consequence of it. The most common disorder of pregnancy with hypertension as a symptom is *preeclampsia*, also known as *pregnancy-induced hypertension* (PIH).

The cause of PIH is unknown. Many theories have been suggested. Whatever the cause it appears to originate in the placenta, because with delivery of the placenta the condition usually resolves. The incidence is difficult to predict because the condition itself is difficult to define and diagnose. However, approximately 10% of women develop PIH, some seriously (Redman 1994). Other signs of PIH are *proteinuria* and marked *oedema*.

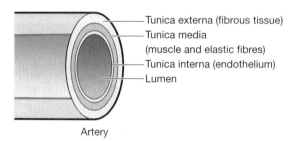

Tunica externa (fibrous tissue)
Tunica media
(muscle and elastic fibres)
Tunica interna (endothelium)
Lumen

Artery

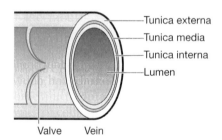

Tunica externa
Tunica media
Tunica interna
Lumen

Valve   Vein

Figure 6.6 Comparison of the structure of an artery and a vein.

Physical factors that affect blood pressure

There are a number of physical factors that affect blood pressure. These are described below.

- *Blood volume.* The total volume of fluid present in the circulatory system affects the pressure it exerts on the walls of the blood vessels. If there is a decrease in blood volume, the pressure exerted will decrease.

- *Viscosity of the blood.* Blood consists of specialised cells suspended in plasma, a fluid containing molecules such as proteins. The number of cells and proteins present in the blood affects the 'thickness' of the blood and the ease with which it can be moved along blood vessels. To move 'thickened' blood, the heart has to increase the strength of its contractions, resulting in an increase in the pressure exerted within blood vessels.

- *Elasticity of the vessel walls.* If the structure of blood vessel walls changes, it may become difficult or impossible for them to stretch to accommodate extra blood when the ventricles contract. This increases the pressure in the blood and hence blood pressure. Structural changes commonly occur when fatty plaques are laid down on the walls of the vessels, as a result of a diet high in fat.

- *Length of the blood vessels.* As blood moves along the length of a blood vessel, blood pressure decreases. In other words, the longer the vessel, the lower the blood pressure becomes.

- *Diameter of the blood vessels.* Pressure in blood vessels increases as their diameter decreases. There may therefore be resistance to the passage of blood through smaller vessels.

Physiological factors that affect blood pressure

As well as physical factors, there are a number of physiological factors which can affect blood pressure. Some of these are outlined below.

- *Alteration to cardiac output.* Changes in cardiac output in response to body function as described above will alter the pressure under which blood enters the circulatory system.

- *Sympathetic nervous system.* The vasomotor centre in the medulla is stimulated by receptors that detect pressure and blood gas levels in the arterial system. This centre then stimulates arterioles to increase or decrease their diameters accordingly, which affects blood pressure as described above. This is a sympathetic nervous system response.

- *Hormonal regulation.* Several hormones are involved in the maintenance of blood pressure by influencing cardiac function, blood volume or the diameters of blood vessels. Adrenaline and noradrenaline from the adrenal gland influence cardiac output, and control vessel diameter. Angiotensin II induces vasoconstriction and water balance by controlling the amount of aldosterone released. Antidiuretic hormone is released from the posterior pituitary gland at times of great blood loss and brings about vasoconstriction to maintain an adequate blood pressure.

● *Autoregulation*. Many organs have the ability to control blood vessel diameter locally to meet the needs of their cells. This is especially vital in organs and tissues such as the heart, muscles and local areas of the brain where cellular activity can alter dramatically. The level of oxygen in the tissues is often the determining factor in vessel diameter.

Return of blood to the heart

Blood moves from the heart, through the arterial system as a result of the blood pressure exerted by the heart's contractions, through the capillary bed where nutrients, wastes and gases are exchanged, then through the venous system, which takes it back to the heart. Blood pressure is the driving force behind this movement of blood through the circulatory system. In the venules and veins, however, blood pressure is very low. Nevertheless there is a decreasing pressure gradient from venules (20 mmHg) to the right atrium of the heart (0 mmHg). This, coupled with the fact that in the healthy person venous resistance is low, means that venous return keeps pace with output from the left ventricle. Three other factors assist the blood's return:

1. when skeletal muscles contract, there is an increase in pressure in the veins enclosed by these muscles
2. the presence of venous valves, which are opened or closed by the action of the skeletal muscles, helps to prevent back flow (Fig. 6.7, Box 6.3).
3. During respiration the diaphragm moves down, increasing pressure in the abdominal cavity, and decreasing it in the thoracic cavity. This pressure difference results in movement of blood towards the heart.

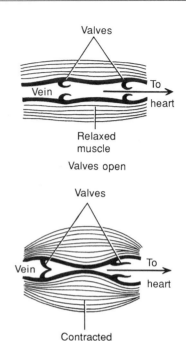

Figure 6.7   The effect of muscular activity on the valves in veins. (Reproduced with permission from Wilson K J W, Waugh A 1996 Ross and Wilson Anatomy and Physiology in Health and Illness. Churchill Livingstone, Edinburgh)

Circulation of the blood

There are three main circulatory routes through which blood can be directed:

1. through the systemic circulation
2. through the hepatic–portal system
3. through the pulmonary circulation.

Systematic circulation

When blood leaves the heart through the left ventricle it is directed to all tissues and organs, except the pulmonary arteries (Fig. 6.8). The *aorta* is the largest artery involved and from this artery, smaller arteries branch off to supply body organs. Once the blood has been through the capillary networks of the body tissues and organs, it is returned to the right atrium through the largest vein, the *vena cava*. The route of blood flow in the systemic circulation is: artery–arteriole–capillary–venule–vein – except in the gastro-

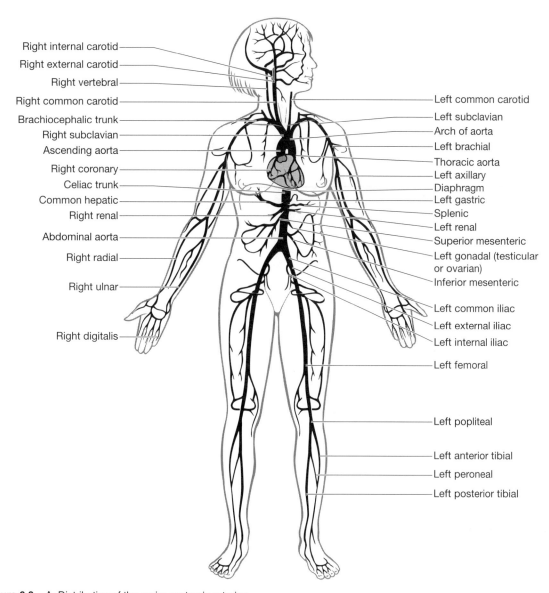

Right internal carotid
Right external carotid
Right vertebral
Right common carotid
Brachiocephalic trunk
Right subclavian
Ascending aorta
Right coronary
Celiac trunk
Common hepatic
Right renal
Abdominal aorta
Right radial
Right ulnar
Right digitalis

Left common carotid
Left subclavian
Arch of aorta
Left brachial
Thoracic aorta
Left axillary
Diaphragm
Left gastric
Splenic
Left renal
Superior mesenteric
Left gonadal (testicular or ovarian)
Inferior mesenteric
Left common iliac
Left external iliac
Left internal iliac
Left femoral
Left popliteal
Left anterior tibial
Left peroneal
Left posterior tibial

Figure 6.8   A: Distribution of the major systemic arteries.

intestinal system, where a hepatic–portal system operates.

The hepatic–portal system

In this system blood passes through the gastro-intestinal organs and then through the liver before returning to the heart (Fig. 6.9). The route of blood flow is: capillaries–veins–capillaries. This allows nutrients and toxins taken into the body through the gastrointestinal tract to be stored or removed before entering the general circulation.

Pulmonary circulation

Deoxygenated blood leaving the heart from the right ventricle goes via the pulmonary arteries to the lungs (Fig. 6.10). Here the blood exchanges

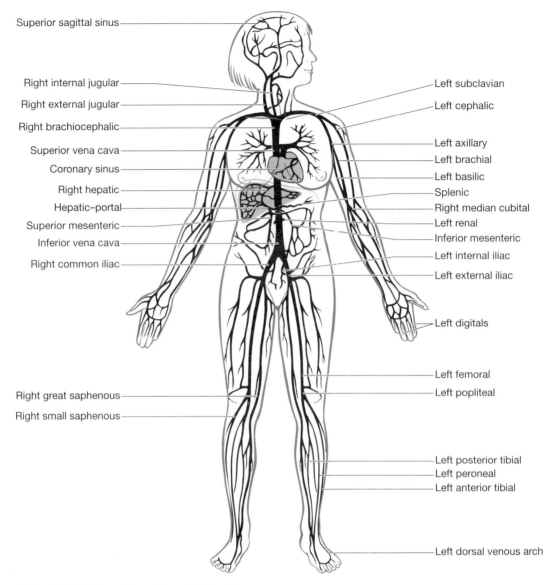

Figure 6.8 B: Distribution of the major systemic veins.

oxygen and carbon dioxide with air within the lungs. Oxygenated blood then returns to the left atrium of the heart before entering the systemic circulation, rich in oxygen.

Fetal circulation

In the fetus the circulation is altered to encompass the placenta, through which the fetus obtains nutrients and oxygen, and removes carbon dioxide and waste products. The circulation is therefore also altered to bypass the lungs and send less blood to the liver (see Ch. 17).

BLOOD

The circulatory system carries in its vessels a fluid in constant motion: blood. *Blood* consists of

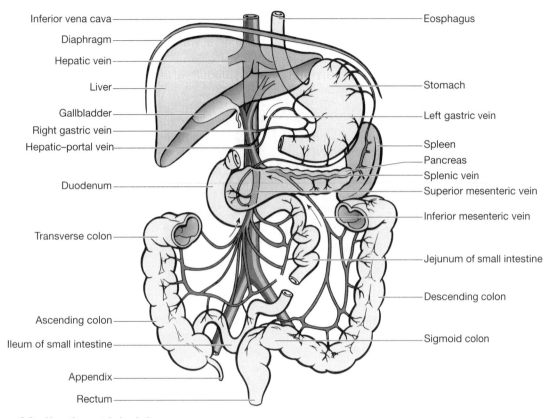

Figure 6.9 Hepatic–portal circulation.

a fluid in which several types of molecules and specialised blood cells are suspended (Fig. 6.11). It circulates round all parts of the body, transporting substances from one area to another. It also plays an important role in temperature control by carrying heat away from highly active tissues to cooler areas of the body.

Plasma

The fluid portion of blood is called *plasma*. This is a straw-coloured substance, similar in composition to interstitial fluid. Plasma makes up approximately 55% of blood volume, and is essential for the maintenance of homeostasis. It is composed of 90% water, plus dissolved or suspended substances, including proteins, nutrients, wastes, gases, electrolytes and the products of cell metabolism.

Plasma proteins play many important roles.

They contribute, for example, to the maintenance of osmotic pressure in the circulatory system. *Albumin* is a protein to which substances such as drugs can bind and be transported in the blood. Other proteins, *globulins*, are antibodies that protect the body from microorganisms. They also assist in transporting nutrients around the body. *Fibrinogen* is a protein which is essential in blood clotting.

Nutrients are carried round the body for distribution to all cells in the form in which they are absorbed in the gastrointestinal tract, i.e. as *amino acids, glucose, fatty acids* and *glycerol*. Wastes include *urea, creatinine* and *bilirubin* produced during the breakdown of nutrients in the gut.

Most *oxygen* is transported from the lungs to all body cells attached to red blood cells, but some is transported dissolved in plasma. *Carbon dioxide* is principally found dissolved in plasma, and is

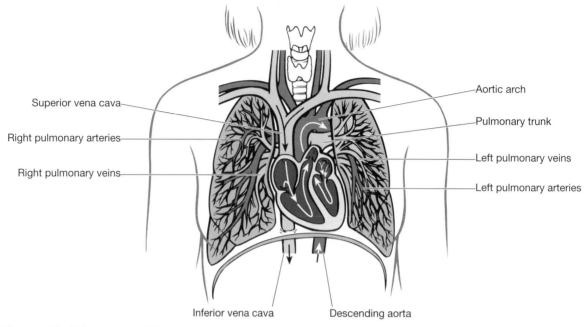

Figure 6.10 Pulmonary circulation.

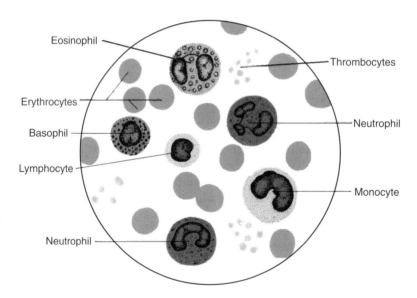

Figure 6.11 Blood cells present in plasma. (Reproduced with permission from Wilson K J W, Waugh A 1996 Ross and Wilson Anatomy and Physiology in Health and Illness. Churchill Livingstone, Edinburgh)

taken from the body cells to the lungs and other organs of excretion for removal from the body. *Nitrogen* is also carried in plasma, but it has no role in metabolism.

Electrolytes are carried round the body in plasma to supply body cells and also to maintain fluid and electrolyte balance. Products of metabolism such as *hormones* and *enzymes* are transported from producing cells to their sites of action.

Blood cells

The remaining 45% of blood is formed by blood cells. There are three main types of blood cell:

1. erythrocytes
2. leucocytes
3. thrombocytes.

Blood cells are formed by a process termed haemopoiesis. In the adult, *haemopoiesis* is carried out in the red bone marrow found in certain bones such as the humerus, femur, vertebrae and pelvis. All blood cells are derived from stem cells which then differentiate into specific cells when acted on by specific substances. For example, *erythropoietin* from the kidneys produces erythrocytes, and *thrombopoietin* produces thrombocytes.

Erythrocytes

Erythrocytes are commonly known as red blood cells (RBCs). They make up 99% of blood cells and are responsible for transporting oxygen from the lungs to all parts of the body. RBCs are circular, biconcave discs measuring less than 8 µm in diameter. Their design allows them to squeeze through capillaries, the smallest blood vessels, whose diameter is only 3 µm. They contain few organelles and no nucleus, and so are not capable of cell division. The lifespan of a RBC is limited to 120 days. The RBC membrane contains antigens which are responsible for cell recognition. These form the basis of blood groups.

RBCs contain the pigment *haemoglobin* which gives the blood its red colour. Haemoglobin is responsible for the transportation of oxygen. As RBCs pass along the capillaries surrounding the alveoli of the lungs, oxygen diffuses through the cell walls and becomes attached to the haemoglobin molecules to form *oxyhaemoglobin*. Each haemoglobin molecule consists of a protein, *globin*, and four polypeptide chains containing a pigment *haem* with an ion of *iron* (Box 6.5) to which one molecule of oxygen can become

---

Box 6.5   Iron deficiency anaemia

Anaemia is a deficiency in either the quality or quantity of red blood cells in the blood, leading to a decrease in the amount of oxygen available in the blood for metabolic processes. Oxygen is carried in the red blood cells attached to haemoglobin. In *iron deficiency anaemia*, insufficient haemoglobin is formed. Most normal diets will supply all the nutrients required to ensure adequate haemoglobin production, but during pregnancy the demand is increased and, if inadequate iron stores are available, anaemia may occur.

In the pregnant woman, the common causes of iron insufficiency are:

● inadequate amounts of iron in the diet
● loss of iron due to excessive vomiting
● excessive demand for red blood cells, e.g. as a result of multiple or frequent pregnancies, chronic infections such as urinary tract infection, or chronic or acute blood loss such as previous heavy periods or bleeding in pregnancy.

If a diagnosis of physiological anaemia is excluded, the treatment of iron deficiency anaemia is iron supplementation and advice about increasing foods rich in iron, such as red meat, wholemeal products and eggs (Day 1997). Low haemoglobin levels in pregnancy pose a danger: any excessive blood loss before, during or after delivery may result in the rapid development of *shock*. Even if no haemorrhage occurs, the anaemic pregnant or postnatal woman may suffer from *tiredness* and *dizziness* and this may spoil the enjoyment of pregnancy and parenthood (Paterson et al 1994).

---

attached. Each molecule of haemoglobin can therefore carry four molecules of oxygen.

Once a RBC reaches an area where the concentration of oxygen is low, the oxygen molecules become detached from the haemoglobin molecule, diffuse out of the RBC into the interstitial fluid, then into the body cells. Haemoglobin also carries approximately 25% of the carbon dioxide that is present in blood by binding it to the globin protein.

With a lifespan of only 120 days new RBCs must be produced constantly. In an adult there are approximately 5 million RBC/mm^2. To maintain this level, 2 million new RBCs must be produced every second.

Blood groups

There are two important methods of classifying blood groups which both depend on identifying genetically determined antigens on the cell membranes of erythrocytes. These are:

1. the ABO system, based on the presence or absence of antigens A and B
2. the rhesus system, based on the presence or absence of the rhesus factor.

The ABO system

There are four blood groups in the ABO system:

1. group A
2. group B
3. group AB
4. group O.

Blood of one group contains naturally occurring antibodies in the plasma, which can react against the cells of other groups. This is significant in cases of blood transfusions: foreign antibodies from the transfused blood may interact with the antigens of the host blood, leading to the erythrocytes sticking together. The host erythrocytes will be identified by the body's defence system as potential threats, and so will be destroyed, with potentially fatal consequences.

Table 6.1 shows which blood groups can and which cannot be used in transfusions for people with blood groups O, A, B and AB.

The rhesus factor

The rhesus factor is also determined genetically and distinguished as an antigen on the surface of the erythrocyte (Box 6.6). There are several rhesus factors, but the one most commonly identified is that of the antigen denoted D. Over 80% of the population has the rhesus factor in their blood,

> **Box 6.6** Rhesus incompatibility
>
> A mother who is rhesus negative may develop *rhesus antibodies* if rhesus-positive fetal blood cells leak into her circulation during pregnancy or delivery (Roberts 1994). This is a rare event in the developed world as a blood test after delivery can determine if fetal blood cells are present in the mother's bloodstream. If so, an injection of *anti-D immunoglobulin* is administered, which destroys the fetal cells before the antibody response can be initiated (Benbow & Wray 1997).
>
> However, fetal cells may pass into the maternal circulation early in pregnancy due to abortion, hypertension or partial separation of the placenta. As a result, rhesus antibodies develop and pass across the placenta to the fetus, where they begin destroying rhesus-positive cells. This results in *haemolytic disease of the newborn*, which can lead to severe *anaemia* with life-threatening complications. The fetus may require a blood transfusion in utero or immediately after delivery.

but a problem will only arise if a person without the rhesus factor, i.e. who is *rhesus negative*, is given blood from someone who is rhesus positive, i.e. whose blood contains the rhesus factor.

Normally no antibodies to the rhesus factor are found in the plasma of either rhesus-positive or rhesus-negative individuals. However, transfusing rhesus-positive blood into a rhesus-negative person will result in the production of antibodies, which destroy rhesus-positive cells. With each subsequent transfusion of rhesus-positive blood this response accelerates and transfused blood cells will be rapidly destroyed, again causing a severe reaction.

Leucocytes

Leucocytes, or white blood cells (WBCs), make up approximately 1% of blood cells. They are the largest of the blood cells and contain nuclei. Some have granules in their cytoplasm, and it is the presence or absence of granules that defines the WBC type.

Granulocytes are WBCs that contain granules. There are three types of granulocyte:

1. *neutrophils*, which contain nuclei that are made up of between two and six lobes connected by strands

Table 6.1 The presence of antibodies and antigens in an individual's blood, indicating compatible and incompatible blood groups

Blood group	O	A	B	AB
Antigen	–	A	B	A/B
Antibody in plasma	a/b	b	a	–
Compatible donor	O	A, O	B, O	A, B, AB, O
Incompatible donor	A, B, AB	B, AB	A, AB	–

2. *basophils*, which have irregular-shaped nuclei
3. *eosinophils*, which have nuclei with two lobes.

Neutrophils are responsible for protecting the body from foreign cells that invade tissues, and for removing debris. Any host cells that are damaged at the site of an infection release *chemotaxins* which attract neutrophils in large numbers. The neutrophils move out of blood capillaries by amoeboid movement, surround the invader and release destructive enzymes called *lysosomes* from the granules in their cytoplasm.

Basophils contain heparin and histamine which enable other cells to reach their sites of action. Eosinophils neutralise histamine and contain lysosomes that act against parasites, and are found in large numbers in areas where body tissues are close to the external environment.

Agranulocytes are WBCs that contain no granules. There are two types of agranulocyte:

1. *lymphocytes*, with a single round nucleus
2. *monocytes*, containing a kidney-shaped nucleus.

Lymphocytes are responsible for identifying foreign or abnormal cells, known as antigens. Lymphocytes are found not only in the blood, but also in interstitial fluid and lymph. On recognising an antigen they reproduce rapidly, releasing an antibody which attacks it, to render it harmless.

Monocytes are found both in the blood and in body tissues. They develop into macrophages and have an active role in immunity and the inflammatory response.

Thrombocytes

Thrombocytes, or *platelets*, are very small fragments of cellular material. Between 200 000 and 400 000 platelets are found in every cubic millimetre of blood. They contain substances essential to blood clotting.

Haemostasis

Being a fluid, blood is easily lost from damaged blood vessels. It is important to limit any loss of this essential substance.

Haemostasis, the stoppage of bleeding, is achieved by a range of measures:

● *Vasoconstriction*. This is the narrowing of blood vessels locally to restrict blood flow into the area. When thrombocytes (platelets) come into contact with a damaged blood vessel they release *serotonin* which, along with other chemicals released by the damaged cells, causes local vasoconstriction of the vessel.

● *Formation of a plug*. Platelets clump together, and release substances such as ADP, which attract many more platelets to the site, adding to the size of the temporary plug formed.

● *Coagulation of the blood*. A permanent clot can be formed, to seal the blood vessel by the production of fibrin. This is a complex process which involves the production of a series of chemicals (Fig. 6.12). In summary, strands of *fibrin* are synthesised by a plasma protein, *fibrinogen*, which combine with water and solutes to form a gel in which blood cells become trapped. This creates a blood clot. As further chemicals become involved this clot hardens and seals the

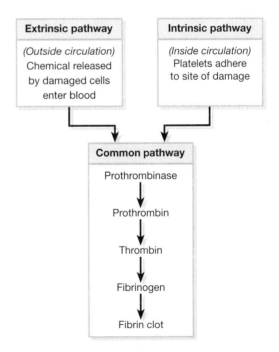

Figure 6.12 Coagulation of the blood.

blood vessel, and also acts as scaffolding for the repair of the damaged blood vessel.

- *Fibrinolysis*. Whilst the repair is being carried out on the damaged blood vessel, the fibrin clot is gradually broken down.

PHYSIOLOGICAL CHANGES THROUGH THE CHILDBEARING YEAR

Pregnancy

During pregnancy the cardiovascular system must meet the increasing demands of both the pregnant woman and the growing fetus. The altered hormone levels of pregnancy also affect the functioning of the system. As a result there is some alteration to the anatomy and physiology of the cardiovascular system.

In the heart, cardiac output rises by up to 40% (de Swiet 1991). Both stroke volume and heart rate contribute to this. These increases occur gradually over the first and second trimesters with little or no further increase after then. The raised cardiac output enables blood to flow through the added circulation formed in the enlarging uterus and the placental bed, and also to meet the extra needs of other organs of the mother's body.

The blood vessels increase in number and length to supply the placenta. Vasodilation occurs as a result of the action of the hormone progesterone on the smooth muscle of the vessel walls. This results in a *decrease in blood pressure* during the second trimester, but levels usually return to prepregnancy values during the third trimester (Blackburn & Loper 1992).

In the blood, the volume of plasma rises by up to 50% and the number of red blood cells by approximately 18% (Thomson 1993). Plasma volume increases gradually in the first trimester, with a greater increase in the second trimester. The rise in the number of red blood cells occurs in the second and third trimesters. These changes compensate for the apparent loss of blood volume – thought to be equivalent to 1 L – resulting from the presence of extra blood vessels and vasodilation.

Other changes that occur in the circulatory system are:

- a slight increase in the numbers of leucocytes
- a decrease in the immunoglobulins IgA, IgG and IgM, possibly due to the immuno-suppressed state of the pregnant body
- an increase in clotting factors, fibrinogen and platelets (Cashion 1995).

For the pregnant woman there is usually little obvious change in the functioning of the cardiovascular system. However, she may experience some symptoms that are due to these changes. The decrease in blood pressure during the second trimester may cause her to feel *faint* when rising suddenly. This may be aggravated, if she lies on her back, by pressure from the weight of the uterus on the major blood vessels in the abdomen. A decrease in blood pressure caused in this way is called *supine hypotension* (Sweet 1997).

The increase in plasma volume is greater than that of red blood cells. This results in haemodilution, which may be seen as an apparent anaemia, *physiological anaemia* (Mahomed & Hytten 1989). Iron supplements prescribed for this condition often aggravate the discomforts of pregnancy, such as gastric upsets and constipation. However, the increase in red blood cell production means that extra iron will be required. If iron stores are insufficient, a *true anaemia* may be present, in which case the woman may find *tiredness* and *apathy* a problem in her pregnancy.

The increase in the amount of plasma in proportion to the number of blood cells and proteins in the bloodstream may result in the loss of fluids into the interstitial fluid compartment in the capillary bed. This may lead to a generalised *oedema* in many pregnant women.

Labour

During labour, the increased metabolic demands of the body are supplied by the circulatory system of the healthy pregnant woman. After delivery, the increased levels of clotting factors, fibrinogen and platelets are available to begin the process of occluding the circulation in the uterus at the placental site. Given the increased blood volume, blood loss at delivery can be compensated for, provided it is within normal limits – usually considered to be less than 500 ml.

Postnatal

During the puerperium, the circulatory system gradually returns to its prepregnancy state. This is aided by a *diuresis* – increased production of urine – during the first 48 hours after delivery.

The neonate

During intrauterine life, the fetus obtains both nutrients and oxygen from the placenta, and so the circulatory system is adapted to pass through the placental site and bypass the lungs. Well before term, however, all the structures are present for a normal circulatory route.

Fetal haemoglobin has an altered composition, with a greater affinity for oxygen. This is to attract oxygen across the increased layers that divide the blood in the placenta from maternal blood (Llewellyn-Jones 1994).

With delivery and the cutting of the umbilical cord, the blood supply to the placenta ceases. A rapid change to an adult circulatory route is needed to allow the essential exchange of gases to take place in the lungs. This is usually completed within a few hours of birth.

Fetal haemoglobin is no longer required and it is replaced with adult haemoglobin. Excess haemoglobin is present in most neonates, so some *haemolysis* may take place.

The by-products of this destruction are excreted, although if liver enzymes are not present in sufficient quantities, a *physiological jaundice* may occur.

REFERENCES

Benbow A, Wray J 1997 Recommendations for the use of anti-D immunoglobulin for RhD prophylaxis. British Journal of Midwifery 6(3):184–186

Blackburn S T, Loper D L 1992 Maternal, fetal and neonatal physiology. A clinical perspective. W B Saunders, Philadelphia, p 206–207

Cashion K 1995 Maternal physiology during the postpartum period: In: Bobak I M, Lowdermilk D L, Jenson M D (eds) Maternity nursing, 4th edn. Mosby, St Louis, p 445

Comport K A, Seng J K 1997 Aortic stenosis in pregnancy: a case report. Journal of Obstetric, Gynecologic and Neonatal Nursing 26(1):67–77

Day L 1997 Iron supplementation in pregnancy: can it be justified? British Journal of Midwifery 6(3):180–183

De Swiet M 1991 The cardiovascular system. In: Hytten F, Chamberlain G (eds) Clinical physiology in obstetrics. Blackwell Scientific, Oxford, p 5–7

Forfar J O, Arneil G C 1984 Textbook of paediatrics. Churchill Livingstone, Edinburgh, p 632

Kelnar C J H, Harvey D, Simpson C 1995 The sick newborn baby, 3rd edn. Baillière Tindall, London, p 264

Kennedy B B 1995 Cardiac disease in pregnancy. Journal of Obstetric, Gynecologic and Neonatal Nursing 24(5):406–412

Kwast B E 1991 The hypertensive disorders of pregnancy. Their contribution to maternal mortality. Midwifery 7(4):157–161

Llewellyn-Jones D 1994 Fundamentals of obstetrics and gynaecology, 6th edn. Mosby, London, p 26–27

Mahomed K, Hytten F 1989 Iron and folate supplementation in pregnancy. In: Chalmers I, Enkin E, Keirse M J N C (eds) Effective care in pregnancy and childbirth. Oxford University Press, Oxford, p 301–302

Paterson J A, Davis J, Gregory M 1994 A study of the effect of low haemoglobin on postnatal women. Midwifery 10(2):77–86

Redman C 1994 Update on the 'sick placenta syndrome' pre-eclampsia: still a difficult disease. Professional Care of the Mother and Child 4(1):7–9

Roberts A 1994 Systems of life. Blood 5. Nursing Times 90(41): 39–42

Silverton L 1993 The art and science of midwifery. Prentice Hall, New York, p 88–89

Sinclair A 1995 Haemorrhoids. Professional Care of the Mother and Child 5(6):161–162

Sweet B (ed) 1997 Mayes' midwifery. A textbook for midwives 12th edn. Baillière Tindall, London, p 222

Thomas S 1992 Congenital defects of the heart. Nursing Standard 6(18):44–49

Thomson V 1993 Psychological and physiological changes of pregnancy. In: Bennett V R, Brown L K (eds) Myles textbook for midwives, 12th edn. Churchill Livingstone, Edinburgh, p 98

7

The lymphatic system

All body cells need a constant supply of oxygen and nutrients in order to carry out their metabolic processes. These are brought to the area by the circulatory system and then diffuse out either directly into cells or, usually, firstly into tissue fluid surrounding the cells, interstitial fluid. Along with these nutrients, fluid also moves into these spaces, to enhance diffusion, and then returns to the circulatory system. However not all fluid that leaves the circulatory system is immediately returned to it, and this is one function of the lymphatic system.

A second vital function of the lymphatic system is to provide lymphocytes, which fight invaders such as bacteria, and remove dead and damaged cells.

In the pregnant woman the lymphatic system alters little in function, although its workload increases. This is because of an increase in tissue fluid, caused by the relaxation of the walls of blood vessels under the influence of progesterone, and the resulting slowdown of venous flow. The immune response of the lymphatic system is adjusted in pregnancy however, to prevent rejection of the fetus, whilst retaining its ability to fight infection.

The lymphatic system is fully functional at birth, however the neonate is immunologically naive. The neonate receives immunoglobulins from the mother to give some resistance to infection until its own immune system matures.

The lymphatic system is composed of:

- lymphatic capillaries, which retrieve excess fluid from around cells

- lymphatic vessels, which transport lymph back into the circulatory system
- lymphatic tissue, which cleans and filters lymph before returning it to the circulatory system, and stores lymphocytes to fight microorganisms
- two lymphatic ducts, which return lymph to the circulatory system.

LYMPHATIC CAPILLARIES

Lymphatic capillaries are fine hair-like vessels found in the interstitial spaces between cells (Fig. 7.1). They are similar in structure to blood capillaries, with a basement membrane, endothelium and porous walls that allow many substances to move freely into the vessel. This flow is one-way only, because the endothelial cells generally overlap when the pressure in tissue fluids is low, so preventing the loss of lymph from the capillary into the tissues.

When external fluid pressures increase, the endothelial cells separate, allowing fluid and its constituents in. The separated cells are like pores, and they can open wider than those in blood capillaries, to allow proteins and cell debris to pass through. *Lymph* has a similar composition to interstitial fluid but includes larger molecules such as proteins and particles. Lymphatic capillaries are blind-ended tubes gathering fluid from around cells. The flow of lymph is always towards the heart.

LYMPHATIC VESSELS

Lymphatic vessels have a very similar structure to veins, with an outer fibrous covering, a middle

layer of elastic and muscle tissue and an inner endothelium. *Lymphatic vessels* are finer and more numerous than veins, however, and have numerous cup-shaped *valves* to ensure lymph moves in the correct direction. These are essential as there is no pump (such as the heart) to push lymph under pressure towards the circulatory system.

Lymphatic vessels are found in most tissues, except those of the central nervous system, and are particularly numerous in subcutaneous tissues. Lymph is directed through one or more lymph nodes before reaching a lymphatic duct.

LYMPHATIC TISSUE

Lymphatic tissue is collected into *nodes* that vary from the size of a pinhead to that of an almond. Lymphatic tissue is also found in two organs: the spleen and the thymus gland.

Lymph is passed through at least one lymph node before returning to the circulation. It is in the node that the lymph is cleaned, and any unwanted particles are removed. Lymph is taken into nodes by several vessels, called *afferent vessels*. There is usually only one lymphatic vessel which leaves the node, an *efferent vessel*. From the node, lymph either passes directly into a lymphatic duct or flows through one or more other nodes first.

Lymph nodes are composed of a fibrous capsule with extensions which dip into the substance of the node forming compartments (Fig. 7.2). Within these compartments there is connective tissue containing *reticular fibres* and *macrophages*, responsible for the cleaning and filtering of the lymph, and *lymphocytes*, involved in the immune response.

Lymph nodes are found in groups around the body at sites where many lymphatic vessels can converge. For example lymph from the head and neck pass through cervical nodes, whereas lymph from the breast passes through the axillary nodes.

Areas where there are large nodes of lymphatic tissue include the tonsils, small intestine, appendix and spleen. In these areas lymph is not filtered, but lymphocytes and macrophages are

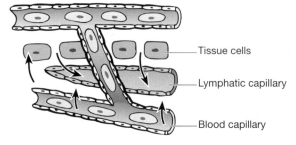

- Tissue cells

- Lymphatic capillary

- Blood capillary

Figure 7.1 Collection of lymph from interstitial spaces.

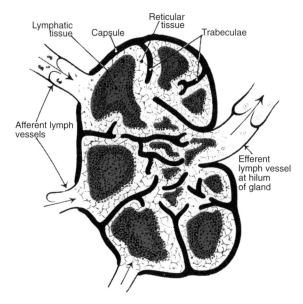

Lymphatic tissue Capsule Reticular tissue Trabeculae
Afferent lymph vessels
Efferent lymph vessel at hilum of gland

Figure 7.2 Internal structure of a lymph node. (Reproduced with permission from Wilson K J W, Waugh A 1996 Ross and Wilson Anatomy and Physiology in Health and Illness. Churchill Livingstone, Edinburgh)

readily supplied to protect the respiratory and gastrointestinal tracts from harmful micro-organisms and foreign materials taken into the body.

LYMPHATIC DUCTS

After passing through lymph nodes, lymph is returned to the circulatory system through two ducts: the thoracic duct and the right lymphatic duct (Fig. 7.3).

The *thoracic duct* is approximately 450 mm long and runs from a dilated section of lymph vessel, the cysterna chyli, situated in front of the second lumbar vertebrae, to the neck, where it empties into the left internal jugular vein. This duct drains lymph from the lower half of the body and the left side of the thorax, neck, head and left arm.

The *right lymphatic duct* is only 10 mm long and empties into the right subclavian vein in the neck. This duct drains lymph from the right side of the upper body.

PHYSIOLOGY OF THE LYMPHATIC SYSTEM

The physiology of the lymphatic system can be summarised as follows:

- Lymphatic vessels *collect excess fluid* from tissues and return it to the circulatory system (Box 7.1). This allows fresh fluid with nutrients and oxygen to bathe body cells.
- *Proteins* that have accumulated in the tissue spaces are also collected and returned to the bloodstream.
- Lymphatic tissue, particularly that found in nodes, *filters out* and *destroys cell debris* from the lymph.
- Lymph nodes contain *lymphocytes*, which *destroy microorganisms*. Lymphocytes also perform this function in the circulatory system and the body as a whole.

Box 7.1 Breast engorgement

The constituents of breast milk are obtained from the blood capillaries that surround the alveoli of the breasts. In the early days of lactation, blood flow to the breasts increases dramatically to enable milk to be produced. This increase may overwhelm the ability of the venous and lymphatic systems to return the blood to the heart and, as a result, fluid may accumulate in breast tissue (Renfrew et al 1990). This causes *engorgement* of the breasts, usually around the 3rd day of the puerperium. Engorgement can be very painful and can make it difficult for the newborn baby to latch on to the breast.

The role of the midwife at this time is to reassure the mother that this a temporary situation which will soon ease once the circulation of blood and lymph become acclimatised to the demands of lactation. Adequate analgesia is essential, particularly prior to breast-feeding, as the added increase in milk flow during the 'let-down' increases the discomfort. Warm flannels on the breasts can encourage both venous return and the flow of milk. If the baby finds it difficult to latch on, a small amount of milk expressed from the ampulla behind the nipple may soften the breast sufficiently to enable the baby to suckle (Smale 1992). However, expressing milk in this way will not succeed in softening the breast overall, because the engorgement is not caused by milk stasis.

Engorgement with milk may occur in later weeks if the baby sleeps through a feed or only takes one breast when he usually takes both. The only solution to this is to encourage the baby to take a good feed as soon as possible.

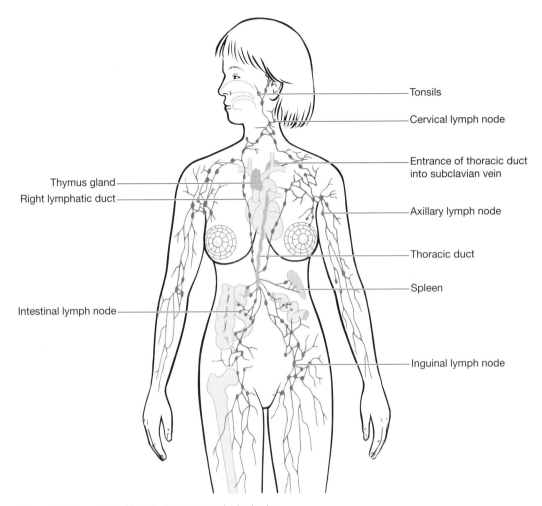

Figure 7.3   Location of lymphatic structures in the body.

- Lymphatic vessels around abdominal organs assist in the *transportation of digested food*, particularly fats.

Circulation of lymph

Circulation of lymph is maintained by a combination of *valves* and pressures from other structures. *Suction* is an important component of circulation: because lymph is emptied into the circulatory system close to the heart, each contraction of the heart creates negative pressure, pulling lymph through the lymphatic ducts and into the veins.

Pressure is also exerted on lymph vessels in a similar way to veins, by muscular contraction and pulsating arteries. This external pressure further contributes to driving the lymph towards the ducts – helped by valves which prevent backflow.

THE SPLEEN

The *spleen* is a gland-like organ composed of a large mass of lymphatic tissue. It lies behind the stomach, in the left hypochondriac region of the abdominal cavity (Fig. 7.3). It is deep purple in colour and is composed of an outer capsule

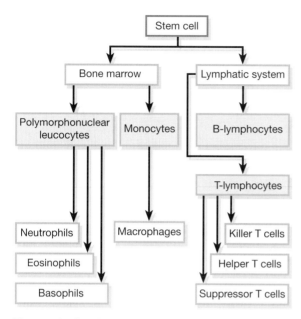

Figure 7.4   Development of immune system cells.

of fibrous tissue, with fibres throughout the gland giving a supporting structure. The spaces enclosed by the fibrous network are filled with *splenic pulp*, lymphoid tissue in which lymphocytes and antibodies are produced.

Physiology of the spleen

Blood entering the spleen travels along sinuses which have large pores that enable the blood to come into contact with the splenic pulp. Two types of cells are present there, whose function is to cleanse the blood:

1. *B-Lymphocytes*, that destroy microorganisms and enter the circulatory system
2. *phagocytes*, which destroy worn-out erythrocytes.

Erythrocytes can also be produced and stored at times of great demand. During fetal life the spleen is an important source of erythrocyte production.

THE THYMUS GLAND

The *thymus gland* is situated beneath the thyroid gland in the neck, and extends down through the upper mediastinum (Fig. 7.3). It is large and at its most active in childhood up until puberty, when it is gradually replaced by fat and connective tissue. The thymus gland consists of two lobes enclosed in a fibrous capsule, which dip into the substance of the gland forming compartments. These compartments contain epithelial cells and lymphocytes.

The function of the thymus gland is to *mature lymphocytes* that have been produced elsewhere.

THE IMMUNE RESPONSE

The immune response is the result of the interaction of components of both the circulatory and lymphatic systems (Fig. 7.4). It is physiologically complex – necessarily so to be able to deal with the variety of organisms and foreign materials that enter the body. The immune system undergoes a considerable adjustment during pregnancy in order to prevent rejection of the fetus, which is in part made up of foreign material. At the same time, it must continue to protect the pregnant body against disease.

Human immunity is controlled by a complex series of processes, which are generally divided into specific and non-specific mechanisms. These mechanisms function simultaneously, are interdependent, and act synergistically. *Specific immunity*, also called acquired immunity, is aimed at specific infectious agents and cells, and is often gained through exposure to that specific infection. *Non-specific responses* are general processes by which the body responds to infection.

Specific immunity

The specific immune response involves the identification of invading microorganisms, and the manufacture of specific cells to fight these organisms. If the same microorganisms invade the body on a subsequent occasion, they are instantly recognised and the immune system can destroy them rapidly. On first exposure, therefore, the response to an invader is delayed and the infection causes symptoms. On second and subsequent invasions, however, the response is much more rapid, so much so that the invaders are often destroyed before they can have any significant effect on the body.

On entering the body, foreign material triggers a series of events designed to seek out and destroy the invading cells. Specific immune responses are thought to work by distinguishing between self (the body) and non-self. Protein molecules 'mark' the cell membranes of all cells. The cells of the immune system recognise the body's own markers, but do not recognise the different markers of foreign cells (Box 7.2). It is in this way that invading cells are identified.

Specific immune responses are of two types:

1. humoral
2. cell-mediated.

Box 7.2   Autoimmune diseases

In rare instances the immune system can show an inability to distinguish between self and non-self. It appears to overreact and damages the body rather than protecting it. This can manifest itself as an allergic reaction to a foreign agent, or as an autoimmune disorder such as *systemic lupus erythematosus* (SLE).

SLE is a chronic multisystem inflammatory disease of connective tissue, mostly affecting young women. It is characterised by autoimmune antibody production, which sets up an inflammatory immune response causing widespread organ damage. SLE can occur very suddenly for no apparent reason, though it can be triggered by some antibiotics, stress or infection. The cause is unknown, but as it is more common in women between puberty and the menopause, it is thought to have a hormonal component (Leach 1998). It is also thought to be hereditary: relatives of an individual with SLE often have other connective tissue disorders such as rheumatoid arthritis or rheumatic fever.

The symptoms of SLE include painful joints, fever, fatigue, lymphatic involvement and loss of hair. Skin ulceration frequently occurs, and many organs, such as the kidneys, liver, heart and nervous system, can become inflamed.

Women with SLE can have a successful pregnancy and delivery (Crofts & D'Cruz 1997). Often however, the pregnancy is complicated by an increased incidence of abortion or preterm labour (Classen et al 1998). Pregnancy-induced hypertension and chronic renal disease are also more common. SLE does not increase the risk of fetal abnormality, but drugs taken for the condition may be teratogenic, i.e. they may induce the formation of congenital defects.

Humoral immunity

B-lymphocytes are responsible for *humoral immunity*. They patrol the body seeking out specific antigens and synthesising antibodies to them. An *antigen* is any non-self protein molecule marking a cell membrane. Several types of cells can be found in the body carrying antigens:

- foreign material, such as bacteria or pollen
- abnormal cells, such as cancer cells
- transplant cells
- cells which have been invaded by viruses.

Antibodies are glycoproteins that are manufactured by the B-lymphocytes to bind with and destroy specific antigens or their products. Antibodies bind to the target cells enabling them to be recognised by phagocytes, which destroy them. These antibodies are called *immunoglobulins*, and are divided into different classes according to their function: IgA, IgD, IgE, IgG and IgM. There are many of these immunoglobulins, and each one has a specific function. IgG is the only immunoglobulin from the mother that crosses the placenta, giving the neonate some initial immunity whilst he builds up his own immune system. IgA is found in breast milk and so provides the infant with immunity from his mother against other antigens.

Cell-mediated immunity

Cell-mediated immunity is initiated by T-lymphocytes (Box 7.3). There are three main types of T-lymphocytes:

1. helper T-cells
2. cytotoxic or killer T-cells
3. suppressor T-cells.

Helper T-cells are activated first in response to the presence of an antigen. They secrete *cytokines*, which stimulate the production of other defence cells such as B-lymphocytes, cytotoxic T-cells and macrophages. *Cytotoxic T-cells* directly destroy cells which contain the antigen markers. *Suppressor T-cells* mediate the immune response, limiting its action. Other lymphocytes have a role in memory and allergic response.

Box 7.3 HIV

Human immune deficiency virus (HIV) is a retrovirus that is taken into the nucleus of cells where it changes the genetic material (Johnstone 1996). HIV has a great affinity for T-lymphocytes, particularly helper T-cells, and is found in all the body fluids of an infected person. Antibodies to HIV develop slowly because the virus hides inside cells and so evades the normal recognition processes. Over a long period of time such a person develops a deficient immune system, and so becomes susceptible to opportunist infections such as tuberculosis, thrush and persistent diarrhoea.

The symptoms of HIV are slow to appear and an individual may not be aware he is HIV positive. The virus is spread by any exposure to infected body fluids such as blood, when sharing needles as an intravenous drug user, or semen during unprotected sexual activities (Scattergood 1995). The recipient of the body fluids has no way of knowing the risk because the HIV-positive person may not display any symptoms.

Once the disease becomes established, acquired immune deficiency syndrome (AIDS) usually develops within 10 years. Death will follow from progressive loss of motor function, nervous system degeneration, or from the opportunist infection. Recent advances in therapy with the development of anti-retroviral drugs have slowed down this process and improved life expectancy (National AIDS Trust 1999).

HIV has infected 33 million people world wide in the 20 years since it first appeared. Of these 14 million have died and it is estimated that 16,000 people become infected every day. 20% of these people are infected during unprotected heterosexual activities (National AIDS Trust 1999). 5000 women have become infected with HIV in the UK and in some parts of London it is thought at least 1 in 420 births are to infected women (Watson 1998). Of these more than 75% are unaware of their infection until their babies develop symptoms of AIDS. The risk of transmission of HIV to the fetus is considerable; HIV can cross the placenta (Lewis et al 1990), be transmitted during delivery (Ehrnst et al 1991) or through breast milk (Dunn 1992).

The midwife deals with body fluids constantly whilst caring for a woman before, during and after delivery. There is considerable debate about testing pregnant women during pregnancy for HIV both because of the risks to health professionals and to her unborn child (Grant & Roth 1998). However many midwives are poorly trained to undertake pre and post test counselling (Allanach 1998).

The risk of the midwife becoming infected is very low; the principal transmission route would be through a break in the natural barrier to infection, the skin. To prevent this it is essential that the midwife uses universal precautions when dealing with women where body fluids are involved. These will protect the midwife from both HIV and other serious diseases transmitted by the same route such as hepatitis B (Morley 1994).

Non-specific response

The *non-specific response* involves physical barriers such as the *skin* and *mucous membranes*, chemical barriers such as *gastric enzymes, lysozyme* and *pH*, and various white blood cells. The three main cell types involved in the non-specific response are:

1. neutrophils and macrophages
2. complement proteins
3. natural killer cells.

Neutrophils and macrophages ingest and destroy any bacteria that invade the body. *Neutrophils* initiate this phagocytic response by damaging the bacteria, releasing chemicals from inside the cell. This is *chemotaxis*. *Macrophages* are attracted by these chemicals and engulf and digest the bacteria.

The *complement system* is a protein cascade, which produces chemicals that break down cells. The proteins of the complement system circulate in the bloodstream until needed. The complement system is initiated in response to markers on the surfaces of invading cells. It is also activated as a specific response to IgG or IgM antibodies binding to an antigen and 'complements' this specific response.

Natural killer cells destroy cancer cells or cells which have been invaded by viruses. Cytokines enhance this process.

Vaccination

Immunity to infection can be achieved by the body's natural processes, such as those described above, or by deliberately exposing the body to the infective agent in a controlled way through vaccination. *Vaccines* are used to stimulate the first immune response and so prevent the damaging effects of the first exposure to the invading organism. There are three types of vaccine:

1. killed vaccines
2. attenuated vaccines
3. toxoid vaccines.

In a *killed vaccine* the damaging organism is dead, but the antigen markers on the cell membranes remain, provoking a response from the immune system. This is a very stable vaccine but must be administered in large doses with frequent boosters, because the organism is dead and so cannot reproduce to confer long-term immunity. Examples of diseases vaccinated against using killed vaccine include whooping cough and cholera.

An *attenuated vaccine* contains the live organism, but it lacks virulence. It therefore produces no disease process, although some local response can occur. A single low dose is all that is required as the organism can replicate normally and so continually stimulates an immune response. Polio and rubella vaccines are both attenuated vaccines (Box 7.4).

A *toxoid vaccine* contains a bacterial toxin which has been chemically modified to be nontoxic. The toxoid will stimulate a weak response from the immune system. Examples of this type of vaccine are those against diphtheria and tetanus.

Box 7.4   Rubella immunity

Because of the risks associated with rubella infection, it is UK policy for all children aged 10–11 to be vaccinated (with parental consent) against the disease. The rubella vaccine had been considered to protect the individual for life, but over recent years an increasing number of women have been found to be *susceptible to rubella* during pregnancy, despite having had the vaccination. It has been estimated that 5% of those vaccinated do not have an antibody response sufficient to confer immunity (Parker 1996). It is essential, therefore, for any woman planning to have a baby to check her immunity to rubella before embarking on the pregnancy. Many women do not plan their pregnancy and, if they are found to be susceptible to rubella, they are offered the vaccination immediately after delivery. They are then advised against pregnancy for at least 3 months.

Vaccines confer *active immunity*, as they stimulate the body to produce its own antibodies. If a person has already been exposed to, and possibly started to show symptoms of, a dangerous infection, then *passive immunity* can be conferred. This is only temporary, and is achieved by injecting the person with ready-made antibodies in the form of immunoglobulins. The risks of having the infection must outweigh the risks of being given the immunoglobulin. The neonate whose mother has caught chickenpox towards the end of pregnancy may be given immunoglobulins, as this disease can be extremely dangerous in the newborn (Storr 1997).

PHYSIOLOGICAL CHANGES THROUGH THE CHILDBEARING YEAR

Pregnancy

The lymphatic system has an increased workload during pregnancy because of the greater volumes of blood plasma and tissue fluid. Progesterone acts on the smooth muscles of the blood vessels causing an increase in the amount of tissue fluid. This slows down venous return, especially in the lower limbs and commonly leads to *oedema* during the later stages of pregnancy.

The immune response shows marked alterations during pregnancy, designed to prevent rejection of the fetus whilst maintaining the woman's defence against infection. *B-lymphocytes* increase, allowing the rapid production of relevant immunoglobulins in the specific response to the presence of antigens. T-lymphocytes however decrease in number. Specific immunoglobulin production varies: levels of *IgG decrease*, whereas levels of *IgA, IgE, IgM* and *IgD remain stable* or show a *slight increase* during gestation. The number of *white blood cells increase*, enhancing the non-specific mechanism for destroying invading bacteria (Priddy 1997). *Complement proteins* are present in greater numbers (Blackburn & Loper 1992), but *natural killer cells* are reduced to protect the fetus and placenta from rejection. This balance leaves the maternal immune system intact, but more vulnerable to viral and opportunist infections (Priddy 1997).

Labour

Lymph flow alters with changes in circulating fluid as labour progresses. The number of white blood cells continues to rise during labour and the puerperium.

Postnatal

The increase in white blood cells continues for a few days after delivery, enabling the body to fight the variety of organisms that may gain entry at this vulnerable time. Levels return to normal however within 4–7 days. The decreased levels of T-lymphocytes continue for several months.

Both colostrum and breast milk are rich in immune factors (Sweet 1997). Leucocytes are present in abundance: macrophages synthesise complement and lysozyme, which destroys the cell membranes of invading bacteria; B- and T-lymphocytes facilitate the production of the immunoglobulins IgA, IgG and IgM. Of these IgA is the most abundant and has a role in protecting the gastrointestinal tract from invasion by microorganisms (Stirrat 1991). This may provide some protection against allergies. Lactoferrin is also present. This prevents the growth of some bacteria and fungi by restricting their access to the iron they require.

These, and the many other immune factors present in colostrum and breast milk, mean that breast-feeding confers an added advantage on the neonate, protecting him from infection until his own immune response is mature (Perry 1995).

The neonate

The neonate is particularly *susceptible to infection* for two principal reasons:

1. the natural barriers to infection may be breached by damage to the skin and mucous membranes – the gastrointestinal tract, for example, is immature and has limited gastric secretions to act as defence mechanisms
2. the immune response is itself immature.

For the first 3 months the neonate has to rely on passive immunity from the mother. The fetus does not manufacture IgA, which plays a leading role in the defence of the respiratory and gastro-intestinal systems, but breast milk provides it in large amounts, so conferring further passive immunity (Kelnar et al 1995). The neonate will have received IgG from his mother, giving him resistance to some of the diseases she has been exposed to. It is vital that he be exposed mainly to the mother at birth, so that her commensals take a hold in his organs before those from the environment (Odent 1992).

The preterm neonate is particularly vulnerable to infection because of his underdeveloped immune system and because he will have received less IgG from his mother.

REFERENCES

Allanach V 1998 Far too little and too late. Nursing Standard 12(36):18
Blackburn S T, Loper D N 1992 Maternal, fetal and neonatal physiology. A clinical perspective. W B Saunders, Philadelphia, p 439–490
Classen S R, Paulson P R, Zacharias S R 1998 Systemic lupus erythematosus: perinatal and neonatal implications. Journal of Obstetric, Gynecologic and Neonatal Nursing 27(5):493–500
Crofts P, D'Cruz D 1997 Management of systemic lupus erythematosus: part 1. Nursing Standard 11(43):39–42
Dunn D T, Newell M L, Ades A E, Peckham C S 1992 Risk of human immunodeficiency virus type 1 transmission through breast feeding. Lancet 340:585–588
Ehrnst A, Lindgreen S, Dictor M 1991 HIV in pregnant women and their offspring: evidence for late transmission. Lancet 339:203–207

Grant J, Roth C 1998 Antenatal HIV testing. Time for a change in practice. The Practising Midwife 1(6): 16–19
Johnstone F D 1996 HIV and pregnancy. British Journal of Obstetrics and Gynaecology 103(12):1184–1190
Kelnar C J H, Harvey D, Simpson C 1995 The sick newborn baby, 3rd edn. Baillière Tindall, London, p 344–370
Leach M 1998 Signs and symptoms of systemic lupus erythematosus. Nursing Times 94(13):50–52
Lewis S H, Reynolds-Kohler C, Fox H E 1990 HIV-1 in trophoblastic and villous Hofbauer cells and haemotological precursors in eight week fetuses. Lancet 335:565–568
Morley D 1994 Midwives and HIV: the case for continuing education. Nursing Times 90(36):48–49
National AIDS Trust 1999 http://www.nat.org.uk/
Odent M 1992 The nature of birth and breastfeeding. Bergin & Harvey, Connecticut, p 72–73

Parker C 1996 Rubella vaccination: why vigilance must continue. Professional Care of the Mother and Child 6(1):2–3

Perry S E 1995 Newborn nutrition and feeding. In: Bobak I M, Lowdermilk D L, Jenson M D (eds) Maternity nursing, 4th edn. Mosby, St Louis, p 417

Priddy K D 1997 Immunologic adaptations during pregnancy. Journal of Obstetric, Gynecologic and Neonatal Nursing 26(4):388–394

Renfrew M, Fisher C, Arms S 1990 Bestfeeding: getting breastfeeding right for you. Celestial Arts, California, p 123

Scattergood S 1995 The impact of human immunodeficiency virus infection on midwifery. In: Murphy-Black T (ed) Issues in midwifery. Churchill Livingstone, Edinburgh, p 223–252

Smale M 1992 The National Childbirth Trust book of breastfeeding. Vermillion, London, p 46

Stirrat G 1991 The immune system. In: Hytten F, Chamberlain G (eds) Clinical physiology in obstetrics, 2nd edn. Blackwell Scientific, Oxford, p 127–128

Storr J 1997 Chickenpox. Professional Nurse 12(12):869–871

Sweet B (ed) 1997 Mayes midwifery. A textbook for midwives, 12th edn. Baillière Tindall, London, p 802

Watson S 1998 New guidelines for pregnant women. Nursing Standard 13(12):6

8

The respiratory system

Oxygen is required continuously by every cell in the body to fuel metabolic processes. Carbon dioxide is produced as a by-product of these chemical reactions. The respiratory system is responsible for obtaining oxygen from the external environment and removing carbon dioxide from the body constantly so that all body cells can continue to function. This is carried out in tandem with the circulatory system, which is responsible for transporting the oxygen to the cells and the carbon dioxide away, to prevent the build-up of toxic levels.

During pregnancy, labour and the postnatal period the demand for oxygen is greater than normal, due to the increased workload, and there is a corresponding increase in the amount of carbon dioxide needing to be removed. The healthy respiratory system is able to cope with these extra demands.

In the fetus the functions of the respiratory system are carried out by the placenta. It is not until after birth that the respiratory organs take over this role. As pregnancy progresses, the fetal respiratory system becomes prepared to function fully. However the fetus that is delivered preterm may suffer from respiratory distress because the lungs are not fully mature.

The main features of the respiratory system are (Fig. 8.1):

● the air passages – the nose, nasal cavity, pharynx, larynx, trachea, bronchi and bronchioles – through which air is warmed, filtered and moistened

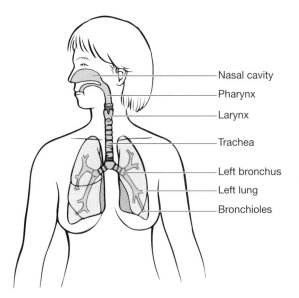

Figure 8.1 Gross structure of the organs of the respiratory system.

- the two lungs, in which gaseous exchange with the circulatory system takes place.

THE AIR PASSAGES

The nose and nasal cavity

The *nose* contains a large irregular-shaped cavity, the *nasal cavity*, divided by a *septum* to form two passages (Fig. 8.2). The cavity is formed by a hollow in the facial bones and the roof of the mouth. The surface area of the mucous membrane lining the nasal cavity is increased by the presence of *conchae*, shelf-like projections from the lateral walls.

When the air enters the nose, it is warmed, cleaned and filtered as it passes over the mucous membrane, which is composed of a highly vascular *ciliated columnar epithelium*, containing *goblet cells*. The vascular content of the epithelium

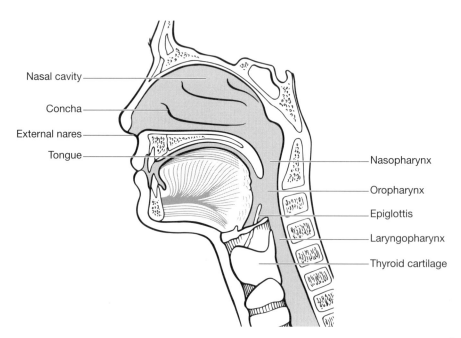

Figure 8.2 Structure of the upper respiratory air passages.

warms and humidifies the air, larger particles of dirt and dust are trapped by the cilia, whilst smaller particles are trapped by the mucus and wafted into the pharynx, where they are removed by coughing or swallowing (Box 8.1).

The nasal cavity also has the function of sensing smell. Nerve endings situated in the lining of the cavity are stimulated by chemical substances released by odorous material (see Ch. 4).

The nasal cavity has four openings: two *external nares*, or nostrils, through which air enters the air passages, and two *posterior nares*, which open into the *pharynx*.

The pharynx

The pharynx (Fig. 8.2) can be divided into three parts:

1. the nasopharynx
2. the oropharynx
3. the laryngopharynx.

Box 8.1   Smoking in pregnancy

Smoking has been widely publicised as being a major cause of adult mortality and morbidity. Yet smoking in pregnancy is still common, despite its significant harmful effects on both the pregnant mother and the fetus.

Smoking in pregnancy decreases the amount of oxygen reaching the fetus. This is because carbon monoxide from the cigarette smoke crosses the placenta and binds with haemoglobin to produce carboxyhaemoglobin, reducing the number of binding sites available for the transportation of oxygen (Chappell & Lilley 1994).

Smoking in pregnancy has been associated with *spontaneous abortion* and *preterm labour*. *Placenta praevia* and *placental abruption* are also more common in women who smoke (Lumley & Astbury 1989). The fetus is at risk from *intrauterine growth retardation*, resulting in a lower birth weight (McGreal 1995).

Postnatally, *sudden infant death syndrome* has been strongly linked with homes in which members of the family smoke (Gilbert et al 1995). *Upper respiratory infections, asthma* and *ear infections* have also been shown to be more common where children are exposed to passive smoking (Cullinan & Taylor 1994, Whatling 1994).

The *nasopharynx* lies behind the nasal cavity and extends down to the level of the soft palate of the mouth. It contains:

- the openings to the middle ear – the *Eustachian or auditory tubes* – which equalise air pressure between the middle ear and the external environment
- the *pharyngeal tonsils* or *adenoids*, made of lymphoid tissue.

The *oropharynx* is situated at the level of the mouth and contains two folds of lymphoid tissue, called the *palatine tonsils*. It is separated from the oral cavity (mouth) by the *Pillars of Fauces* and the *uvula*.

The *laryngopharynx* is the lowest section of the pharynx and is continuous with both the oesophagus, into which food is directed, and the larynx, through which air passes.

The pharynx is a tube approximately 130 mm long, composed of mucous membrane and muscle. It provides a passage for air and food, and acts as a resonance chamber for sound. The presence of lymph tissue provides a local source of antibodies for protection against infection. Nerve endings are present in the pharynx to detect taste.

The larynx

The *larynx* is commonly known as the voice box. It is a short passageway that connects the pharynx with the trachea, and it contains the vocal cords which produce sound.

Within the walls of the larynx are four significant sections of cartilage (Fig. 8.3):

1. the *thyroid cartilage*, also known as the Adam's apple, which is larger in males than females
2. the *cricoid cartilage*
3. the *arytenoid cartilage*, which influences the length and tension of the vocal cords, so altering the sound produced
4. the *epiglottis*, a flap of elastic cartilage attached to the trachea which, during swallowing, closes the entrance to the trachea to prevent food or fluids from entering the respiratory passages.

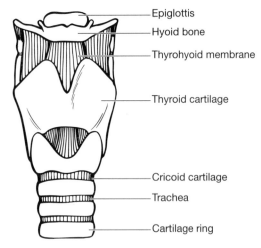

- Epiglottis
- Hyoid bone
- Thyrohyoid membrane
- Thyroid cartilage
- Cricoid cartilage
- Trachea
- Cartilage ring

Figure 8.3 External structure of the larynx and upper trachea.

The *vocal cords* are two folds of mucous membrane situated at the entrance to the trachea. Air passing over them can cause them to vibrate, producing sound waves. The vocal cords of the male tend to become thicker after puberty due to the influence of male hormones, so the sounds produced are lower in pitch than in the female.

The trachea

The *trachea* or windpipe is a tube approximately 120 mm long situated in front of the oesophagus (Fig. 8.4). It is composed of 16–20 incomplete rings of cartilage stacked one on top of the other. The function of this cartilage is twofold:

1. to prevent the closure of the trachea whilst a bolus of food passes down the oesophagus

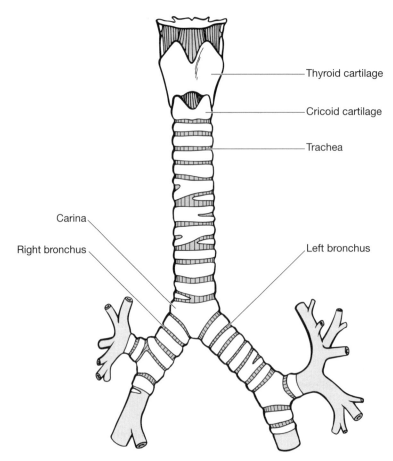

- Thyroid cartilage
- Cricoid cartilage
- Trachea
- Carina
- Right bronchus
- Left bronchus

Figure 8.4 Structure of the bronchi.

2. to allow slight expansion of the oesophagus during swallowing.

At the point where the trachea divides to form the two bronchi, there is a ridge of highly sensitive tissue called the *carina*. This area is associated with the cough reflex, which prevents the entry of foreign material into the lungs.

The bronchi

The trachea bifurcates into two air passages called bronchi (Fig. 8.4), which lead to the lungs (Box 8.2). The right bronchus is shorter and wider than the left, and leaves the trachea at a more vertical angle, due to the position of the heart on the left side. As a result, any inhaled particles are more likely to lodge in the right bronchus than the left.

Box 8.2 Asthma

Asthma is a condition in which the bronchi are narrowed inappropriately by chemical or emotional stimuli such as pollen, house dust, or distress. The mucous membranes lining the airways become inflamed and thickened. During an asthma attack the airways become constricted. Inspiration is normal, but complete expiration is difficult. Air becomes trapped within the alveoli.

Signs of asthma include *dyspnoea* (breathlessness) and *wheezing*. If not treated the condition can worsen to a severe acute condition, known as *status asthmaticus*. The patient will become cyanosed and exhausted. Bronchodilators and anti-inflammatory drugs are commonly prescribed for asthma.

The woman with asthma should be advised before starting a pregnancy to ensure that the medication she has been prescribed will not harm the fetus. She must also be closely monitored to ensure that the medication is appropriate to prevent asthmatic attacks during pregnancy, as these will prevent sufficient oxygen reaching the fetus. She should continue this treatment throughout pregnancy, labour and the puerperium.

Asthma complicates 1% of pregnancies (Reihill 1994). Of these cases, 10–15% will be hospitalised for recurrent asthma attacks. However, many women experience fewer attacks during pregnancy, possibly due the effect of progesterone, which relaxes and dilates the air passages. There is some evidence to suggest that pregnant women with asthma are more likely to develop hyperemesis (excessive vomiting) or preeclampsia (Moore-Gillon 1994).

The structure of the bronchi is similar to that of the trachea, with incomplete rings of cartilage keeping the airways wide open, i.e. maintaining their *patency*.

Bronchioles

The bronchi divide into progressively smaller passages:

- *bronchioles*
- *terminal bronchioles*
- *respiratory bronchioles*
- and finally *alveoli ducts*, that lead into the air sacs, the alveoli.

As these passages become smaller, the rings of cartilage become replaced with smooth muscle. The muscle is under autonomic nervous control allowing the diameters of the bronchioles to be altered to regulate the amount of air admitted to the lungs.

THE LUNGS

The lungs are two cone-shaped structures that lie in the thoracic cavity (Fig. 8.5). They are separated by the mediastinum, which contains the heart. The lungs extend from above the clavicles, superiorly, down to the diaphragm, which divides the thoracic cavity from the abdominal cavity. Laterally the lungs extend to the rib cage. The lungs are enclosed in two layers of pleural membrane: the outermost membrane is attached to the wall of the thoracic cavity, the inner membrane covers the lungs themselves. Between the two layers is a potential space containing a lubricating fluid which allows limited movement of the lungs without friction.

Macrostructure

The right lung is divided into three distinct lobes, the left into only two, due to the space taken up by the heart. The concave inferior section of each lung is known as the *base*, the superior section as the *apex* and the area close to the mediastinum as the *hilum*. The bronchi, blood, lymphatic vessels, and nerves enter and leave the lungs through the *hilum*.

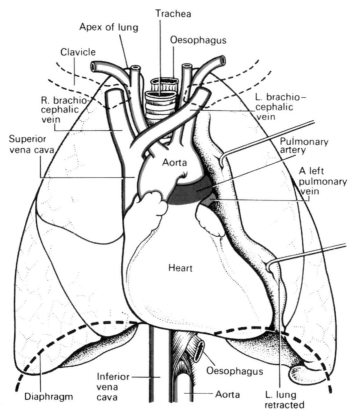

Figure 8.5   External anatomy of the lungs, showing the relative position of the heart. (Reproduced with permission from Wilson K J W, Waugh A 1996 Ross and Wilson Anatomy and Physiology in Health and Illness. Churchill Livingstone, Edinburgh)

Microstructure

The substance of the lungs is divided into lobules that contain collections of air sacs known as *alveoli*. There are some 750 million alveoli in the lungs. Surrounding the alveoli is a network of blood capillaries. Both alveolar and capillary walls are composed of a single layer of epithelium through which oxygen and carbon dioxide can pass by diffusion. This is called gaseous exchange, and involves oxygen passing from the alveoli across into the capillaries, to used in the body, and carbon dioxide passing in the opposite direction, to be exhaled. Within the alveolar walls are cells that secrete a fluid to keep the alveoli cells moist. This fluid contains a substance known as *surfactant*, which reduces surface tension and prevents the alveoli walls collapsing and sticking together.

ASSOCIATED STRUCTURES

Some muscle groups are essential to the functioning of the respiratory system. These are:

1. the intercostal muscles
2. the diaphragm.

Intercostal muscles

There are eleven pairs of *intercostal muscles* occupying the spaces between the ribs. There are two layers to each muscle, called external and internal intercostal muscles. The first rib is fixed to the skeleton so that when these muscles are stimulated to contract, each pulls the rib towards the one above. Due to the shape of the ribs this action results in movement outwards as well as upwards, so the thoracic cavity increases in volume, drawing air into the lungs.

The diaphragm

The *diaphragm* is a large dome-shaped muscle that separates the thoracic and abdominal cavities. It is attached to the lower ribs. When stimulated to contract, the diaphragm becomes flattened, which also increases the volume of the thoracic cavity, so drawing more air into the lungs.

BLOOD SUPPLY AND LYMPHATIC DRAINAGE

The right and left pulmonary arteries bring deoxygenated blood to the respiratory structures. Oxygenated blood is returned to the heart via four pulmonary veins. Oxygenated blood needed for pulmonary cell function is provided by the right and left bronchial arteries that branch directly from the aorta. Most of this blood returns via the pulmonary veins, but some drains into bronchial veins.

Lymph is drained into nodes situated around the trachea and the bronchi.

NERVE SUPPLY

Nerve supply for the respiratory system comes from the autonomic nervous system. This controls the dilation and constriction of the smaller air passages, and the ventilation (i.e. breathing) rate.

PHYSIOLOGY OF RESPIRATION

The main purpose of the respiratory system is to constantly supply all body cells with oxygen and to remove carbon dioxide. This function can be divided into three main processes:

1. ventilation – movement of air into and out of the lungs
2. external respiration – gas exchange between the alveoli and the blood
3. internal respiration – gas exchange between the blood and body cells.

Ventilation

Ventilation, the movement of air into and out of the lungs, occurs as a result of a difference in pressure between the air outside the body and the air in the lungs. Movement of air into the lungs is termed inspiration; movement out of the lungs is expiration.

Breathing in or *inspiration* is an active process which occurs as follows:

1. The diaphragm and the intercostal muscles contract, increasing the volume of the thoracic cavity.
2. The pleural membranes, which surround the lungs, are attached to the inside of the thoracic cavity and the outside of the lungs. So, as the thoracic cavity expands, the lungs expand too.
3. As the volume of the lungs increases, so the pressure of the air inside them decreases. This means the pressure of the air in the lungs becomes lower than the air pressure outside the body.
4. Boyle's law states that whenever a pressure difference or *gradient* is set up between two areas of gas, a volume of gas will move from the area of high pressure to the area of lower pressure in order to equalise pressures.
5. Air therefore moves from the area of higher pressure (i.e. outside the body) to the area of lower pressure (i.e. inside the lungs). In other words, air is drawn into the lungs.

Breathing out or *expiration* is a passive process which occurs as follows:

1. The diaphragm and intercostal muscles relax.
2. As a result, the volume of the thoracic cavity decreases.
3. This causes the volume of the lungs to decrease too.
4. As lung volume decreases, the pressure of the air in the lungs increases.
5. Once the air pressure is higher in the lungs than outside the body, Boyle's law dictates that the air will flow out of the lungs, in order to equalise the pressure.

Following each inspiration and expiration there is a pause before the ventilation cycle begins again. The healthy adult will complete an average of 12 ventilation cycles, commonly known as respirations, every minute. Each respiration moves approximately 500 ml of air into and out of the lungs. Of the 500 ml that enters the lungs, however, only 350 ml reaches the alveoli; the remainder only gets as far as the airways.

Factors that affect ventilation

The two main factors that affect ventilation are:

1. compliance
2. airway resistance.

Compliance is a term which describes the 'stretchability' of lung tissue and the chest wall. When the elastic fibres in the lungs encourage good expansion and contraction of lung tissue, the compliance is said to be high. However, if these fibres are damaged due to mechanical or disease processes, the elastic recoil of the lungs is impaired, i.e. compliance is reduced.

Airway resistance depends on the diameter of the small muscular airways. Healthy lungs give little physical resistance to the movement of air into the alveoli. However, chemical or nervous interference can decrease the diameter of airways, so increasing resistance.

Control of ventilation

Ventilation is normally under involuntary control, i.e. there is no conscious awareness of the need to inspire and expire. However, control can be exerted if required, for example when speaking, singing, swimming under water or entering a smoke-filled room. This control is limited, and once carbon dioxide levels disrupt homeostasis, ventilation resumes whatever the environmental conditions.

Ventilation is under nervous and chemical control.

Nervous control. The respiratory centre is situated in the brain stem. It is composed of groups of cells that control the rate and depth of ventilation.

Chemical control. Central chemoreceptors on the surface of the medulla oblongata detect very slight increases in carbon dioxide levels resulting in nerve impulses to the respiratory centre. This responds rapidly by altering the rate and depth of ventilation.

Peripheral chemoreceptors are found in the arch of the aorta and in the carotid bodies, where they react rapidly to increases in carbon dioxide levels by sending impulses to the respiratory centre. They also respond to changes in blood pH or in H^+ and stimulate the respiratory centre to alter ventilation to return pH to normal values.

Both central and peripheral chemoreceptors detect decreases in oxygen levels, but respond more slowly than to carbon dioxide. Increases in carbon dioxide levels are primarily responsible for initiating changes in ventilation rate and depth.

External respiration

External respiration is the movement of gases across the membranes that separate the alveoli and the blood capillaries (Fig. 8.6). It is governed by the temperature, composition and partial pressures of the gases involved.

Temperature. Air is warmed as it enters the lungs, because body temperature is (usually) higher than that of atmospheric air. Gas molecules that are warmed become more mobile, causing an increase in pressure (Charles' law).

Composition and pressure. Air is a mixture of gases. In a mixture each gas acts independently to exert its own partial pressure on the total

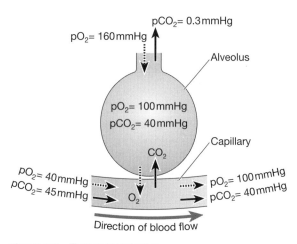

Figure 8.6 External respiration.

mixture (Dalton's law of partial pressures). The total pressure of the mixture is that of all the partial pressures added together. So, atmospheric pressure is created by the sum of all the partial pressures of the gases found in the air. Normal atmospheric pressure at sea level is 760 mmHg (101.3 kPa).

Alveolar air, however, contains increased water vapour, because it is moistened as it passes through the air passages. It also contains decreased oxygen and increased carbon dioxide levels, because gas exchange is independent of ventilation. Thus, the partial pressures of the individual gases in alveolar air differ from atmospheric pressures.

The partial pressure of oxygen (pO_2) in atmospheric air is approximately 160 mmHg. Once the air has entered the alveoli this pressure drops to 100 mmHg. In venous blood pO_2 is 40 mmHg. In other words, a pressure gradient has been set up. Oxygen diffuses through the alveolar cell membrane and capillary cell membrane into the bloodstream to equalise this pressure difference.

An opposite carbon dioxide (CO_2) pressure gradient exist: in the veins pCO_2 is 45 mmHg, in the alveoli it is 40 mmHg and in atmospheric air it is 0.3 mmHg. Carbon dioxide therefore diffuses out of the bloodstream into alveolar air and is removed from the body.

Efficiency

The efficiency of external respiration depends on several factors:

- partial pressure
- surface area
- diffusion distance
- depth and rate of ventilation.

Partial pressure. Atmospheric pressure decreases as height above sea level increases. Assuming that the composition of the air is unchanged, this means that partial pressures also decrease. If the decrease is sufficient to bring partial pressures down towards or below alveolar pressures, then diffusion of gases will not take place. Symptoms of lack of oxygen, e.g. shortness of breath and dizziness, result.

Conversely, atmospheric pressure increases as altitude decreases. Below sea level the pressure increases to above normal levels. This results in increasing partial pressures that enable gases not usually involved in gas exchange to diffuse into the bloodstream. The presence of nitrogen in the bloodstream from diffusion at these increased pressures results in the condition known as 'the bends', which divers can experience as they return to the surface.

Surface area. A large surface area is normally available for gas exchange due to the large number of alveoli in the lungs. If this number is reduced significantly, e.g. by disease, then insufficient oxygen will be able to move into the bloodstream for full cell metabolism to take place.

Diffusion distance. The total thickness of the membranes separating an alveolus and a blood capillary is normally 0.5 μm. Any increase in this distance, such as would occur when extra fluid is present (a condition termed pulmonary oedema), slows the rate of gas exchange.

Depth and rate of ventilation. The depth and rate of ventilation is controlled by the autonomic nervous system. If this system is disrupted, e.g. by drugs, the resulting diminished air flow into the lungs may provide insufficient oxygen for the cells.

Internal respiration

Internal respiration, sometimes known as tissue respiration, is the process by which oxygen and carbon dioxide diffuse between blood capillaries and body cells (Fig. 8.7). The driving force behind this process is again the pressure gradient set up by the differences in partial pressures of the

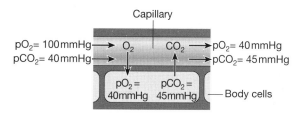

Figure 8.7 Internal respiration.

gases, which works in a similar way to that described for external respiration.

In arterial blood reaching the cells pO_2 is 100 mmHg; pO_2 in body cells is 40 mmHg. Oxygen therefore flows down the pressure gradient from the blood into the cells. Conversely, pCO_2 in cells is 45 mmHg, and in arterial blood, 40 mmHg. Again, a pressure gradient is present and so carbon dioxide diffuses from the cells into the bloodstream. This results in deoxygenated blood having a pO_2 of 40 mmHg and a pCO_2 of 45 mmHg, which ensures that the pressure gradient is in place when the blood returns to the lungs.

PHYSIOLOGICAL CHANGES THROUGH THE CHILDBEARING YEAR

Pregnancy

The demands placed on the body by pregnancy increase the cells' need for oxygen by approximately 20% (de Swiet 1991). There is a corresponding increase in the amount of carbon dioxide to be removed. These demands are met by an increase in tidal volume i.e. in the amount of air moving into and out of the lungs during one ventilation. There is usually no increase in ventilation rate.

Throughout pregnancy the increased levels of hormones, particularly progesterone, result in minor changes to the respiratory system that are usually annoying rather than debilitating. *Flaring of the ribs* occurs from early in pregnancy (Sweet 1997). Increased capillary engorgement due to the larger circulatory volume of blood makes *nose breathing difficult* (Thomson 1993). This may lead to difficulty in intubation for surgery, especially if compounded by oedema, caused by raised blood pressure (Silverton 1993).

Progesterone can also cause a relaxation of the bronchioles, which restricts the efficient movement of air into and out of the lungs, and can result in a mild degree of *dyspnoea*. This is aggravated later in pregnancy by the enlarging uterus pressing up on the base of the lungs, which means less air reaches the alveoli in the base of the lungs.

The increase in tidal volume, however, results in an overall decrease in pCO_2 in the bloodstream. For the pregnant woman, the effect of this is minimal, but for the fetus this enhances the removal of carbon dioxide across the placenta (de Swiet 1991).

Labour

The demands of labour are met by the ability of the lungs to increase ventilation rate and depth, and also by increased dissociation of oxygen from haemoglobin in areas such as the uterine muscles where activity has greatly increased. However, if uterine contractions occur too frequently, with little time in between for relaxation, the muscles will become starved of oxygen, a condition known as *hypoxia*, which causes increased pain (Moore 1997).

Postnatal

After delivery, respiratory function rapidly returns to normal. Hormonal levels return to normal and the alveoli at the base of the lungs are once again available for respiration.

The neonate

During intrauterine life the lungs are filled with fluid produced by alveolar epithelial cells. Gas exchange is carried out for the fetus by the placenta. In the later stages of pregnancy the fetus makes small *respiratory movements* which cause small amounts of amniotic fluid to enter the air passages. Respiratory movements are thought to stimulate the development of lung tissue (Blackburn & Loper 1992).

At the onset of labour alveolar epithelial cells actively remove the lung fluid in readiness for air breathing. As the fetus is squeezed through the vagina during delivery any remaining amniotic fluid present in the air passages is removed. The stimuli of delivery – change in temperature, bright lights, loud noises – shock the newly-delivered neonate into taking a deep breath, and the remainder of the fluid in the lungs is absorbed. The first breath is also stimulated by the small increase in pCO_2 that usually occurs during the stress of labour and by the cutting of the umbilical cord. Occasionally, however, the respiratory centre in the medulla of the brain is depressed by narcotics given during labour for pain relief (Dickerson 1989). In such cases an antidote can be given, and respiration quickly begins.

With the first deep breath after delivery the alveoli that have been closed during intrauterine life inflate. A substance that has been produced in the lungs since the 23rd week of gestation, *surfactant*, prevents the wet surfaces in the alveoli sticking together when they meet again during expiration. In neonates that are born before sufficient surfactant has been produced, the alveoli will thus collapse with each expiration and the neonate will quickly become tired and develop respiratory distress (Box 8.3).

In the full-term healthy neonate, however, the initiation of respiration and the cutting of the umbilical cord stimulate changes in both the pulmonary and cardiovascular systems, which redirect blood into the pulmonary circulation to allow gaseous exchange to take place.

Box 8.3 Respiratory distress syndrome

The respiratory structures are not functional in the fetus until birth. Before then, the placenta fulfils their roles. Whilst in utero, the fetal lungs are filled with fluid and the alveoli are collapsed. When the first breath is taken after birth, the lungs and alveoli expand and most of the fluid is squeezed out by the process of birth. For the lungs and alveoli to expand successfully, one essential substance is required: surfactant.

Surfactant is a phospholipid which lowers surface tension within the alveoli, ensuring that the alveoli do not collapse during expiration. Surfactant is produced from the 23rd week of pregnancy, and by the 28th week it is usually present in sufficient quantities to prevent alveolar collapse in a newborn. The baby who is born before 28 weeks' gestation, however, will have difficulty respiring: with each expiration, the alveoli are likely to collapse. The effort required to inspire when there is deficient surfactant is greatly increased – each breath taken is similar to the first breath taken after birth, and the baby quickly runs out of energy (Kelnar et al 1995). This condition is known as *respiratory distress syndrome* (RDS).

Treatment for RDS is by ventilator support, which provides continuous pressure in the lungs to ensure that the alveoli do not collapse. Artificial surfactant has been developed for administration to babies that are deficient in the substance (Halliday 1994).

REFERENCES

Blackburn S T, Loper D L 1992 Maternal, fetal and neonatal physiology. A clinical perspective. W B Saunders, Philadelphia, p 288

Chappell C, Lilley G 1994 Effects of smoking on the fetus and young children. British Journal of Midwifery 2(12):587–591

Cullinan P, Taylor A J N 1994 Asthma in children: environmental factors. British Medical Journal 308:1585–1586

De Swiet M 1991 The respiratory system. In: Hytten F, Chamberlain G (eds) Clinical physiology in obstetrics. Blackwell Scientific, Oxford, p 87–97

Dickerson K 1989 Pharmacological control of pain during labour. In: Chalmers I, Enkin E, Keirse M J N C (eds) Effective care in pregnancy and childbirth. Oxford University Press, Oxford, p 916

Gilbert R E, Wigfield R E, Fleming P J, Berry P J, Rudd P T 1995 Bottle feeding and the sudden infant death syndrome. British Medical Journal 310:888–890

Halliday H 1994 New hope for respiratory distress syndrome. Recent advances: surfactant replacement therapy. Part 2. Professional Care of Mother and Child 2(5):136–138

Kelnar C J H, Harvey D, Simpson C 1995 The sick newborn baby, 3rd edn. Baillière Tindall, London, p 168

Lumley J, Astbury J 1989 Advice for pregnancy. In: Chalmers I, Enkin E, Keirse M J N C (eds) Effective care in pregnancy and childbirth. Oxford University Press, Oxford, p 242

McGreal I E 1995 Smoking and the pregnant woman. Midwives 108(1290):218–221

Moore S 1997 Understanding pain and its relief in labour. Churchill Livingstone, Edinburgh, p 40–43

Moore-Gillon J 1994 Asthma in pregnancy. British Journal of Obstetrics and Gynaecology 101(8):658–660

Reihill C 1994 Asthma in pregnancy; reassurance is justified. Professional Care of the Mother and Child (4)7:198

Silverton L 1993 The art and science of midwifery. Prentice Hall, New York, p 427

Sweet B (ed) 1997 Mayes' midwifery. A textbook for midwives, 12th edn. Baillière Tindall, London, p 130

Thomson V 1993 Psychological and physiological changes of pregnancy. In: Bennett V R, Brown L K (eds) Myles textbook for midwives, 12th edn. Churchill Livingstone, Edinburgh, p 100

Whatling, J 1994 Childhood asthma and passive smoking. Nursing Standard 8(46):25–27

9

The musculoskeletal system

The musculoskeletal system is responsible for supporting, protecting and moving the body. The skeleton provides a framework for the structure of the body and protects vulnerable internal organs from damage. The muscles – with the aid of joints, ligaments and tendons – enable the bones of the skeleton to move.

During pregnancy, the skeleton itself alters very little, but it is expected to support the increasing weight of the growing fetus and the adapting maternal body. Certain joints are affected by the increased levels of hormones released in pregnancy. They become more flexible, in preparation for the birthing process, but this flexibility results in some related discomforts. Labour requires sustained muscular effort to achieve delivery. Postnatally, the musculoskeletal system slowly returns to normal, adapting as it does so to the different demands made on the body by the constant care of a newborn baby.

The newborn baby itself is born with a fully functional musculoskeletal system, which is able to increase in size along with the vast changes that occur during maturation into childhood and early adulthood.

The musculoskeletal system consists of:

- 206 bones, which provide a framework for movement of the body and for the protection of internal organs
- joints which allow two- or three-dimensional movement of the body
- muscles which enable movement of both the body and the internal organs

- tendons and ligaments, which provide attachments between bones and muscles.

THE BONY SKELETON

Bones are formed of a connective tissue composed primarily of water, organic materials such as collagen, and inorganic materials, principally calcium and phosphate. These combinations produce one of the hardest materials in the body.

The development of bone

Two types of cells are involved in the development of bone:

1. *osteoblasts*, which produce bone
2. *osteoclasts*, which remodel bone.

During embryonic life, the skeleton is mostly made up of cartilaginous models that roughly resemble the bones of the adult. *Cartilage* is a fibrous connective tissue which is less dense than bone. It is found in adults in areas where it gives support or provides shape, such as in the pinna of the ear and the symphysis pubis. Like bone, cartilage is composed of water and collagen, but it differs in that it has not been calcified. Not all bones develop from cartilage. Some are formed directly from fetal tissue.

Bone development begins in fetal life, and continues throughout childhood into adulthood (Fig. 9.1). Blood vessels infiltrate the cartilage of the fetus and osteoblasts develop in centres of ossification. They use minerals to form bone cells which replace the cartilage – a process termed calcification. The osteoblasts become trapped inside the calcified tissue, where they become *osteocytes*, responsible for maintaining the bone. Osteoblasts are also active around the outside of bone, increasing its thickness. Eventually most of the cartilage is replaced by bone, creating a rigid structure. Areas of cartilage remain strategically placed to allow growth. Once these cartilaginous plates are converted to bone no further growth is possible. However, the osteocytes retained in the bone continually break down and replace existing bone tissue throughout life.

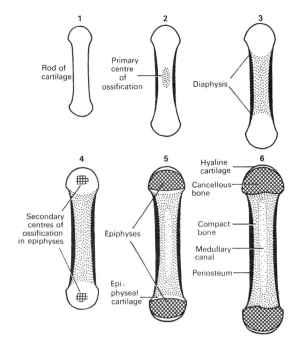

Figure 9.1 Stages in the development of bone. 1: Cartilage model. 2–3: Primary centre of ossification develops. 4: Secondary centre of ossification develops. 5: Calcified bone with cartilaginous plate. 6: Growth ceases. (Reproduced with permission from Wilson K J W, Waugh A 1996 Ross and Wilson Anatomy and Physiology in Health and Illness. Churchill Livingstone, Edinburgh)

Hormones control the growth and mineral content of bone. Growth hormone and the thyroid hormones ensure normal development of the skeleton during childhood. Oestrogen and testosterone are produced during puberty, and influence the development of the adult form. The thyroid and parathyroid glands are involved in the homeostasis of calcium in blood and bone tissue.

Microstructure

All bones contain two types of tissue, which vary in proportion and position depending on the type of bone. These tissues are:

1. compact bone
2. cancellous bone.

Compact bone tissue is very hard and dense (Fig. 9.2). It is composed of sheets of bone – *lamellae* – arranged as concentric cylinders called

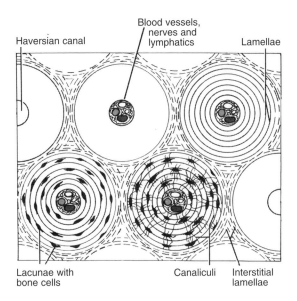

A. Cross section.

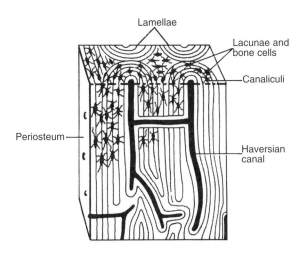

B. Longitudinal section.

Figure 9.2 Three-dimensional structure of compact bone. (Reproduced with permission from Wilson K J W, Waugh A 1996 Ross and Wilson Anatomy and Physiology in Health and Illness. Churchill Livingstone, Edinburgh)

Haversian systems. At the centre of these cylinders are *Haversian canals* that carry blood vessels, bringing nutrients and removing waste products. Bone cells (osteocytes) lie on and within the sheets of bone, in hollows or *lacunae*. Radiating in all directions from the lacunae are minute canals, which form an interconnecting network of *canali-*

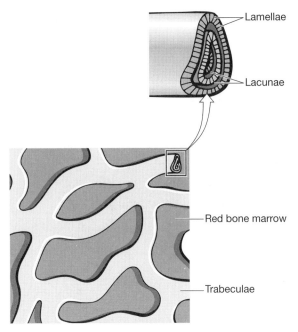

Figure 9.3 Structure of cancellous bone.

culi, passages for the movement of nutrients which nourish osteocytes.

Cancellous bone is made up of an irregular honeycomb of thin plates of bone called *trabeculae* (Fig. 9.3). Lacunae also lie within these plates of tissue. Red bone marrow, which produces red blood cells, is found within cancellous bone.

Macrostructure

Bones are commonly classified according to their shape.

There are five main types:

1. long bones
2. short bones
3. flat bones
4. irregular bones
5. sesamoid bones.

Long bones consist of a shaft or *diaphysis* composed of compact bone, with two extremities – the *epiphyses* – containing cancellous bone. Surrounding the entire structure is a dense white highly vascular covering, the *periosteum*, which protects the bone from injury and provides an attachment for tendons and ligaments. Underneath the periosteum of the diaphysis is a layer containing special bone cells – osteoblasts – which produce new tissue for the shaft of the bone. At the two extremities, *hyaline* or *articular cartilage* replaces periosteum on the surfaces involved in moveable joints. Within the diaphysis of the bone is a central medullary canal containing yellow bone marrow. Examples of long bones are the femur, humerus and phalanges.

Short bones are composed of cancellous bone with a thin layer of compact bone on the surface. They tend to be cube-shaped. Examples of these are bones of the wrist and ankle.

Flat bones are made up of two parallel plates of compact bone surrounding a layer of cancellous bone. Their large surface areas protect inner organs, and allow muscle attachment. The cranial bones, sternum and scapula are all flat bones.

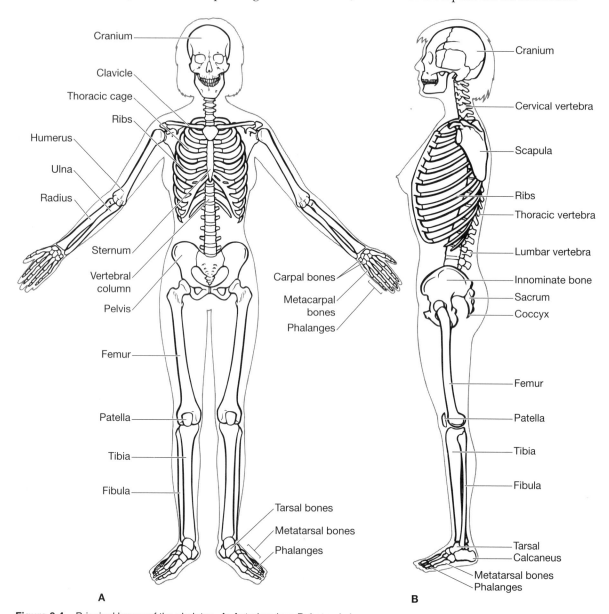

Figure 9.4 Principal bones of the skeleton. A: Anterior view. B: Lateral view.

Irregular bones have complex shapes and are varied in composition. They include the vertebrae and facial bones.

Sesamoid bones are very small and are found in tendons in places where a lot of pressure is exerted. They are often sited over a joint, for example, the patella.

Physiology of the bony skeleton

Bones provide a framework for the body, and provide attachments for muscles, tendons and ligaments. They also protect vital organs, such as the brain, spinal cord and liver, and make speech, hearing and movement possible. Joints between bones allow posture to be altered and movements to be made. The principal bones of the body are shown in Figure 9.4.

Within red bone marrow, blood cells are produced and within bone itself, minerals are stored, particularly calcium, phosphorus and sodium. These are removed for use in vital functions such as blood clotting, muscle contraction and metabolic processes. Diet replaces these minerals when available.

Bone healing

Bones can be fractured by trauma or by disease processes. A *simple fracture* involves a clean break, with the broken ends kept within the body. In a *compound fracture*, the broken ends protrude through the skin.

Healing takes many weeks to complete and goes through a number of stages (Fig. 9.5):

1. A haematoma forms around the broken ends of bone.
2. Macrophages are stimulated to go to the area. These remove small particles of loose bone and phagocytose both the haematoma and any inflammatory exudate.
3. New granulation tissue and blood vessels are formed.
4. Large numbers of osteoblasts develop and lay down disorganised bone tissue, forming a callus.
5. Osteoclasts reshape the bone and remove the callus, forming a central medullary canal.

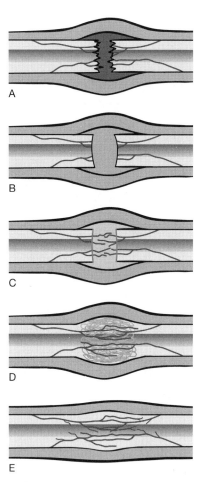

Figure 9.5 Stages of bone healing. A: Haematoma forms. B: Macrophages phagocytose debris. C: New granulation tissue is laid down. Blood vessels proliferate. D: Callus forms. E: Remodelling by osteocytes reshapes bone structure.

JOINTS

A *joint* is formed where two bones meet. In many cases the joint makes free movement possible, enabling the body to adopt many different postures. However, not all joints allow movement. There are three types of joint:

1. fibrous or fixed joints
2. cartilaginous joints
3. synovial joints.

In *fibrous* or *fixed joints*, adjacent bones are held firmly together by tough collagen fibres. The bones of the skull are examples of this type of immoveable joint.

Cartilaginous joints are slightly moveable joints. The bony surfaces at these joints are covered with hyaline cartilage and held together by tough fibrous tissue embedded into the cartilage. These joints occur, for example, between the two pubic bones in the pelvis (the symphysis pubis) and between the vertebrae.

Synovial joints are the most common type of joint, and they allow a great deal of movement. A synovial joint is completely surrounded by a fibrous capsule lined with *synovial membrane* (Fig. 9.6). This membrane secretes synovial fluid into the joint space, which nourishes and lubricates the joint. The surfaces of the bones of the joint are covered with hardwearing hyaline cartilage. Synovial joints are prevented from dislocating by surrounding muscles that prevent extreme movements, and by support from strong ligaments.

There are five types of synovial joint:

1. *hinge* joints, which allow movement in one direction only, e.g. the elbow and knee
2. *pivot* joints, which allow rotation, e.g. the distal joint of the radius and ulna

---

Box 9.1 Congenital dislocation of the hip

Congenital dislocation of the hip (CDH) occurs in approximately 1 in 1500 births (Sweet 1997). This is a condition in which the acetabulum in the pelvis is abnormally formed, so the head of the femur cannot be held securely in place (Way 1991). It is generally the result of a genetic defect, but may be caused by a breech presentation or by oligohydramnios, i.e. abnormally low amniotic fluid volume, leading to the fetus having difficulty moving in utero (Brunnar & Suddarth 1991).

Screening for congenital dislocation of the hip should be carried out soon after birth, when the neonate is given his first examination. If the condition goes undetected, it can lead to significant disability (Fowlie & Forsyth 1995). Usually the diagnosis is suspected when undertaking flexion and abduction of the hips – Ortolani's or Barlow's test. A click is felt or heard as the head of femur moves into and out of the acetabulum. Diagnosis is confirmed by X-ray or ultrasound.

Treatment of CDH may be unnecessary if the condition is thought to be transitory. However in most cases, it is treated by placing the hips in an abducted and flexed position in a splint which is worn continuously for 3 months. This is usually totally successful.

---

3. *ellipsoidal* joints, which allow movement in two directions without rotation, e.g. the wrist.
4. *ball and socket* joints, which allow rotation and movement in two directions, e.g. the joints of the shoulder and hip (Box 9.1)
5. *gliding* joints, which allow bones to slide over one another, e.g. the carpels and tarsals.

MUSCLES

Muscle accounts for half the weight of a typical adult. Although bones and joints provide the framework and pivot system necessary for movement, it is the *muscles* that move the bones at the joints, by contracting and relaxing. Muscles may be attached directly to bone or, where this bulk would interfere with function, may be attached by tendons.

Muscles are tissues whose cells have the ability to contract. However, muscle fibres do not contract partially: they either contract fully or, if the stimulus is insufficient, not at all. To contract, muscle fibres require:

- an *adequate blood supply* to provide nutrients and remove waste

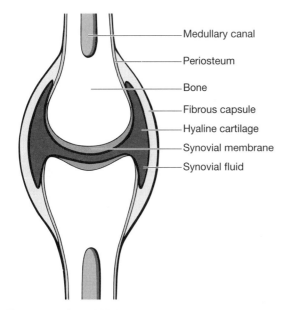

Medullary canal
Periosteum
Bone
Fibrous capsule
Hyaline cartilage
Synovial membrane
Synovial fluid

Figure 9.6 Synovial joint.

- sufficient glucose in the form of stored glycogen
- calcium.

If insufficient glucose is available from glycogen it will be formed by anaerobic processes, which create lactic acid as a by-product. Most of this lactic acid is converted to energy, but some will be retained in the muscle. The presence of large quantities of lactic acid in muscle causes *cramp*.

Three types of muscles can be identified (Fig. 9.7):

1. skeletal muscle
2. involuntary muscle
3. cardiac muscle.

Skeletal muscle

Skeletal muscle is also known as voluntary or striated muscle, the latter name being due to its striped appearance, formed by the two main types of filament: actin and myosin. Actin and myosin interact with each other in such a way that when stimulated to contract, the filaments slide into each other and pull the ends of the muscle together. Skeletal muscle is made up of fibres that vary in length from a few millimetres to 300 mm or more. The fibres are arranged longitudinally as unbranched cylinders, known as

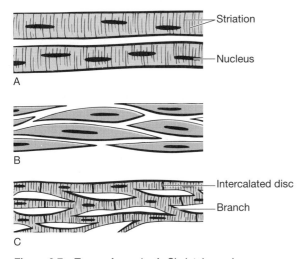

Figure 9.7   Types of muscle. A: Skeletal muscle. B: Involuntary (smooth) muscle. C: Cardiac muscle.

myofibrils. Each muscle cell has many nuclei and is supported by connective tissue. Three layers of connective tissue can be identified in skeletal muscle:

1. the *epimysium*, which encircles the whole muscle
2. the *perimysium*, which surrounds bundles of muscle fibres
3. the *endomysium*, which surrounds and separates individual muscle cells.

Skeletal muscle is under voluntary control and contracts strongly when stimulated. It also tires very quickly, and so requires a good blood supply to bring the nutrients necessary to maintain contraction. Movement of a part of the body is achieved by the coordinated contraction and relaxation of opposing groups of muscles.

Muscle coordination is learned. It involves sensory and motor neurones from the cortex of the brain. The impulses from motor neurones originate in the cerebral cortex, synapse in the spinal cord and travel to the muscles. Because there are many unconnected muscle fibres, each neurone branches extensively so an impulse can reach all relevant muscle fibres. These may be as few as ten fibres in the eye, and as many as 500 fibres in the larger muscles of the body.

Involuntary muscle

Involuntary muscle is also known as smooth or visceral muscle. It forms the walls of internal organs such as the uterus, bowel, bladder and blood vessels. The cells of this muscle are spindle-shaped and each contains one nucleus. The cells are bound together by connective tissue and are linked by gap junctions that enable contractions to be coordinated. Actin and myosin filaments are present throughout these cells.

Involuntary muscle is under the control of the autonomic nervous system, which means it contracts without the conscious intervention of the individual. Involuntary muscle works more slowly than voluntary muscle, and so is able to maintain a contraction over a longer period of time. Involuntary muscle is stimulated to contract by nerve fibres that run along the length of the muscle cells, releasing neurotransmitters at intervals that excite the muscles to contract in a regular pattern.

Cardiac muscle

Cardiac muscle is found only in the heart wall. It is highly specialised in order to perform a precise function. Like involuntary muscle, it too is controlled by the autonomic nervous system. It is formed from short, cylindrical, branched fibres whose cells each contain one nucleus. The branched cells and their interconnections, called intercalated discs, cause cardiac muscle cells to contract and relax in rhythm, enabling the efficient contraction of the heart as a whole. The rate of these rhythmic contractions is normally controlled by the heart's pacemaker, the sinoatrial node, which is under the control of the autonomic nervous system.

Cardiac muscle cells are stimulated to contract by specialised cells which have an inbuilt ability to initiate a contraction regularly and to conduct these contractions along specific routes through the heart muscle.

Functions of muscles

Muscles carry out a number of functions, including:

- making movement possible
- maintaining posture
- producing heat.

Movement may be in the form of whole-body activities such as walking and running, or finer tasks such as grasping objects or making gestures. Involuntary actions such as the beating of the heart, movement of chyme (digesting food) through the gastrointestinal tract, and contraction of the uterus are also muscle functions.

To maintain correct *posture* and balance, muscle groups are constantly readjusted. This is principally carried out without conscious thought by the individual.

All muscle action produces *heat*. Whenever muscles contract, the metabolic processes generate heat as a by-product, which helps to maintain body temperature within normal limits. A large amount of muscle action, however, may result in more heat being produced than the body needs, and it can be difficult to dissipate this heat rapidly.

LIGAMENTS AND TENDONS

The bones of most joints are joined together by *ligaments*, which are bundles of dense irregular connective tissue arranged in parallel bundles to resist strain. They are attached to the periosteum of a bone and run from one bone to another, across or within a joint. Ligaments allow movement but are strong, inelastic and rich in sensory nerve fibres and so protect the joints from excessive movement and strain.

Tendons are extensions of the dense connective tissue that covers and runs through muscle fibres to strengthen and protect skeletal muscle. Tendons attach the muscle to the periosteum of a bone, where direct muscle attachment is not possible.

PHYSIOLOGICAL CHANGES THROUGH THE CHILDBEARING YEAR

Pregnancy

During pregnancy, relaxin and progesterone act on the cartilage and connective tissue of the many joints, allowing them more movement (Russell & Reynolds 1997). This is useful in the pelvis because it gives slightly *larger diameters* for the passage of the fetus (Symonds & Symonds 1998), but it can lead to some discomfort for the pregnant woman, particularly later in pregnancy when levels of these hormones are at their highest. It also partly accounts for the *change in gait* that can be observed in many women, but this is also caused by the change in her centre of gravity.

Backache may result from the relaxation of the sacroiliac joint, and is aggravated by the change in posture (Parsons 1994). The midwife can advise the pregnant woman to wear low-heeled shoes and to limit her physical activity to minimise this pain. Other diagnoses such as

---

Box 9.2 Symphysis pubis dysfunction

Severe pain in the pelvis and perhaps the thighs and lower back during pregnancy can be the result of a condition in which the mobility of the symphysis pubis joint is increased to such a degree that the pubic bones can grind against each other. This condition is commonly called *separation of the symphysis pubis* or diastasis of the symphysis pubis. Its cause is not known, although there appears to be a genetic link (Davidson 1996).

The symphysis pubis joint normally loosens in pregnancy to leave a space of up to 9 mm, due to the affect of relaxin on collagen fibres in ligaments. Separation of the symphysis pubis is considered to be significant if the gap is 10 mm or more (Shepherd & Fry 1996). The incidence of this condition is unknown, but it appears to have been increasing in recent years.

Separation of the symphysis pubis may occur during pregnancy and also during or after labour. In pregnancy, the woman usually begins to feel pain during the second or third trimester. Pain is felt over the symphysis pubis and often down the thighs and into the lower back. Walking and climbing in and out of bed is difficult and painful. Treatment for the remainder of the pregnancy may be the use of walking aids and pelvic support in the form of a broad elastic bandage or special belt. Adequate analgesia is essential. Much support will be required at home to minimise physical exertion. Labour will depend on the degree of hip abduction that is possible, and a physiotherapist should be involved in planning for the event (Fry et al 1997). Separation of the symphysis pubis may occur as a result of labour, in which case complete bed rest will be necessary until the acute pain subsides.

Postnatally care will need to be continued, with exercises designed to encourage normal return of function. Full recovery may take weeks or even months. The mother will require much extra support to care for her new baby.

---

urinary tract infection must also be considered, however, when a woman complains of lower backache.

Pain on physical exertion that can be severe can indicate involvement of the symphysis pubis (Box 9.2).

Relaxation of the sacrococcygeal joint enables the coccyx to bend backwards during delivery, to allow the fetus to pass through the pelvis more readily.

Abdominal muscles become greatly stretched during pregnancy. This may cause the rectus abdominis muscles to separate in the third trimester. This can aggravate backache and poor posture if the uterus tilts forwards, a condition known as a *pendulous abdomen*. Pendulous abdomen may predispose to a malpresentation of the fetus for delivery (Matthew 1993). The use of a well-fitting maternity corset will minimise discomfort from this condition, and postnatally exercises can be taught by the physiotherapist to correct the problem (Sheppard 1996).

Cramp is a very uncomfortable condition frequently associated with pregnancy. Its cause is unclear – the role of dietary imbalances such as calcium and phosphorus is still being debated (Bracken et al 1989). No treatment is known to be successful, but extension of the leg when cramp occurs, and raising the foot of the bed, appear to be of some benefit.

Labour

Successful delivery depends on the coordinated functioning of uterine muscles during labour. Uterine muscles have the unique property of *retraction after contraction* that results in the dilatation of the cervix and the movement of the fetus down the birth canal. With each subsequent labour this process may become more efficient, shortening the length of labour.

Pelvic floor muscles are greatly stretched during a vaginal birth, and may be damaged during the process.

Postnatal

The musculoskeletal system can take up to 3 months to revert to its prepregnancy condition. Pelvic floor and abdominal muscles may regain their tone more readily if the mother undertakes regular *postnatal exercises* (Bishop et al 1992).

The neonate

Early in fetal development, muscles are involved in movement of limbs (Box 9.3). The pregnant woman will be reassured by the sensation of movement felt from around 18 weeks in a first pregnancy and from 16 weeks in subsequent pregnancies (Silverton 1993). These movements ensure that *fetal muscle tone* will be present at delivery, allowing the neonate to resist the force of gravity.

Box 9.3 Fetal activity charts

Fetal activity can be a useful indicator of the health of the fetus in utero. Fetal movement is felt from early in pregnancy and reaches a peak at around 30 weeks' gestation. From this time space becomes limited, but movement is still felt regularly. When the fetus is in a compromised state, there is diminished fetal movement, which ceases altogether if fetal death is imminent (Kelnar et al 1995).

In cases where the fetus requires closer monitoring, women may be asked to complete fetal activity charts, noting down the number of movements over a fixed period of time, or how long it takes for a fixed number of movements to occur. If fewer movements are felt than expected she can notify the midwife who can run a cardiotocograph to determine fetal wellbeing. In most cases the fetus will be shown to be healthy. If, however,

the fetus continually appears less active than is considered the norm, the obstetrician may consider running other tests to assess the fetus, such as a biophysical profile.

Fetal activity charts are useful because they are non-invasive and most women find them reassuring. However, they may not be totally accurate, because individual fetuses show great variation in the amount they move (Grant & Elbourne 1989). Also, women feel movements in very different ways: some consider a series of movements to be one movement, while others attempt to count each individual movement separately. Additionally, some women feel fetal movements more easily then others. So this method of assessing fetal wellbeing can be very subjective, and must be interpreted with care (Marnoch 1992).

In the last weeks of pregnancy, the fetus moves into the pelvis in preparation for delivery. In the normal cephalic presentation, the fetal head will move into the pelvis, and then through it during delivery. The fetal skull is the largest diameter to pass through the pelvis, and the ability of the fetal skull bones to override each other aids its passage.

At birth the full-term infant has a functional musculoskeletal system, but muscle function will be largely meaningless until the motor system of the brain matures. Many *reflexes* are present in the neonate, which enable him to react to the external environment. These will change as the infant develops and are a useful indication of correct neurological development (Johnston 1994).

At birth, *bones* have not completed ossification. This does not happen until the child is 12–15 years old, to allow growth to take place. For the infant this is advantageous when learning to move around the external environment, which involves many knocks and falls.

REFERENCES

Bishop K R, Dougherty M, Mooney R, Gimotty P, Williams B 1992 Effects of age, parity, and adherence on pelvic floor response to exercise. Journal of Obstetric, Gynecologic and Neonatal Nursing 21(5):401–406

Bracken M, Enkin M, Campbell H, Chalmers I 1989 Symptoms in pregnancy. In: Chalmers I, Enkin E, Keirse M J N C (eds) Effective care in pregnancy and childbirth. Oxford University Press, Oxford p 508–509

Brunnar L S, Suddarth D S 1991 The Lippincott manual of paediatric nursing, 3rd edn. Harper Collins, London, p 445

Davidson M R 1996 Clinical practice exchange. Examining separated symphysis pubis. Journal of Nurse-Midwifery 41(3):259–262

Fowlie P, Forsyth S 1995 Examination of the newborn infant. Modern Midwife 5(1):15–18

Fry D, Hay-Smith J, Hough J, McIntosh J, Polden M, Shepherd J, Watkins Y 1997 National clinic guideline for the care of women with symphysis pubis dysfunction. Midwives 110(1314):172–173

Grant A, Elbourne D 1989 Fetal movement counting to assess fetal well being. In: Chalmers I, Enkin E, Keirse M J N C (eds) Effective care in pregnancy and childbirth. Oxford University Press, Oxford, p 440–454

Johnston P G B 1994 Vulliamy's the newborn child. Churchill Livingstone, Edinburgh, p 49–52

Kelnar C J H, Harvey D, Simpson C 1995 The sick newborn baby, 3rd edn. Baillière Tindall, London, p 399

Marnoch A 1992 An evaluation of the importance of formal, maternal fetal movement counting as a measure of fetal well being. Midwifery 8(2):54–63

Matthew J T 1993 Structural abnormalities affecting pregnancy. In: Bennett V R, Brown L K (eds) Myles textbook for midwives, 12th edn. Churchill Livingstone, Edinburgh, p 379

Parsons C 1994 Spinal strain and pelvic joint pain in pregnancy. Modern Midwife 4(8):10–12

Russell R, Reynolds F 1997 Back pain, pregnancy, and childbirth. British Medical Journal 314:1062–1063

Shepherd J, Fry D 1996 Symphysis pubis pain. Midwives 109(1302):199–201

Sheppard S 1996 Management of postpartum gross

divarication recti. Journal of Association of Chartered
Physiotherapists in Women's Health 79:22–24

Silverton L 1993 The art and science of midwifery. Prentice
Hall, New York, p 136

Sweet B (ed) 1997 Mayes' midwifery. A textbook for
midwives, 12th edn. Baillière Tindall, London, p 918

Symonds E M, Symonds I M 1998 Essential obstetrics and
gynaecology, 3rd edn. Churchill Livingstone, Edinburgh,
p 131

Way S 1991 Screening for congenital dislocation of the hip.
Nursing Times 87(13):36–38

10

The digestive system

The functioning of the human body depends entirely on the chemical processes carried out by the individual cells that make up every tissue and organ. These chemical processes require energy and nutrients that are largely derived from the food and fluids taken into the body. The digestive system is responsible for:

- breaking down ingested food and fluids into molecules small enough to be absorbed into the bloodstream
- removing waste products from the body.

During pregnancy, the functioning of the digestive system is altered by the increased levels of hormones in the body. These physiological changes do not normally prevent sufficient nutrients from reaching the cells, but they can lead to discomfort for the pregnant woman, which is aggravated by the congestion caused by the enlarging uterus in the abdomen.

In the fetus nutrients are obtained via the placenta. The digestive organs, however, are patent and become functional after birth.

The anatomical structures that make up the digestive tract are (Fig. 10.1):

- The mouth, pharynx and oesophagus, through which nutrients enter the system and the process of digestion begins
- The stomach, in which food is mixed and divided into small portions and digestion continues
- The small intestine, in which digestion continues and nutrients are absorbed

117

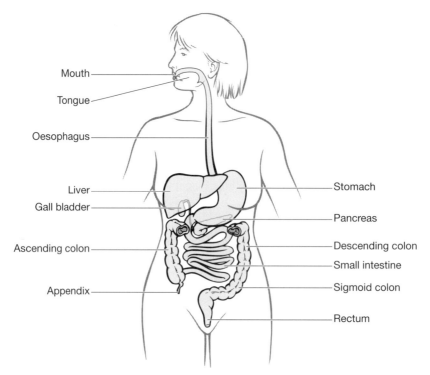

Figure 10.1 Position of the organs of the digestive system.

- The large intestine, which continues the processing
- The rectum and anal canal, through which waste is evacuated from the body
- Accessory glands, which provide and store digestive secretions that aid the chemical breakdown of food.

THE MOUTH

The *mouth*, also called the oral cavity, is formed by the muscular cheeks (the sides), the hard and soft palates (the roof), and the tongue (the floor). The entrance to the mouth is surrounded by fleshy folds, the *lips*. Behind the lips are ridges of the *maxilla* and *mandible*, covered with a mucous membrane called the *gingiva* or gum, surmounted with teeth.

Teeth

Two sets of *teeth* develop in the maxilla and mandible in the course of a lifetime. The 20 *decid-*

uous, or *milk*, teeth erupt into the oral cavity from around the 6th month of life. From the age of 6 these are gradually pushed out, and by the age of about 24 they will have been replaced by 32 *permanent* teeth. There are two main types of teeth:

1. *incisors* and *canines*, which are shaped into sharp edges for cutting and biting
2. *premolars* and *molars* that have broad flat surfaces for grinding and chewing.

The general structure of all teeth is similar (Fig. 10.2). The *crown* protrudes from the gum and the *root* is embedded into the gum. The *neck* is the narrowed area between the two. Within the tooth is a pulp cavity containing blood, lymph vessels and nerve cells. Surrounding this is a dense substance called *dentine*, and covering the entire crown is a very hard enamel layer. *Enamel* is the hardest tissue in the body, and once formed it cannot be replaced. The root is covered with a cement which holds the tooth in its socket in the gum.

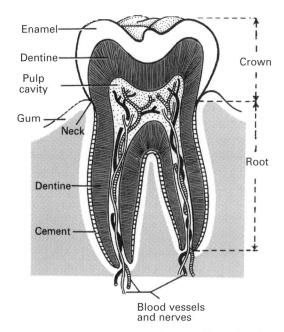

Figure 10.2 Internal structure of a tooth. (Reproduced with permission from Wilson K J W, Waugh A 1996 Ross and Wilson Anatomy and Physiology in Health and Illness. Churchill Livingstone, Edinburgh)

The palate

The *hard palate* is situated at the front of the roof of the mouth. It is formed by the maxilla and palatine bones. The back of the roof of the mouth is the *soft palate*, which is composed of muscle. The soft palate is continuous with the pharynx. At the rear of the soft palate is a muscular protrusion called the *uvula*, to either side of which are folds of mucous membrane. The anterior fold is the palatoglossal arch, the posterior one the palatopharyngeal arch. These folds are also known collectively as the *pillars of fauces*. Between these arches the palatine tonsils can be seen, which are collections of lymphoid tissue.

The tongue

The *tongue* is a large muscular structure occupying the floor of the mouth. It is attached posteriorly to the hyoid bone and inferiorly, by a fold of mucous membrane called the frenulum, to the floor of the mouth. The surface of the tongue is covered with stratified epithelium containing minute projections, or papillae, some of which contain taste-sensitive nerve endings, i.e. *taste buds*. These nerve endings extend into the soft palate, pharynx and epiglottis. Glands are also found on the surface of the tongue that secrete digestive enzymes.

The muscular action of the tongue enables food to be chewed, shaped and swallowed. The shape and size of the tongue can be altered to aid speech.

Opening into the mouth are ducts from the salivary glands.

SALIVARY GLANDS

Three pairs of compound exocrine glands empty their productions of digestive enzymes into the mouth. These *salivary glands* are:

- The *parotid* glands, situated beneath and slightly to the front of the ears. The parotid ducts terminate close to the second upper molar teeth.
- The *submandibular* glands, situated beneath the angle of the jaw. The ducts open into the mouth beneath the tongue to either side of the frenulum.
- The *sublingual* glands, which lie above the submandibular glands. A number of ducts leave the gland and open into the floor of the mouth.

Saliva is made up of the combined secretions of the six salivary glands and small mucus-secreting glands found scattered around the mouth. It contains 99.5% water and 0.5% chemical solutes such as sodium and potassium ions. Also present are organic substances including mucus, immunoglobulin and the enzymes lysozyme and salivary amylase. The functions of saliva are:

- to dissolve foods so that their taste can be determined
- to keep the mouth moist
- to lubricate food for easier swallowing
- to begin the chemical breakdown of the food.

The presence of lysozyme and immunoglobulin helps to prevent tooth decay and infection in the mucous membranes of the mouth. The mucus aids lubrication of the food so that it can be more easily chewed and swallowed.

Secretion of saliva is under the control of the autonomic nervous system. The amount secreted usually varies between 1–1½ L each day. A small amount is secreted constantly to keep the mucous membranes of the mouth, pharynx and oesophagus lubricated. With the presence, smell or even thought of food, production is increased. Production continues for some time after eating to clean the mouth and remove any irritating substances that remain.

THE PHARYNX

The *pharynx* is described in depth as part of the respiratory system (Ch. 8). Two sections of the pharynx, the *oropharynx* and *laryngopharynx*, are associated with the digestive tract. Food passes from the mouth to the pharynx and then to the oesophagus as a continuous process. The pharyngeal walls contain smooth muscle which is involved in the swallowing process.

Digestive functions of the mouth and pharynx

Food taken into the mouth is manipulated into position by the cheeks and tongue so that it can be chewed and mixed with saliva to form a soft mass. Saliva contains the enzyme *salivary amylase* which begins to break down starch. This mass, or *bolus*, of food can then be swallowed. Swallowing proceeds in three phases involving the mouth, pharynx and oesophagus:

1. Voluntary movement of the bolus of food to the rear of the mouth by the action of the tongue against the palate.

2. Involuntary passage through the pharynx. The soft palate rises to occlude the nasopharynx; the tongue and pharyngeal folds close the way back into the mouth; the larynx is lifted upwards and forward so that the epiglottis covers the opening into the respiratory passages. In this way the bolus is moved into the oesophagus. During this process, which is coordinated by the deglutition centre in the brain stem, breathing is interrupted for a few seconds.

3. Peristaltic action moves the bolus of food down the oesophagus into the stomach.

Salivary amylase is unable to complete the breakdown of disaccharides and polysaccharides in the mouth, but its action continues until it is neutralised by gastric acids in the stomach.

MICROSTRUCTURE OF THE DIGESTIVE TRACT

The organs of the digestive tract from the oesophagus to the anus are composed of four basic layers (Fig. 10.3):

1. the mucosa
2. the submucosa

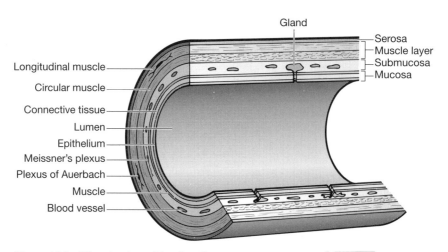

Figure 10.3 Microstructure of the digestive tract.

3. the muscle layer
4. the serosa.

These are examined below.

The mucosa

The *mucosa* is the innermost layer of the digestive tract. It consists of a lining of epithelium supported by connective tissue and a layer of smooth muscle. The epithelial cells contain mucus-secreting cells. In areas where there is the likelihood of damage, e.g. the oesophagus and anal canal, the epithelium is stratified. In selected areas of the digestive tract, the epithelium contains glands which secrete the hormones that control digestion. The layer of connective tissue contains blood vessels, which transport absorbed substances round the body, nerve cells, which innervate the tract and lymph vessels which protect the body from organisms that may have entered with the food.

The submucosa

The *submucosa* consists of connective tissue, and contains blood vessels, nerves and lymphoid tissue. The nerve plexus *Meissner's plexus* (also known as the submucosal plexus) is located in this layer, and has an important role to play in controlling the release of gastric secretions.

The muscle layer

The *muscle* layer is composed of two layers of smooth muscle:

- an inner layer of circular fibres
- an outer layer of longitudinal cells.

Involuntary muscular action breaks up the food, mixes it with digestive secretions and propels it along the tract by peristaltic action. In this layer is the *plexus of Auerbach*, or the mesenteric plexus, which contains autonomic nerve fibres. This plexus is responsible for the degree of contraction or relaxation of the muscles of the digestive tract, i.e. for its motility.

The serosa

The outermost layer of the digestive tract, the *serosa*, consists of connective tissue and epithelium which, in the majority of the tract, is a continuation of the *peritoneum*. The peritoneum is considered to consist of two layers:

1. the *parietal* layer, which lines the abdominal cavity
2. the *visceral* layer, which covers the organs and supports their position.

The cavity between the parietal and visceral peritoneum is a potential space containing serous fluid, which makes it possible for the two layers to slide over one another without friction.

THE OESOPHAGUS

The *oesophagus* is a thin-walled muscular tube approximately 240 mm long, which runs from the pharynx to the superior portion of the stomach (Fig. 10.4). It passes through the diaphragm at the *oesophageal hiatus* and bends sharply upwards before entering the stomach. This latter anatomical feature is thought to prevent the regurgitation of stomach contents into the oesophagus.

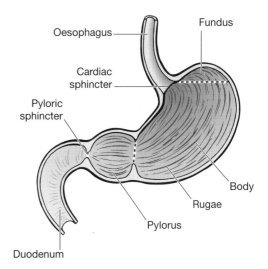

Figure 10.4 Structure of the oesophagus and stomach.

Two sphincters are situated at either end of the oesophagus:

1. superiorly the *cricopharyngeal* sphincter prevents air entering the oesophagus during inspiration
2. inferiorly the *cardiac* sphincter prevents the regurgitation of gastric contents.

Boluses of food are transported through the oesophagus by peristalsis.

THE STOMACH

The *stomach* is an enlarged J-shaped section of the digestive tract (Fig. 10.4). It is continuous with the oesophagus above and the duodenum below. It is commonly described in three parts:

1. the *fundus*, above the level of the cardiac sphincter
2. the *body*, which makes up the greater portion of the stomach
3. the *pylorus*, the lower end which leads to the duodenum.

The fundus and body walls contain little muscle and are used as a reservoir for food. The walls of the pylorus contain more muscle and in this region strong muscular contractions churn up the food and mix it with gastric juices. Food is then removed from the stomach by peristalsis through the pyloric sphincter into the duodenum.

The size of the stomach varies according to the amount of food present. The walls of the fundus and body are arranged in folds or *rugae* and are therefore capable of great distension.

Gastric secretions, commonly called gastric juices, are produced in the stomach to continue the process of digestion. Approximately 2–3 L of gastric juice are produced daily, composed of water to liquefy the food, mucus to further lubricate it, and the following specialised secretions released by the numerous gastric glands in the epithelium:

● Hydrochloric acid, which makes the stomach contents highly acidic (pH 1.5–3.5) and is a major defence against ingested harmful microorganisms. It also enables enzymes to begin the process of protein digestion, by denaturing the proteins and activating the enzymes.

● Pepsinogen, the precursor of pepsin responsible for the breakdown of proteins.
● Intrinsic factor, required for the absorption of vitamin B_{12}.

Digestive functions

Once food enters the stomach, gentle mixing waves break it up, mix it with gastric secretions and reduce it to a semi-fluid mass known as *chyme*. This wavelike movement, *peristalsis* (Fig. 10.5), is created by the alternate contraction and relaxation of portions of the stomach wall. As digestion proceeds the waves become stronger and they move the contents down towards the pylorus. The pyloric sphincter remains almost closed, allowing only small fluid portions to leave the stomach at a time. The majority of the chyme reaching the sphincter is rolled back into the body of the stomach, where chemical and mechanical breakdown continue.

Gastric secretions and muscular contractions are controlled by both hormonal and nervous stimulation. Before the ingestion of food, during the *cephalic stage*, the sight and smell of food stim-

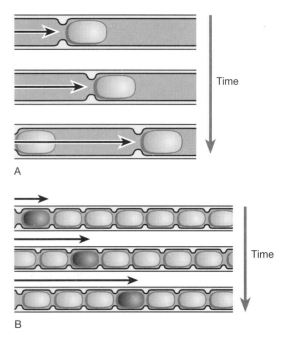

Figure 10.5 Movement of a bolus of food. A: By peristalsis. B: By segmentation.

ulate the autonomic nervous system to begin peristalsis and the production of gastric secretions. Once food reaches the stomach, distension and a rise in pH stimulate the production of the hormone gastrin, which further stimulates gastric secretions. This phase is known as the *gastric phase* and continues until the stomach is emptied and the pH falls to 1.5. Finally, during the *intestinal phase*, the presence of food in the duodenum stimulates the production of three hormones:

1. gastric inhibitory peptide, which inhibits both gastric secretions and gastric motility
2. secretin, which inhibits gastric secretions
3. cholecystokinin (CCK), which inhibits stomach emptying, preventing over-distension of the duodenum, and allowing more time for gastric digestion. The *enterogastric reflex*, a neural reflex, also affects this process.

It takes 2–6 hours after eating a meal for the stomach to be emptied of food. Proteins stay in the stomach for the longest period of time, whilst carbohydrates are moved on more quickly into the small intestine. The stomach wall is impervious to most of the substances that are ingested, so absorption of nutrients generally does not begin until chyme enters the small intestine. However water, alcohol, some electrolytes and certain drugs such as aspirin are absorbed from the stomach.

THE SMALL INTESTINE

The pyloric sphincter leads into the *small intestine*, which is approximately 6.5 m long. It is situated centrally in the abdominal cavity and opens into the large intestine. Most digestion and absorption takes place in the small intestine.

Anatomically the small intestine is divided into three parts (Fig. 10.6):

1. the duodenum
2. the jejunum
3. the ileum.

The *duodenum* is the shortest section of the small intestine, measuring about 250 mm. At

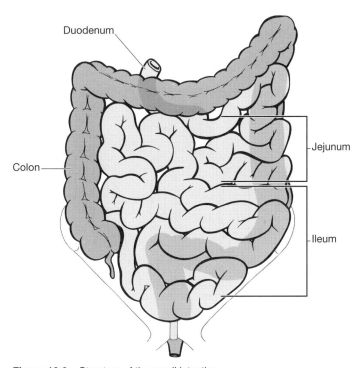

Figure 10.6   Structure of the small intestine.

its midpoint, two openings enter, one from the common bile duct and the other from the pancreas. The pylorus empties into the duodenum, which in turn empties into the jejunum.

The *jejunum* is the middle section of the small intestine, measuring approximately 2.5 m. It empties into the ileum.

The *ileum* is the final section of the small intestine, and is about 3.6 m long. It joins the large intestine at the ileocaecal sphincter.

Microstructure

The microstructure of the small intestine follows the general four-layer pattern of the digestive tract. However, both the mucosal and submucosal layers are modified to facilitate both digestion and absorption.

The mucosal layer is folded, to increase the surface area available for absorption. The surface layer of epithelial cells are further folded to produce *villi* surmounted with hair-like projections, *microvilli*. This is known as the *brush border* (Fig. 10.7). A network of blood capillaries and lymph vessels are present in each villus to transport absorbed substances around the body. Interspersed throughout the epithelial layer are goblet cells secreting mucus.

The submucosal layer contains *intestinal glands* and provides cells to renew the epithelium, and digestive enzymes to complete the digestion of carbohydrates, fats and proteins.

The small intestine continuously secretes intestinal juice at a pH of approximately 7.5 which contains water, mucus and the digestive enzyme enterokinase. Each day, 2–3 L of intestinal juice are produced.

Digestive functions

Chyme enters the small intestine from the stomach and is mixed with intestinal juice, bile and pancreatic juice. As this mixture passes over the brush border of the intestinal lining, further enzymes are secreted from the epithelial layer. All these contribute to the breakdown of proteins, carbohydrates, and fats into amino acids, monosaccharides, fatty acids and glycerol respectively, which is completed as the chyme moves through the length of the small intestine. Approximately 90% of these substances are absorbed into the bloodstream during this process, along with electrolytes, vitamins and most of the water ingested, or released as part of the digestive process.

The rate at which chyme is emptied from the

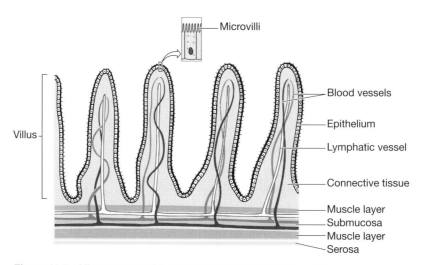

Figure 10.7 Microstructure of the brush border of the small intestine.

stomach governs its passage along the small intestine, which is brought about partly by peristalsis but predominantly by segmentation (Fig. 10.5). Both of the processes are controlled by the autonomic nervous system.

In *segmentation*, a localised contraction of the intestinal wall results in the chyme being separated into small parcels. Subsequent relaxation of the wall at this point, at the same time as contraction of the wall around the centre of the parcels, mixes the food thoroughly, allowing digestive enzymes to work efficiently. It takes 3–5 hours for chyme to pass through the small intestine.

THE LARGE INTESTINE

The *large intestine* extends from the ileum to the rectum and is about 1.5 m long (Fig. 10.8). It has a larger lumen than the small intestine and is divided into two anatomical sections:

1. the caecum
2. the colon.

The caecum

The *ileocaecal sphincter* separates the ileum from the *caecum*, the first section of the large intestine. It is here that the *appendix* is attached (Box 10.1).

Box 10.1 Appendicitis

Whilst caring for a young healthy pregnant female, the midwife must be alert for symptoms of a condition unrelated to pregnancy. *Appendicitis* is one such condition that occurs more frequently in pregnant than non-pregnant women of childbearing age (Blackburn & Loper 1992). The symptoms include abdominal pain and vomiting – both of which could, wrongly, be put down to the pregnancy (Mayberry et al 1986).

Other conditions that may occur in pregnancy with similar symptoms are peptic or duodenal ulcers, gastro-enteritis and brain tumours. Other symptoms such as pyrexia and diarrhoea may also be present. It is important to be able to distinguish between different disorders that share common symptoms. This is called making a *differential diagnosis*.

The appendix is a small tube with a blind end that leads from the caecum. It is similar in structure to the caecum, but contains additional lymph tissue. The caecum is a dilated section of the large intestine that is continuous with the ascending colon.

The colon

The *ascending colon* is situated on the right side of the abdomen and ascends to a point beneath the liver where it bends towards the left, forming the *transverse colon*. This section of the colon passes

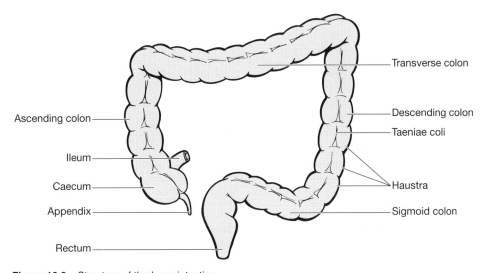

Figure 10.8 Structure of the large intestine.

around the base of the spleen and in front of the duodenum to the left side of the abdomen, where it bends downwards to form the descending colon. The *descending colon* passes down the left side of the abdomen until it enters the pelvis, where it becomes known as the sigmoid colon. The *sigmoid colon* is S-shaped, and moves towards the midline to join the rectum.

Microstructure

The microstructure of the large intestine is similar to the general structure of the digestive tract in most respects. However, one principal way in which it differs is in the structure of the muscle layer. Portions of the longitudinal layer are thickened to form three bands, the *taeniae coli*, located at regular intervals around the length of the large intestine. These bands of muscle are slightly shorter than the overall length of the colon and give the colon a puckered appearance. The walls of the large intestine therefore form pouches known as *haustra*.

Digestive functions

By the time chyme reaches the large intestine the majority of the nutrients have been absorbed. However, more water is absorbed here, as are some further electrolytes and vitamins.

Mucus is secreted by the large intestine but no enzymes are produced. Bacteria are found as commensals, which play a role in the production of certain B vitamins and vitamin K. They also prepare the chyme for its elimination in the form of faeces.

Any remaining carbohydrates are fermented by the bacteria present and produce hydrogen, carbon dioxide and methane. These gases are the constituents of flatus present in the colon. Further bacteria break down the bile pigment bilirubin to urobilinogen, which gives faeces their colour. The colon empties these faeces into the rectum for storage until elimination.

As in the small intestine, movement of chyme through the large intestine is principally governed by the rate of gastric emptying. As food enters the large intestine, it is moved up the ascending

colon by the contraction of the muscle layer in each individual haustrum as it is filled. Peristalsis only occurs at a very slow rate, except after the ingestion of food, which initiates a strong wave of peristalsis from the middle of the transverse colon to the rectum. This results in *mass movement* of chyme whenever food is eaten.

THE RECTUM AND ANUS

The final 200 mm of the digestive tract consists of a dilated portion, the *rectum*, and a short canal leading to the exterior of the body, the *anus*. Both structures are of a similar construction to the rest of the digestive tract. The anus contains two sphincters which are responsible for the elimination of faeces from the body:

1. the *internal sphincter*, under involuntary control
2. the *external sphincter*, under voluntary control.

Defecation

The rectum is normally empty, but mass movement of chyme in the colon moves *faeces* into it. Distension of the rectum stimulates stretch receptors in the rectal walls, initiating the *defecation reflex*. The internal sphincter relaxes, but as the external sphincter is under voluntary control, the defecation reflex can be inhibited, in which case the faeces are fed back into the colon until the next episode of mass movement.

When a voluntary decision is made to allow defecation, the external sphincter relaxes and, with increased intra-abdominal pressure from the abdominal muscles and the lowering of the diaphragm, defecation occurs.

SUPPORTING STRUCTURES

The main supporting structures of the digestive tract are extensions of the peritoneum, which are arranged in folds to hold the organs closely together, near the walls of the abdomen. These folds carry many of the blood, nerve and lymph vessels that supply the tract. They also provide protection, particularly where they fold over the transverse colon and down over the small intestine. This is known as the *greater omentum* and it contains large quantities of fatty tissue, so forming a protective apron beneath the anterior abdominal wall, which acts as a heat insulator, and prevents friction between abdominal organs.

BLOOD SUPPLY AND LYMPHATIC DRAINAGE

The blood supply to the abdominal digestive organs comes from the coeliac artery, and superior and inferior mesenteric arteries. The coeliac artery supplies the stomach, duodenum, liver, gall bladder and pancreas. The superior mesenteric artery supplies the small intestine and the large intestine from the caecum to the transverse colon. The inferior mesenteric artery supplies the remainder of the colon and most of the rectum. Rectal arteries supply the remaining rectum and anus.

Venous return is via the hepato-portal system. Veins from each of the structures of the abdominal digestive organs join to form the portal vein, which then passes through the liver before returning the deoxygenated blood to the heart via the hepatic veins and the inferior vena cava.

The blood from the digestive organs is rich in nutrients. As it passes through the liver these nutrients can be converted for storage, and any toxins can be detoxified or modified before they enter the systemic circulation.

Because of the risk of ingesting harmful substances or organisms, there is a plentiful supply of lymph nodes associated with the digestive organs.

NERVE SUPPLY

The enteric nervous system is largely responsible for nervous control of the digestive system. However, the autonomic nervous system also influences digestion. Parasympathetic supply is from the vagus nerve which, when stimulated, initiates smooth muscle contraction and the release of digestive secretions. Sympathetic supply is through many of the nerves leaving the spinal cord which form nerve plexuses controlling the levels of digestive secretions.

ACCESSORY STRUCTURES

Digestion in the small intestine depends on secretions from the small intestine, and on the activities of three accessory structures situated outside the digestive tract. These structures are:

1. the liver
2. the gall bladder
3. the pancreas.

The liver

The *liver* is the largest gland in the body weighing on average 1.5 kg in an adult. It is essential to life, but can continue to function even when a large portion has been damaged. It is situated in the upper right section of the abdominal cavity – the right hypochondriac region – under the diaphragm, partially protected by the lower ribs.

Macrostructure

The liver is enclosed in a dense capsule of connective tissue, and is covered almost completely by peritoneum. It is anatomically divided into right and left lobes by a ligament, the *falciform* ligament (Fig. 10.9). This ligament is attached to the under surface of the diaphragm and holds the liver in position. A second ligament extends from the falciform ligament to the umbilicus. This is the *ligamentum teres*, which is a remnant of the umbilical vein present in the fetus. The *portal fissure* is a structure situated on the posterior surface of the liver, where vessels and nerve fibres enter and leave.

Microstructure

The liver is composed of a large number of hepatic lobules formed from *hepatocytes* (Fig. 10.10). A central sinusoid is situated within each one. The sinusoids carry a mixture of venous and arterial blood which can come into close contact with the hepatic lobules. Situated around the walls of the sinusoids are specialised cells, called *Kupffer cells*, which are hepatic phagocytes. Their function is to destroy worn-out blood cells, bacteria and toxins. Around the circumference of the

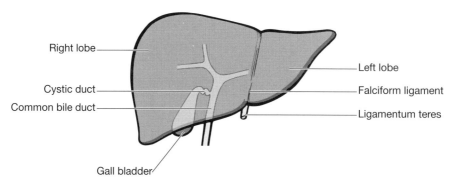

Figure 10.9 External structure of the liver.

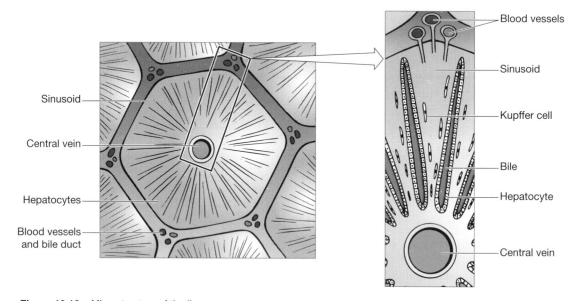

Figure 10.10 Microstructure of the liver.

lobules are portal canals carrying a branch of the portal vein, hepatic artery and a small bile duct.

Bile production

Every day, 750–1000 ml of *bile* are produced by the adult liver, and stored in the gall bladder, situated beneath the liver. Bile is a thick, alkaline, greenish-yellow substance containing water, bile salts, bile pigments and cholesterol. It is released intermittently into the duodenum via the bile duct, and has a role in both digestion and excretion.

Bile aids the digestion of fats in the small intestine. Most of the bile salts are reabsorbed in the ileum and returned to the liver via the portal vein for recycling.

The main bile pigment is *bilirubin*, which is a product of the breakdown of red blood cells. Hepatocytes in the liver process fat-soluble bilirubin produced by haemolysis and change it to water-soluble bilirubin. This is then further broken down in the digestive system and excreted in the faeces as stercobilin, which gives faeces their characteristic colour, or by the renal system in the urine as urobilinogen (Box 10.2).

Box 10.2   Physiological jaundice

Physiological jaundice is common in the neonate between the 3rd and 7th day after delivery. It occurs because the full-term fetus usually has a greater number of red blood cells than required after birth, as a consequence of the need to attract oxygen across the layers separating fetal and maternal blood in the placenta (Sweet 1997). At birth, therefore, an increased number of red blood cells are broken down, producing the orange or yellow bile pigment *bilirubin* as a waste product. Bilirubin is fat-soluble and binds to albumin in the blood, where it is transported to the liver to be conjugated, i.e. made into a water-soluble form, so that it can be excreted through the digestive or renal systems.

In many neonates, particularly those who are ill or preterm, the liver does not have enough of the relevant enzymes to conjugate all the bilirubin in the blood (Hey 1995). The unconjugated bilirubin leaves the blood and is stored in areas of fat such as those beneath the surface of the skin. This accounts for the typical yellow appearance of the skin of a neonate with physiological jaundice.

If the levels of unconjugated bilirubin rise too high there is a danger that it will be stored in fatty areas of the brain, particularly the *basal ganglia*, and cause an irreversible condition called *kernickterus*, which causes brain damage (Kelnar et al 1995). The neonate is therefore observed carefully to detect inappropriately rising levels of bilirubin in the blood, so that treatment can be initiated if needed.

There are also pathological conditions which give rise to jaundice in the neonate. These include, rhesus incompatibility, abnormalities of the bile ducts and metabolic disorders, all of which can be detected by careful observation.

Functions of the liver

The liver has three principal functions in the digestive process:

1. metabolism
2. storage
3. secretion.

Metabolism. The liver *regulates blood sugar levels* within very fine limits by converting glucose to glycogen in response to insulin, and glycogen back to glucose in response to glucagon.

The liver also mobilises *stored fat* for use by body cells. Proteins are broken down, and their waste products are prepared for excretion, while the useful molecules are used in the production of other proteins, blood-clotting factors, and antibodies and antitoxins.

Additionally, the liver plays an important role in the *detoxification of drugs* and poisons, as well as deactivating hormones no longer required by the body.

Heat is produced as by-product of all these metabolic activities, and it plays a vital role in maintaining core temperature which is necessary for metabolism to proceed at an optimum rate.

Storage. The liver stores vitamins A, B_{12}, D, E and K. It also stores the elements iron and copper, as well as glucose in the form of glycogen.

Secretion. Bile is produced by the liver and secreted from the gall bladder into the digestive tract to aid the breakdown of fats. Urea is formed in the liver from waste products such as ammonia and carbon dioxide, and is excreted in urine.

Blood and nerve supply

The hepatic artery supplies the liver with oxygenated blood, and the portal vein brings nutrient-rich blood directly from the digestive organs. Hepatic veins drain into the inferior vena cava. The autonomic nervous system controls the liver function.

The gall bladder

The *gall bladder* is a pear-shaped structure situated beneath the liver (Fig. 10.11). It is approximately 100 mm long and is attached to the liver by connective tissue. Its structure, though similar to that of the digestive tract generally, has no submucosal layer. The epithelial layer is arranged in rugae.

Bile enters the gall bladder from the liver through the *cystic duct*, and exits by the same route. Secretion of bile from the gall bladder into the duodenum is controlled both neurally and hormonally: stimulation of the vagus nerve by autonomic impulses during the cephalic phase of digestion, and the release of the hormones secretion and CCK when fats are present in chyme entering the duodenum, combine to cause the gall bladder to contract and secrete bile into the small intestine.

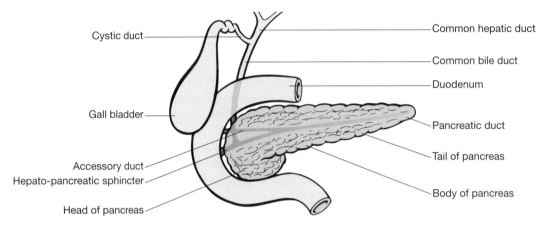

Figure 10.11 Position of the gall bladder and related structures.

Functions

The main function of the gall bladder in the digestive process is to absorb water from the bile, making it 10 times more concentrated than when it was produced in the liver. Mucus is secreted into the bile, which is stored until required by the digestive tract.

Bile ducts

The hepatic ducts leave the liver through the portal fissure and join to form the *common hepatic duct*. The cystic duct from the gall bladder joins the common hepatic duct to form the *common bile duct* which passes behind the head of pancreas. This then joins the main pancreatic duct before it enters the duodenum through the *hepato-pancreatic sphincter*.

Blood and nerve supply

The cystic artery supplies the gall bladder and bile ducts with oxygenated blood, and the cystic vein drains deoxygenated blood away. Nerve supply is via the autonomic nervous system.

The pancreas

The *pancreas* is a soft, greyish-pink gland about 150 mm long. It lies transversely across the posterior abdominal wall behind the stomach. It consists of an expanded head tucked into the curve of the duodenum, a body, and a narrow tail lying behind the stomach (Fig. 10.11). Secretions from the pancreas are passed along two ducts, one of which joins the common bile duct before entering the duodenum, the other entering the duodenum directly.

Microstructure

The pancreas consists of two types of tissue:

1. exocrine tissue
2. endocrine tissue.

The *exocrine tissue* forms the majority of the pancreas and consists of lobules containing alveoli lined with secretory cells. Each alveolus drains into a duct, which join together to leave the lobules and empty into two central ducts: the *pancreatic duct* and the *accessory duct*. The pancreatic duct joins with the common bile duct before entering the duodenum. The accessory duct enters directly into the duodenum.

Endocrine tissue is found throughout the pancreas as small collections of specialised cells known as the *islets of Langerhans*. These islets contain alpha cells and beta cells. *Alpha cells* secrete glucagon, a hormone which converts glycogen to glucose when blood sugar levels are low. *Beta cells* secrete insulin, a hormone which converts glucose to glycogen when blood sugar levels are high.

Approximately 1500 ml of pancreatic juice are produced daily by the exocrine glands. This juice contains water, salts, sodium bicarbonate and enzymes. The sodium bicarbonate gives pancreatic juice an alkaline pH, necessary for the pancreatic enzymes to act on the chyme in the duodenum. Regulation of the production of pancreatic juice is both hormonal and neural.

Function

The exocrine glands in the pancreas produce pancreatic juice which contains enzymes responsible for the breakdown of proteins, carbohydrates and fats e.g.:

- trypsin and chymotrypsin digest proteins
- pancreatic amylase digests carbohydrates
- pancreatic lipase digests fats.

Blood and nerve supply

Splenic and mesenteric arteries and veins supply and remove blood from the pancreas. Nervous control is by the autonomic nervous system.

PHYSIOLOGICAL CHANGES THROUGH THE CHILDBEARING YEAR

Pregnancy

Physiological changes in the digestive tract are commonly associated with many of the minor disorders experienced by pregnant women. Although described as 'minor', they can make life very uncomfortable. The physiological changes that occur are largely the result of the relaxation of smooth muscle, caused by the increased levels of progesterone.

Morning sickness is the nausea with vomiting sometimes associated with early pregnancy. It is often the first symptom of pregnancy, and occurs in many women up to the 16th week of pregnancy. Its cause is not known (Anderson 1994).

Heartburn is caused by the regurgitation of stomach contents, which occurs because of the relaxation of the cardiac sphincter (under the influence of progesterone) at the entrance to the stomach. This can be a problem throughout pregnancy and may be aggravated in later months by the mechanical displacement of the stomach by the enlarging uterus.

Constipation is another uncomfortable side effect of the increased levels of progesterone: relaxation of smooth muscle causes the movement of chyme in the large bowel to slow, with an increased reabsorption of water (Anderson 1996).

Other common minor discomforts include *gingivitis* (higher levels of oestrogen cause increased vascularity in the gums), *increased salivation* and *food cravings* (Hytten 1991). Most women also experience an increase in appetite, which will ensure that sufficient nutrients are available for fetal growth and maternal stores (Box 10.3). It is estimated that an extra 300 kcal are required daily during the second and third trimesters of pregnancy to meet these needs.

Labour

The increase in intra-abdominal pressure during labour leads to a slowdown in gastric emptying. This means the acidity of the stomach contents

---

Box 10.3   Folic acid

Changes in hormones in pregnancy lead to enhanced uptake of the nutrients required by the mother and her baby. The nutritional wellbeing of the mother affects the development of the fetus, especially in the first 3 months of pregnancy (Thompson 1993). Women should consider their diet before conception – waiting until pregnancy has been confirmed is leaving it too late (Rennie 1991).

One recent campaign has encouraged women to take folic acid before becoming pregnant, in order to reduce the risks of having a baby with a neural tube defect. Neural tube defects have been found to occur because of both genetic and environmental factors. Research has shown that folic acid can reduce the risks of fetal defects in all women embarking on a pregnancy, including those with a previous history of neural tube defect (Hibbard 1993). Folic acid is found in fortified breads and cereals, sprouts, broccoli, spinach, cauliflower and oranges. However, diet alone is unlikely to provide sufficient folic acid, so it is recommended that women take a folic acid supplement (0.4 mg a day, or 4 mg if there is a previous history) from before conception until 12 weeks of pregnancy (Anderson 1995).

rises (Hytten 1990). The use of narcotics for pain relief and the presence of fear and anxiety will further affect gastric emptying.

The benefits and risks of feeding women in labour have been thoroughly investigated in recent years, due to the risk of Mendelson's syndrome during general anaesthesia (Box 10.4). Yet if oral nutrition is withheld, the body may need to call on reserves of energy from the breakdown of body fat, which can also lead to complications in labour. Nutrients may need to be administered intravenously (Johnson et al 1989).

Postnatal

With the decrease in circulating levels of progesterone, the digestive system quickly returns to normal functioning. Immediate *weight loss* can be up to 5 kg and within 3–6 months the body may return to its prepregnancy weight. *Constipation* may continue in the first few days, but this will probably be associated with the trauma of delivery.

The neonate

During intrauterine life, the fetus obtains all its nutrients through the placenta. The digestive system is fully functional by the end of pregnancy (Box 10.5), so at birth the full-term baby is able to carry out all processes needed to digest breast milk. Absorption of formula feeds is less complete, as can be seen in the increased production of bulky stools.

The first stools passed by the neonate consist of *meconium*. This is a thick, soft, greenish-black substance which has formed during intrauterine life. It contains epithelial cells, waste products such as bile salts, fatty acids, mucus and amniotic fluid. It is usually passed from the digestive tract within the first 48 hours, changing gradually to the typical yellow stool of a breast- or bottle-fed baby within 4–5 days of birth. Meconium passed during labour is an indication of stress in the fetus (Grant 1989).

Box 10.4 Nutrition in labour

Despite the increased demands of labour on the body's metabolism, it has become normal policy in many obstetric units to starve women in labour (Michael et al 1991). This is to prevent a condition called *Mendelson's syndrome*, or acid aspiration syndrome, from occurring, should the woman need to be given a general anaesthetic.

During labour there is delayed emptying of the stomach, with a corresponding increase in the acidity of the stomach contents. With the administration of a general anaesthesia, these acid stomach contents may be regurgitated through the relaxed cardiac sphincter and pass down the trachea into the lungs. This is Mendelson's syndrome, and it causes damage to the alveoli of the lungs and carries a high maternal mortality risk (Pearson & Rees 1989).

The administration of antacids to all women in labour has reduced this risk. The recent introduction of local anaesthesia such as epidural or spinal anaesthesia for operative deliveries has lessened the risk further. Despite these changes, there is lively professional debate about, and continued research into, the risks of feeding women in labour (Baker 1996, Lewis 1998).

Box 10.5 Inborn errors of metabolism

In rare instances, a baby is born who is unable to break down foods, due to a deficiency in one or more digestive enzymes. One of the most well-known conditions in which an enzyme is absent is *phenylketonuria*, which occurs in 1 in 10 000 births (Laing 1995). In this condition, the enzyme *phenylalanine hydroxylase* is not produced by the body, as a result of an autosomal recessive genetic abnormality. The absence of phenylalanine hydroxylase means that the amino acid phenylalanine cannot be broken down into the amino acid tyrosine. Both of these are essential in the production of proteins required by the body. The levels of phenylalanine rise, whilst there is a deficiency of tyrosine. The resulting phenylketonuria (PKU) is toxic to the brain and so causes brain damage (Gibbings 1994).

The treatment for this condition is a special diet low in phenylalanine, which will ensure minimal brain damage if commenced within 20 days of birth (MRC 1993). Because of the ease of screening for this condition and the effectiveness of treatment, all babies are tested for PKU with the *Guthrie test*, a simple blood test, usually carried out between the 4th and 10th day after birth, or at least 48 hours after milk feeds have started. The Guthrie test also screens for other metabolic disorders such as hypothyroidism and galactosaemia.

REFERENCES

Anderson A 1994 Managing pregnancy sickness and hyperemesis gravidarum. Professional Care of the Mother and Child 4(1):13–15

Anderson A S 1995 Folic acid: the message we're failing to get across. Professional Care of the Mother and Child 5(3):64–66

Anderson A S 1996 Constipation in pregnancy: is your advice on diet effective? Professional Care of the Mother and Child 6(4):87–90

Baker C 1996 Nutrition and hydration in labour. British Journal of Midwifery 4(11):568–572

Blackburn S T, Loper D L 1992 Maternal, fetal and neonatal physiology: a clinical perspective. W B Saunders, Philadelphia, p 395

Gibbings B 1994 Keeping phenylketonuria under control. Modern Midwife 4(10):23–26

Grant A 1989 Monitoring the fetus during labour. In: Chalmers I, Enkin E, Keirse M J N C (eds) Effective care in pregnancy and childbirth. Oxford University Press, Oxford, p 848

Hey E 1995 Phototherapy: a fresh light on a murky subject. Midwifery Digest 5(3):256–260

Hibbard B M 1993 Folates and fetal development. British Journal of Obstetrics and Gynaecology 100(4):307–309

Hytten F 1990 The alimentary system in pregnancy. Midwifery 6(4):201–204

Hytten F 1991 The alimentary system. In: Hytten F, Chamberlain G (eds) Clinical physiology in obstetrics. Blackwell Scientific, London, p 138

Johnson C, Keirse M J N C, Enkin M, Chalmers I 1989 Nutrition and hydration in labour. In: Chalmers I, Enkin E, Keirse M J N C (eds) Effective care in pregnancy and childbirth. Oxford University Press, Oxford, p 830–831

Kelnar C J H, Harvey D, Simpson C 1995 The sick newborn baby, 3rd edn. Baillière Tindall, London, p 304–305

Laing S 1995 The baby with a metabolic or allergic disorder. Professional Care of the Mother and Child 5(5):123–127

Lewis P 1998 Not to our taste, midwives' failure to feed women in labour. The Practising Midwife 1(7/8):4–5

Mayberry J F, Bond A P, Morris J J 1986 Medical disorders in pregnancy. Edward Arnold, London, p 103–110

Michael S, Reilly C S, Caunt J A 1991 Policies for oral intake during labour: a survey of maternity units in England and Wales. Anaesthesia 46:1071–1073

MRC Working Party on Phenylketonuria 1993. Recommendations on the dietary management of PKU. Archives of Diseases in Childhood 68:426–427

Pearson J, Rees G 1989 Technique of caesarean section. In: Chalmers I, Enkin E, Keirse M J N C (eds) Effective care in pregnancy and childbirth. Oxford University Press, Oxford, p 1238

Rennie M 1991 Nutrition in pregnancy. Modern Midwife 7:7–11

Sweet B (ed) 1997 Mayes' midwifery. A textbook for midwives, 12th edn. Baillière Tindall, London, p 873

Thompson J 1993 Nutrition in pregnancy. Nursing Times 89(2):38–40

11

The renal system

The renal system plays an essential role in the elimination of waste from the body, and in fluid and electrolyte balance. It carries out these functions by controlling the composition, volume and pressure of the blood passing through the kidneys. The renal system continually removes and reabsorbs water and the solutes contained in the blood, eliminating any substance not required or which is creating an imbalance in the body, whilst retaining other substances useful to the body.

Throughout pregnancy the functioning of the renal system is altered by factors such as hormone levels, the enlarging uterus and changes in the volume of fluid circulating in the cardiovascular and lymphatic systems. The body is able to function effectively despite these changes, provided the pregnancy remains within normal parameters.

In the fetus, waste products are removed from the blood by the placenta. However, urine is formed, and it contributes to the amniotic fluid surrounding the fetus. After delivery, the renal system is sufficiently mature to remove waste from the blood and to balance fluid and electrolytes within the body.

The anatomical structures that make up the renal system are (Fig. 11.1):

- two kidneys, which form urine
- two ureters, that take the urine to the bladder
- the urinary bladder, which stores urine
- the urethra, through which urine is directed out of the body.

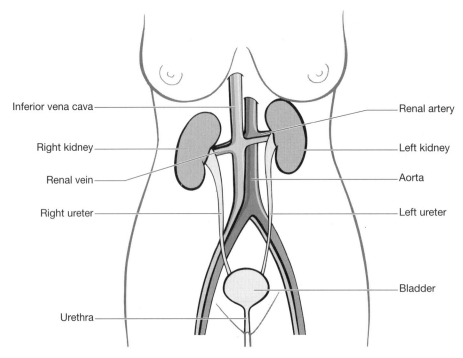

Figure 11.1 Position of the individual organs of the renal system.

THE KIDNEYS

The *kidneys* are paired organs that are situated on either side of the vertebral column, on the posterior wall of the abdominal cavity. They are placed behind the peritoneum at the level of the twelfth thoracic to the third lumbar vertebrae, and are kept in position by a mass of fat. The right kidney is situated slightly lower than the left, because of the position of the liver.

Macrostructure

The kidneys are approximately 100 mm long, 65 mm wide and 30 mm deep. Each kidney weighs about 120 g.

A longitudinal section reveals three main areas in the kidney (Fig. 11.2):

1. the *renal capsule*, which is composed of tough fibrous tissue
2. the *cortex*, which is dark in colour due to the presence of blood vessels
3. the *medulla*, in which cone-shaped areas are

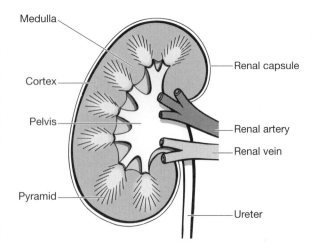

Figure 11.2 Longitudinal section of the kidney, showing its internal anatomy.

present, the pyramids, containing the nephrons along which urine is formed.

At the concave surface of the kidney is the *hilum*, where the blood vessels and nerves enter, and the ureters leave. The area beneath the medulla surrounding the hilum is known as the *renal pelvis*, and this collects the urine from the pyramids and directs it to the ureter.

Microstructure

The adult kidney is composed of approximately 1 million *nephrons* in which urine is formed, and many thousands of *collecting ducts*, which carry the urine to the ureters (Fig. 11.3).

Each nephron is surrounded by a network of blood capillaries which exchanges fluids and solutes as required to produce urine. The nephron can be subdivided into four anatomically and functionally different regions:

1. the *Bowman's capsule*, a cup-shaped region which surrounds a mass of capillaries known as the *glomerulus*
2. the *proximal convoluted tubule*, a twisting portion of the nephron close to the Bowman's capsule
3. The *loop of Henle*, where the tubule dips deep into the medulla of the kidney
4. The *distal convoluted tubule*, a twisting portion of the nephron distant from the capsule, leading into the collecting ducts.

The *collecting ducts* are straight tubules that collect urine from several individual nephrons and direct it to the ureters.

Physiology of urine formation

Urine is formed in the nephrons continuously by three processes:

1. glomerular filtration
2. selective tubular reabsorption
3. tubular secretion.

Glomerular filtration

Filtration is the process by which water and dissolved substances move across a membrane under pressure. In the Bowman's capsule there is a mass of capillaries (the glomerulus), which comes from the renal artery, entering through the hilum of the kidney (Fig. 11.4). The *afferent arteriole* that leads to the glomerulus has a larger diameter than the *efferent arteriole* that leads away from it, producing increased pressure in the glomerulus. This pressure drives plasma and small molecules through the walls of the capillaries and into the capsule. Separating the glomerulus from the Bowman's capsule are the two layers of cell membranes made up of single cells, which aid the filtration process. Only those substances that are small enough to pass through the walls of the arteriole and the capsule are filtered. This normally includes all blood constituents except red and white blood cells and plasma proteins.

In the Bowman's capsule, 10% of all blood that

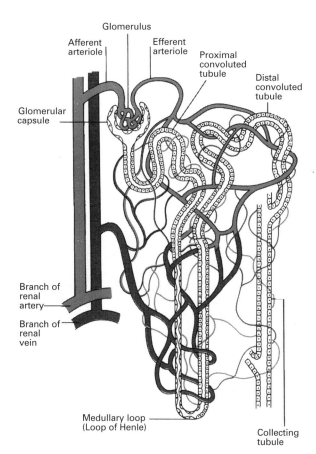

Figure 11.3 Structure of a nephron, with associated blood vessels. (Reproduced with permission from Wilson K J W, Waugh A 1996 Ross and Wilson Anatomy and Physiology in Health and Illness. Churchill Livingstone, Edinburgh)

Labels in figure:
Glomerulus
Afferent arteriole
Efferent arteriole
Proximal convoluted tubule
Distal convoluted tubule
Glomerular capsule
Branch of renal artery
Branch of renal vein
Medullary loop (Loop of Henle)
Collecting tubule

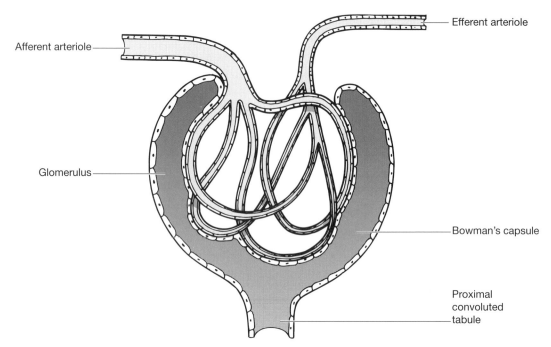

Afferent arteriole

Efferent arteriole

Glomerulus

Bowman's capsule

Proximal convoluted tabule

Figure 11.4 Longitudinal section of a Bowman's capsule, showing the glomerulus.

enters the glomerulus is filtered. The factors that facilitate the filtration process are:

- the large surface area created by the length of the glomerular capillaries
- the very porous and thin (0.1 μm) filter membranes
- the net filtration pressure.

Net filtration pressure is the driving force of glomerular filtration, and is initiated by the difference in diameter of the afferent and efferent arterioles. Three opposing pressures are then set up in the Bowman's capsule:

1. hydrostatic pressure from the arteriole
2. osmotic pressure
3. capsular pressure from the capsule.

These pressures act on each other as shown below to produce the net filtration pressure:

hydrostatic pressure – (osmotic pressure + capsular pressure) = net filtration pressure.

As a result of glomerular filtration, a filtrate is formed that is very dilute and contains many solutes from the blood, some of which require elimination whilst others are of value to the body. To retain the valuable substances, selective tubular reabsorption occurs.

Selective tubular reabsorption

Tubular reabsorption occurs along the entire length of the tubule of nephrons, but it occurs differently in each portion.

Proximal convoluted tubule. In the proximal convoluted tubule (PCT), water and the substances dissolved in it (solutes) are largely reabsorbed back into the bloodstream. Water is absorbed passively by osmosis, whereas the solutes are reabsorbed as required by active and passive processes. 80% of the filtrate is reabsorbed in the PCT.

Normally substances required by the body, such as glucose, are totally reabsorbed in the PCT, but the amount that can be reabsorbed is limited. This is known as the *renal threshold*, and is different for each substance. Exceeding the threshold overloads the process of tubular reabsorption, and so some of the substance is retained in the tubule, and will appear in the urine.

Loop of Henle. The loop of Henle dips deep into the medulla of the kidney then returns to the cortex. The collecting duct runs parallel to this section of the tubule entering the medulla. This sets up a concentrated medullary environment in which most of the valuable solutes that have been filtered can be reabsorbed without too much loss of fluid. It is a method therefore of concentrating the urine.

Distal convoluted tubule. By the time the filtrate reaches the distal convoluted tubule (DCT), 95% of the water and solutes have been reabsorbed into the bloodstream. Further reabsorption occurs in the DCT and the collecting tubule, of substances required by the body. It is also at this site that fluid balance is achieved.

Fluid and electrolyte balance are controlled by two hormones: aldosterone and antidiuretic hormone (ADH). *Aldosterone* brings about sodium reabsorption in the distal tubule and *ADH* controls water reabsorption by increasing the permeability of the DCT and the collecting duct.

Tubular secretion

In tubular secretion, any remaining harmful substances are moved from the tubule into the bloodstream. Thus excess hydrogen and potassium ions, and certain drugs that have escaped the filtration process, are removed from the body in urine. Tubular secretion therefore also plays an important role in maintaining acid-base balance.

The juxtaglomerular apparatus

In each nephron, the final portion of the ascending limb of the loop of Henle comes close to the afferent arteriole of that nephron (Fig. 11.5).

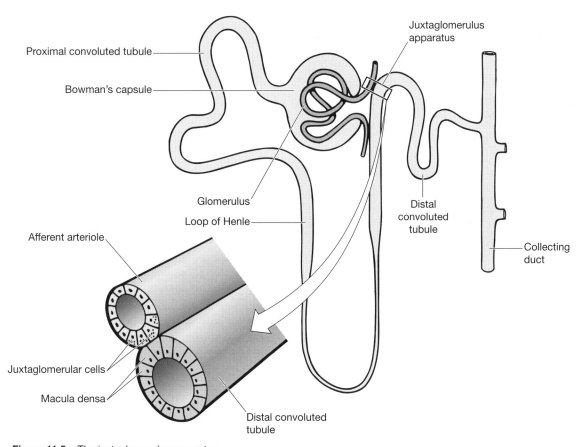

Figure 11.5 The juxtaglomerular apparatus.

The walls of both the afferent arteriole and the nephron contain specialised cells that measure and alter the flow of blood through the arteriole. In the nephron these cells are crowded together to form the *macula densa*, and they measure the amount of sodium passing through the filtrate. The arteriole wall cells are called the *juxta-glomerula cells*, and they contain small muscle fibres and granules containing renin. Together, both these types of cell constitute the *juxta-glomerular apparatus*, which alters the diameter of the afferent arterioles to ensure adequate perfusion of the kidneys when arterial pressure falls.

The composition of urine

As a result of the processes carried out in the nephrons, urine is formed, a concentrated fluid which contains minimal water plus unwanted waste products for removal from the body by urination (Box 11.1). Should these waste products build up, they will cause dysfunction of body systems with subsequent illness and eventual death.

Following its formation, the urine passes into the collecting ducts and then into the pelvis of the kidney, where the ureters direct it into the bladder for storage before being discharged from the body by urination.

Box 11.1   Urinalysis

Because urine is formed directly from the blood, analysis of its constituents gives some indication of the functioning of the body. If metabolism is not operating efficiently, this may be reflected in urinalysis.

During pregnancy, urine is tested regularly because the presence of some abnormal constituents can be an early indication of a pregnancy-related disorder. For example, protein in the urine may suggest the presence of bacteria, a urinary tract infection, or damage to the kidneys from rising blood pressure associated with preeclampsia. The presence of glucose may be an indication that the woman has gestational diabetes. However, it must be remembered that during pregnancy the kidneys may be unable to reabsorb all the glucose in the filtrate, due to the increased volume of circulating blood (i.e. the renal threshold may be exceeded). It is common therefore for some glucose to appear in the urine for this reason.

Other functions of the kidneys

As well as regulating the composition and volume of blood, and removing wastes from the body, the kidneys also carry out additional functions, including:

- the synthesis of glucose during periods of starvation or fasting
- the secretion of erythropoietin to stimulate the production of red blood cells
- the synthesis of vitamin D.

Supporting structures

The kidneys are firmly embedded in fat. Extra support is supplied by the close proximity of other abdominal organs, and by the attachment of the renal artery and vein to the descending aorta and inferior vena cava respectively.

Blood, nerves and lymph

The kidneys receive 25% of cardiac output via the renal arteries, which branch directly from the aorta. An intricate network of arterioles, capillaries and venules surround the nephrons. Venous drainage is into the inferior vena cava.

The nerve supply for the kidneys is from the sympathetic branch of the autonomic nervous system via the renal plexus.

Lymph vessels surround the kidneys, draining into the aortic and lumbar lymph glands.

THE URETERS

The *ureters* are situated in the peritoneal cavity, and pass from the pelvis of the kidney to the bladder. There are two ureters, one for each kidney. They are composed of an outer layer of fibrous tissue, a middle muscular layer and an inner layer of transitional epithelium which is impermeable to water. This layer ensures that no water from adjacent blood vessels can enter the ureters (a possibility because of differences in osmotic pressure).

The ureters enter the bladder at an oblique angle (Fig. 11.6), so when the bladder becomes distended with urine, the openings into the

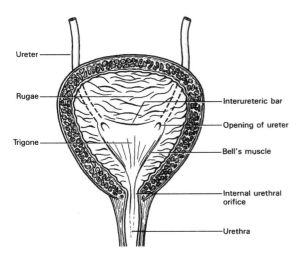

Figure 11.6 Cross-section of the bladder to show its internal structure. (Reproduced with permission from Bennet V R, Brown L K 1999 Myles Textbook for Midwives, 13th edn. Churchill Livingstone, Edinburgh)

ureters are occluded to prevent the backflow of urine into the kidneys.

Urine is passed down the ureters by peristaltic action.

THE BLADDER

The *bladder* is situated in the pelvic cavity but when it is distended by a large amount of urine it will rise into the abdominal cavity, and can be palpated above the symphysis pubis. Behind the bladder lies the uterus in the female, and the bowel in the the male. The ureters enter midway down the body of the bladder. From the base of the bladder, the urethra transports urine to the exterior of the body for disposal.

Macrostructure

The bladder is roughly pear-shaped when empty, but becomes globular as it fills with urine. It can hold up to 600 ml of urine, but the desire to micturate (urinate) will be conveyed to the nervous system once it contains approximately 300 ml. The upper surface of the bladder is known as the *fundus*, and is loosely covered with peritoneum in order to allow it to expand as it fills. The pouch that is formed between the bladder and the uterus is known as the *uterovesicular pouch*.

The base of the bladder is called the neck, and internally it forms a triangle or *trigone* with the openings from the ureters.

Microstructure

The bladder wall is composed of three layers:

1. an outer layer of connective tissue
2. a middle layer of smooth muscle, the *detrusor muscle*, intermingled with elastic fibres to allow the bladder to contract and regain its shape when empty
3. an inner layer of transitional epithelium, arranged in folds called *rugae*, to enable the bladder to distend.

The trigone has an inner layer which is not arranged in folds, thus maintaining the position of the three orifices of the ureters and urethra.

Where the urethra leaves the bladder there is a thickening of the muscle layer to form the *internal sphincter* that controls the passage of urine into the urethra.

Supporting structures

The bladder is kept in position by ligaments that extend from the umbilicus, pelvic cavity lateral walls and pubic bone.

THE URETHRA

The *urethra* leaves the bladder at the base of the trigone and passes through the muscles of the perineum to the urethral orifice. The length of the urethra is different in each sex: in the male it is approximately 200 mm long; in the female approximately 40 mm. Their short urethra predisposes women to ascending urinary tract infections (Box 11.2). The female urethra runs behind the symphysis pubis in front of the vagina to the vestibule of the vulva.

The urethra consists of three layers of tissue:

1. an outer layer of muscle
2. a middle layer of spongy tissue containing blood vessels
3. an inner layer of transitional epithelium.

Box 11.2 Urinary tract infections

The short length of the female urethra predisposes women to ascending infection. During pregnancy, hormones further aggravate this by relaxing the smooth muscle of the urinary tract. *Cystitis*, caused by an ascending infection, results in inflammation of the bladder with painful, frequent voiding of small quantities of urine.

Acute pyelonephritis is an infection of the kidney, pelvis and nephrons, usually resulting from infection lower down the renal tract. This is aggravated by relaxation of the muscle of the ureters under the influence of the hormones of pregnancy and the pressure from the enlarging uterus, which encourages stasis of urine. The condition is characterised by loin pain, pyrexia, headache, nausea and vomiting, and occurs in 1–2% of pregnancies (Enkin et al 1995). The causative organism is often Escherichia coli, a bacterium usually found in the bowel. Pyelonephritis is thought to increase the risk of preterm labour (Plattner 1994).

The urethral orifice is surrounded by a thicker layer of muscle situated between the superficial and deep muscle layers of the pelvic floor, which forms the *external sphincter*. Between the internal and external sphincters lies an area which has a layer of muscle and elastic fibres under both voluntary and involuntary control. This area aids continence during episodes of increased abdominal pressure, such as laughing, coughing or sneezing.

Blood, nerves and lymph

The ureters are supplied with blood from branches of the renal, iliac and vesical arteries draining into corresponding veins. The bladder receives its blood from the superior and inferior vesical arteries, and venous drainage is into vesical veins. The urethral blood supply comes via the inferior vesical artery and vein, and pudendal artery and vein.

Nerve supply is principally from the autonomic nervous system through the mesenteric and pelvic plexuses (ureters and urethra) and via the Lee–Frankenhauser plexus (bladder). Voluntary control of the external urethral sphincter is supplied by the pudendal nerve.

Lymph drainage from the ureters, bladder and urethra is into iliac glands.

PHYSIOLOGY OF MICTURITION

Micturition, the passage of urine, is under both voluntary and involuntary control. When the bladder is distended with approximately 300 ml of urine, stretch receptors in the wall of the bladder are stimulated to send information to the spinal cord, which initiates a spinal reflex to open the internal sphincter in the urethra, allowing urine to enter. This is an involuntary process. If it is not convenient at that time to void urine, voluntary contraction of the external urethral sphincter will prevent micturition. The bladder will continue to fill until such time as the bladder becomes over-distended, at which point voluntary control is overridden and the external urethral sphincter relaxes, i.e. micturition occurs, aided by contraction of the detrusor muscle.

Emptying of the bladder can be aided by the use of the diaphragm and abdominal muscles to increase pressure in the abdominal cavity. Coughing, laughing or sneezing will also increase pressure in the bladder, and for some people, especially women who are pregnant or have had previous pregnancies, this results in the involuntary passage of a small amount of urine, a condition known as *stress incontinence* (MacArthur et al 1991). This is often due to incompetence of the urethral sphincter or nerve damage during delivery (Swash 1988).

PHYSIOLOGICAL CHANGES THROUGH THE CHILDBEARING YEAR

Pregnancy

The increased amounts of circulating hormones, especially progesterone, released during pregnancy result in dilatation of the pelvis and calyces of the kidney causing obstruction of the ureters, particularly on the right. Dilated blood vessels also slow urine flow (Sweet 1997). These factors can predispose pregnant women to *urinary tract infection* with involvement of the kidneys (Box 11.2).

The increasing bulk of the gravid uterus can also have the effect of inhibiting flow throughout the renal system and the storage of large amounts of urine in the bladder (Baylis & Davidson 1991). This results in *frequency of micturition*, both in early pregnancy, due to the presence of the uterus in the pelvic cavity, and towards the end of pregnancy, when the uterus takes up most of the space in the abdominal cavity.

Pregnant women frequently wake at night to pass urine. This is called *nocturia* and is thought to be due to poor venous return whilst upright during the day, causing diminished passage of urine (Blackburn & Loper 1992). Sodium is thus retained in the body. Once venous return is encouraged by lying down at night, the raised levels of sodium in the blood cause a slightly higher production of urine, and so the woman is more likely to need to pass urine.

The increase in circulating fluid in the cardiovascular and lymphatic systems, leads to an increase in the glomerular filtration rate of the kidneys (Baylis & Davidson 1991). As a result, the kidneys are unable to reabsorb totally some substances, and any excess is excreted in the urine. This is a physiological phenomenon of pregnancy, referred to as the *lowering of the renal threshold*. This explains why glucose can be found in the urine of women who have normal blood glucose levels.

Labour

During labour the bladder rises above the symphysis pubis, as the fetus moves deeper into the pelvis. This may lead to restriction of the urethra, causing *retention of urine*. If, as a result, the bladder becomes distended, it may obstruct the progress of labour. It may also become damaged (as may the urethra) during delivery, giving rise to difficulties passing urine postnatally.

Assessment of the condition of the labouring woman includes regular urinalysis to ensure that she is coping with the increased physiological demands. To meet these demands, the metabolic rate increases. The extra energy required comes initially from glucose stores but if, as labour progresses, these stores are not replaced by sufficient nutrition, fat is utilised instead. This creates a condition common in labouring women, called *ketonuria*, in which ketone bodies are passed as waste in the urine (Grant 1990).

Postnatal

Urinary output increases for 7 days after delivery, as the amount of circulatory fluid decreases and the waste products associated with involution of the uterus (i.e. its shrinking to its normal size) are removed. However, bladder function may be slow to return to normal, due to factor such as the length of labour and whether the pelvic floor was damaged during delivery. Psychological fear due to the presence of sutures or bruising can also affect the ability of a woman to urinate normally. A delivery with complications such as haemorrhage may result in more severe damage to the renal system (Box 11.3).

The renal system takes approximately 6 weeks to return to its prepregnancy state. Urinary tract infection occurs in 2–4% of women during the puerperium, particularly in those who were catheterised during labour (Clark 1995).

The neonate

Once delivered, the neonate must begin to eliminate waste in urine and maintain fluid and electrolyte balance. The kidneys are relatively immature at term, although anatomically complete. They are unable to dilute or concentrate urine as effi-

---

Box 11.3 Renal disorders

Acute renal failure may occur after a period of decreased blood pressure caused by massive haemorrhage (e.g. *postpartum haemorrhage*) or circulatory failure (e.g. in *eclampsia*). Whenever the glomerular filtration rate is markedly decreased, the nephrons of the kidney become damaged, although in a brief acute episode such as the examples above, this is usually reversible. Careful observation is made of urinary output after any acute episode when circulatory fluid volume has been compromised. An output of less than 400 ml in 24 hours indicates the possibility of acute renal failure.

Any woman with *chronic renal disease* who becomes pregnant runs the risk of developing *renal failure*. This is a condition in which damage to the nephrons is so severe that 75% of renal function has been lost. Infertility is common in women with chronic renal disease or renal transplant, but improved medical care means an increasing number of them are achieving pregnancy. These women then have a higher risk of complications in pregnancy and perinatal morbidity is increased too (Perry 1994).

ciently as in the adult, but can achieve fluid and electrolyte balance within a narrow range. Any imbalance will occur more rapidly, especially in the neonate who is ill or preterm.

In the healthy full-term infant, passage of urine is expected within 24 hours, to indicate normal functioning of the kidneys and patency of the renal tract.

REFERENCES

Baylis C, Davidson J 1991 The urinary system. In: Hytten F, Chamberlain G (eds) Clinical physiology in obstetrics. Blackwell Scientific, Oxford, p 246–252
Blackburn S T, Loper D L 1992 Maternal, fetal and neonatal physiology. A clinical perspective. W B Saunders, Philadelphia, p 346
Clark R A 1995 Infections during the postpartum period. Journal of Obstetric, Gynecologic and Neonatal Nursing 24(6):542–548
Enkin M, Keirse M, Renfrew M, Neilson J 1995 A guide to effective care in pregnancy and childbirth. Oxford University Press, Oxford, p 114
Grant J 1990 Nutrition and hydration in labour. In: Alexander J, Levy V, Roch S (eds) Intrapartum care: a research-based approach. Macmillan, Basingstoke, p 61
MacArthur C, Lewis M, Knox E G 1991 Health after childbirth. HMSO, London, p 253
Perry L A 1994 A multidisciplinary approach to the management of pregnant patients with end-stage renal disease. Journal of Perinatal and Neonatal Nursing 8(1):12–19
Plattner M S 1994 Pyelonephritis in pregnancy. Journal of Perinatal and Neonatal Nursing 8(1):20–27
Swash M 1988 Childbirth and incontinence. Midwifery 4(1):13–18
Sweet B R (ed) 1997 Mayes' midwifery. A textbook for midwives, 12th edn. Baillière Tindall, London, p 129–130

Reproduction

Part 2 covers the anatomy and physiology of reproduction through the childbearing year. It begins by examining the reproductive systems of both sexes, and moves on through fertilisation, the development of the embryo and fetus, pregnancy, labour and delivery, the puerperium and the neonate.

12

The male reproductive system

The function of the male reproductive tract is to manufacture spermatozoa and transmit them to a female to allow fertilisation to take place. After that, the male need have no more to do with the development, birth and caring of the offspring which results from the mating. However, in the majority of cases, the male continues to play a part in any resulting pregnancy, offering support to his partner through the 9 months of pregnancy. Often he attends the birth of their baby and is involved in the bringing up of the child until adulthood.

At birth, the male neonate will have the basic anatomical structures required for sexual reproduction, but these do not become fully functional until puberty.

The male reproductive system consists of both external and internal organs of reproduction. The external organs are:

- the scrotum, containing two testes which are responsible for the manufacture of spermatozoa, and two epidydimides in which spermatozoa mature and are stored
- the penis, through which spermatozoa are expelled by ejaculation.

The internal organs include:

- ducts that transport spermatozoa from the testes to the end of the penis
- glands that secrete nutrients that support spermatozoa and chemicals that influence their function.

EXTERNAL GENITALIA

The external genitalia (Fig. 12.1) comprise:

- the scrotum
- the testes
- the epididymis
- the penis.

The scrotum

The *scrotum* is a pouch of loose skin situated behind the penis, below the symphysis pubis and in front of the thighs. The scrotum is divided into two sacs, each containing one testis, and is composed of skin lined with an involuntary muscle layer, the dartos muscle. The *dartos muscle* is responsible for maintaining an appropriate temperature for spermatogenesis i.e. the production of mature sperm. This temperature is 3°C lower than core body temperature. The dartos muscle contracts or relaxes according to external temperatures, bringing the scrotum closer to or further away from the groin. The closer it is to the groin, the warmer it will be.

The testes

The *testes*, or testicles, are the male sex organs or *gonads*. They develop from structures high up in

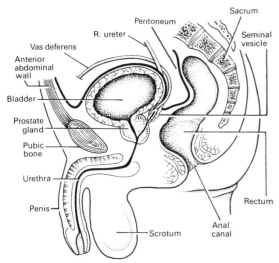

Figure 12.1 The male reproductive organs. (Reproduced with permission from Wilson K J W, Waugh A 1996 Ross and Wilson Anatomy and Physiology in Health and Illness, 8th edn. Churchill Livingstone, Edinburgh)

Box 12.1 Male infertility

In rare instances, the testes do not descend into the scrotum before birth. This condition is called *cryptorchidism*. In the majority of such cases, the testes will descend spontaneously during the first year of life (Perry 1995). Should this not occur, the testes must be brought down into the scrotum as soon as possible. This may be by surgery or, occasionally, by hormonal treatment (Mason 1993). Placement of the testes in the scrotum is essential: if they remain in the pelvic cavity, the higher core temperature there may prevent the initial development of the spermatozoa. Where both testes are undescended, there is a high risk of male infertility (Lee 1996).

Other causes of infertility include the following:

- *Defective spermatogenesis*, which can be characterised by insufficient spermatozoa in each ejaculate, too many abnormal spermatozoa or chemical anomalies in seminal fluids.
- *Obstruction* in ducts or tubules of the genital tract, possibly due to infection, congenital defects, or tumours.
- *Failure to ejaculate*, because of impotence caused by pathological conditions e.g. diabetes, heroin addiction or smoking, or psychological conditions e.g. stress (Quinn & Lowdermilk 1995).

---

the abdomen close to the kidneys and usually descend into the scrotum 2 months before birth (Box 12.1). The testes have two functions:

1. the production of spermatozoa
2. the production of the male hormone testosterone.

Spermatozoa are produced in the mature testes in long convoluted tubules called the seminiferous tubules. Testosterone is manufactured in endocrine cells situated in the tissues between the seminiferous tubules.

The testes are oval in shape, measure 50 mm by 25 mm, and weigh 10–15 g (Fig. 12.2). There are three layers surrounding the testes:

1. the *tunica vaginalis*, the outermost covering, which allows free movement of the testes within the scrotum
2. the *tunica albuginea*, a dense fibrous tissue which divides the substance of the testes into lobules
3. the *tunica vasculosa*, a fine network of capillaries surrounding each lobule.

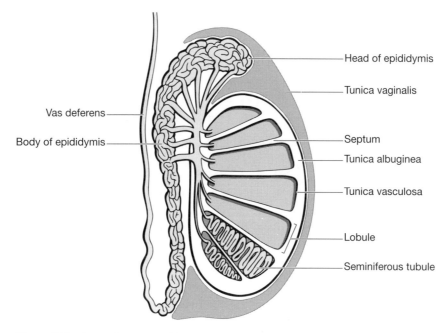

Figure 12.2   Internal structure of the testis and epididymis.

Each testis is divided into 200–300 lobules, each of which contain two or three tightly coiled *seminiferous tubules*, where spermatogenesis takes place. Each tubule is lined with germinal epithelium from which *spermatozoa* are produced regularly from puberty. As they develop, spermatozoa move from the germinal epithelium towards the lumen, which they reach at maturity (Fig. 12.3). It takes 70–80 days to produce mature spermatozoa. From the lumen they move

through efferent ducts to the epididymis and then to the vas deferens.

Sertoli cells develop within the tubules from puberty to nourish the spermatozoa during development. Between the seminiferous tubules are small clusters of endocrine cells called *Leydig cells*, which produce the hormone *testosterone*.

The epididymis

The *epididymis* is a comma-shaped structure that consists of a head, body and tail, and contains a coiled tubule 6 m long situated over the superior surface of the testis. Ciliated epithelium lines the tubule, moving the spermatozoa along its length. Towards the tail of the epididymis, the tubule becomes less convoluted and is called the vas deferens. The *vas deferens* is about 450 mm long and travels along the posterior border of the testis leaving the scrotum along with blood and lymph vessels as the *spermatic cord* (Box 12.2). This cord suspends the testis in the scrotum. The spermatic cord, along with nerve fibres, enters the abdomen through the *inguinal canal*.

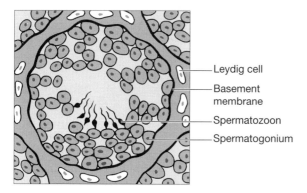

Figure 12.3   Cross-section of a seminiferous tubule.

Box 12.2 Vasectomy

A commonly used male method of contraception is the *vasectomy*. This is an operation in which both the vas deferentia are severed, resulting in sterility without loss of desire or sensation. It is a relatively simple outpatient procedure, usually carried out under local anaesthesia (Cashion & Johnston 1995). Two small incisions are made in the groin, and 20–30 mm of the vas excised. Although spermatozoa will still be produced, the effect of the operation is to interrupt their passage along the vas deferens. Up to 12 weeks will elapse before no spermatozoa are present in ejaculate, because some will have been present in the seminal vesicles and ejaculatory duct at the time of the vasectomy (Alexander 1993). Examination of semen samples determines whether spermatozoa are still present. Male sterilisation cannot be assured until three consecutive samples have shown a complete absence of sperm.

Other methods of male contraception include the use of a barrier such as a condom or spermicidal creams, or withdrawal before ejaculation.

Blood, nerves and lymph

Blood is supplied to the scrotum and testes by the testicular artery, which branches from the aorta. The testicular vein drains blood away to the renal vein (left) or the inferior vena cava (right). Nerve supply is from the tenth and eleventh thoracic nerves. Lymph drainage is into lymph nodes around the aorta.

The penis

The *penis* is a highly vascular organ composed of a root lying in the perineum and a body surrounding the urethra (Fig. 12.1). The *body* is made up of three cylindrical masses of erectile tissue held together by fibrous material and covered with skin. The two lateral columns are the *corpus cavernosa*; surrounding the urethra is a spongy *corpus spongiosum*. Normally, the erectile tissue is honeycombed with empty spaces and the penis is flaccid. However, this tissue has a rich blood supply and when stimulated by the autonomic nervous system it becomes engorged with blood, making the penis erect. The *root* of the penis is attached to perineal muscle, which assists in erection.

The distal end of the penis is slightly enlarged and is known as the *glans penis*. It is covered with a loose fold of skin called the prepuce, or *foreskin*, which protects the delicate glans. The urethra exits the body through the glans penis, at the urethral meatus. At this point both urine and semen are released.

Blood and nerve supply

Blood is supplied to the penis by branches of the internal pudendal arteries and drains into pudendal and iliac veins. Both the central and autonomic nervous systems supply the penis.

INTERNAL GENITALIA

The vas deferens travels into the pelvis, behind the base of the bladder to the prostate gland (Fig. 12.1). There it joins the ducts of the seminal vesicles to form the ejaculatory duct.

Seminal vesicles

The *seminal vesicles* are situated between the base of the bladder and the rectum. They are irregular-shaped sacs 50 mm long. The seminal vesicles act as a reservoir for the spermatozoa, and secrete a nourishing fluid for the spermatozoa to live in.

The ejaculatory duct

The *ejaculatory duct* is 25 mm long and ejects spermatozoa into the urethra, leading from the bladder. The urethra has a dual purpose as a common pathway for urine from the bladder and for spermatozoa from the testes. However, a small sphincter prevents the simultaneous passage of urine and semen and also prevents spermatozoa from entering the bladder.

The prostate gland

Surrounding the upper portion of the urethra is the *prostate gland*. This gland is cone shaped, and measures 40 mm by 30 mm. The prostate gland is composed of glandular tissue and smooth muscle, and aids ejaculation. Secretions from the prostate gland are added to seminal fluid as it passes through the urethra.

Bulbourethral glands

Bulbourethral glands, also known as Cowper's glands, are situated at the root of the penis. These are small glands the size of peas with ducts which empty into the urethra before it enters the penis. These glands add secretions to seminal fluid and also release lubricants into the urethra which aid the entry of the penis into the vagina.

Semen

The result of the addition of secretions from the seminal vesicles, prostate and bulbourethral glands to the passing spermatozoa is the production of *semen*, also called seminal fluid. The average volume of semen at each ejaculation is 2.5–6 ml, and there are 50–150 million spermatozoa in each millilitre. Semen has a pH of 7.2–7.6. It therefore neutralises the acid environment of the male urethra and female vagina.

As well as fluids, nutrients and spermatozoa, seminal fluid also contains enzymes required to activate spermatozoa after ejaculation. These include hyaluronidase, which aids the passage of the spermatozoa through the cervical mucus and assists in breaking down the cell membrane of the ovum.

Spermatozoa are normally produced at a rate of 300 million per day and can survive for 3–4 days in the right environment after ejaculation. Spermatozoa are composed of a head, body and tail (Fig. 12.4). The *head* contains the nucleus and an *acrosome*, a structure in which the enzymes required for penetrating the cell membrane of the ovum are found. The *body* contains numerous mitochondria, the organelles that produce energy. These provide energy for the tail, a single *flagellum*, which is responsible for propelling the spermatozoon on its long journey from the vagina, through the cervix and uterus, and along the length of the uterine tube.

HORMONAL CONTROL

When a boy is around 10–14 years old, *gonadotrophin-releasing hormone (GnRH)* is released by the hypothalamus which stimulates the release of

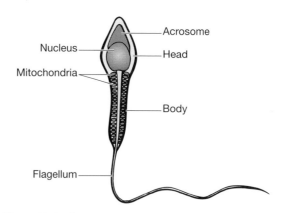

Figure 12.4 A spermatozoon.

follicle-stimulating hormone (FSH) and *luteinising hormone (LH)* from the anterior pituitary gland. In girls, this usually happens a little earlier. In boys, FSH acts on the seminiferous tubules to begin spermatogenesis. LH acts on the Leydig cells in the matrix of the testes to begin testosterone production. *Testosterone* is responsible for the maturation of the boy into a man. Small amounts are present from before birth, having controlled the descent of the testes into the scrotum. At puberty, however, increasing amounts are produced resulting in:

- the development, growth and maintenance of the male reproductive system
- an increase in protein production
- maturation of spermatozoa
- sexual behaviour
- musculoskeletal growth
- the growth of the secondary sex characteristics, i.e. facial, pubic and body hair, and the enlargement of the larynx producing a deeper voice.

In the mature male, a negative feedback system controls the hormones released:

1. GnRH is released from the hypothalamus, which stimulates the anterior pituitary gland to release LH.

2. LH stimulates the production of testosterone from Leydig cells in the testes.

3. Once testosterone reaches a certain level in the blood, it inhibits the release of GnRH by the hypothalamus and LH by the pituitary.

4. Testosterone levels therefore begin to decrease.

5. Once testosterone levels fall below a certain level, GnRH production begins again, stimulating the release of LH.

A second cycle, the FSH-inhibin cycle, controls the production of spermatozoa:

1. Once spermatogenesis has produced sufficient spermatozoa for reproductive needs, the hormone *inhibin* is released from the Sertoli cells in the seminiferous tubules.

2. Inhibin acts on the anterior pituitary gland, causing it to decrease FSH production.

3. Because FSH controls the production of spermatozoa, spermatogenesis slows.

4. However, once spermatogenesis has decreased below a certain level, inhibin levels also drop and so FSH is again released from the anterior pituitary.

SPERMATOGENESIS

Spermatogenesis is the process by which spermatozoa are produced. In most males spermatogenesis is fully functional by the age of 16. Spermatogenesis is a continuous process, resulting in a constant supply of mature spermatozoa. The development of one spermatogonium into a mature spermatozoon takes about 75 days.

Spermatogenesis takes place in the seminiferous tubules of the testes under the hormonal instruction of follicle stimulating hormone (FSH). The process goes through a series of stages:

1. *Spermatogonia* are produced by mitosis from the germinal epithelium of the tubule. These are nourished by Sertoli cells and develop into primary spermatocytes.

2. *Primary spermatocytes* contain the full complement of chromosomes, i.e. 46 in 23 homologous pairs. They move away from the basement membrane of the seminiferous tubule and undergo the first reduction division of meiosis to produce secondary spermatocytes, which contain 23 chromosomes, one from each homologous pair (Box 12.3).

3. *Secondary spermatocytes* then undergo the second meiotic division, resulting in the creation

---

> **Box 12.3** Sex determination
>
> The *sex of a baby* is determined when the spermatozoon and ovum meet at fertilisation. All ova carry an X chromosome in their nucleus, but spermatozoa carry either an X or a Y chromosome. If a spermatozoon containing an X chromosome fertilises an ovum, this will result in an XX baby, i.e. a female. If a spermatozoon containing a Y chromosome fertilises the ovum, an XY baby will result, i.e. a male.

---

of four *spermatids* from the one original spermatogonium. These are situated close to the lumen of the seminiferous tubule.

4. Under the influence of luteinising hormone (LH), mature spermatozoa are formed, ready for fertilisation.

However, these spermatozoa have yet to become motile. They are moved through the epididymides to the vas deferens, and secretions from the seminal vesicles give them some motility. As they pass by the openings to the prostate gland and bulbourethral glands more secretions are added, making the spermatozoa more active. However, it is not until they become deposited in the female vagina that spermatozoa become completely motile.

A normal ejaculation of semen has the following characteristics (WHO 1994):

- a volume of 2–4 ml
- more than 20 million spermatozoa per millilitre
- 40% of the spermatozoa are motile
- 30% are anatomically normal.

PHYSIOLOGY OF SEXUAL INTERCOURSE

Sexual intercourse, or coitus, is a complex physiological and psychological event. Both the male and female require stimulation for the experience to be pleasurable. In the male, sexual intercourse is initiated by anticipation, followed by visual or tactile stimulation which leads to the penis becoming erect. Parasympathetic nerve impulses cause the smooth muscle of the arteries in the penis to relax, allowing blood to enter and fill the spongy tissue of the corpora. These compress the veins, preventing the blood draining back towards the heart, so maintaining the erection. Meanwhile the bulbourethral glands secrete mucus to lubricate the penis and assist entry into the vagina of the female.

Intensive stimulation of the penis follows, by rhythmical movement in the vagina. This causes sympathetic nerve impulses to produce peristaltic contractions of the seminiferous ducts, epididymis and vas deferens to move spermatozoa along the urethra. Similar contractions in the seminal vesicles and prostate add seminal fluid to the spermatozoa and subsequently these are all added to the secretions from the bulbourethral glands. Ultimately skeletal muscles become involved to eject the semen from the urethra into the vagina of the female. This is ejac-ulation. A body-wide response is felt which involves general muscle tension and pleasurable sensations – the male orgasm.

The female is also stimulated by touch or by pleasurable thoughts. As a result, the vagina becomes lubricated with mucus from the cervix and the Bartholins glands. The labia become engorged, allowing easier access to the vagina. The breasts and clitoris also become engorged, enhancing pleasurable sensations. Should female orgasm result, muscular spasms cause the cervix to dip into the vagina, encouraging the passage of spermatozoa into the cervical canal.

Once male ejaculation has been achieved, blood drains from the penis, and so it loses its rigidity and leaves the vagina. Although the female can continue to feel pleasure after orgasm, the male usually needs time to recover before commencing coitus again.

REFERENCES

Alexander J 1993 Family planning. In: Bennett V R, Brown L K (eds) Myles' textbook for midwives, 12th edn. Churchill Livingstone, Edinburgh, p 264

Cashion K, Johnston C L A 1995 Nursing care during the postpartum period. In: Bobak I M, Lowdermilk D L, Jenson M D (eds) Maternity nursing, 4th edn. Mosby, St Louis, p 501–502

Lee S 1996 Counselling in male infertility. Blackwell Science, Oxford, p 23

Mason M C 1993 Male infertility – men talking. Routledge, London, p 34

Perry S E 1995 The newborn. In: Bobak I M, Lowdermilk D L, Jenson M D (eds) Maternity nursing, 4th edn. Mosby, St Louis, p 330

Quinn E B, Lowdermilk D L 1995 Common reproductive concerns. In: Bobak I M, Lowdermilk D L, Jenson M D (eds) Maternity nursing, 4th edn. Mosby, St Louis, p 871–872

WHO (World Health Organization) 1994 Laboratory manual for the examination of human semen and semen–cervical interaction. Cambridge University Press, Cambridge

13

The female reproductive system

Reproduction is essential for the continuation of the human species. The female reproductive system performs the following functions:

- it produces a small number of ova, i.e. mature egg cells
- it provides a suitable site for the fertilisation of an ovum by a spermatozoon
- it subsequently provides the ideal environment in which the resultant embryo can be nourished, and can develop and mature.

The female reproductive system goes through vast changes during pregnancy. The hormones produced both in the reproductive system and elsewhere enable alterations to take place in the body that allow it to accommodate and adapt to the growing fetus. Labour and delivery require the coordination of many body systems. Post-natally, the reproductive organs rapidly regain their non-pregnant status as well as producing nourishment for the neonate.

The neonate is born with the basic anatomical features of the reproductive system, but these do not begin to function until puberty, under the influence of hormones. However, in the female all ova are present at birth in a rudimentary state, and can be damaged during the course of her life by external factors such as radiation, resulting in possible fertility problems. Male spermatozoa are produced constantly after puberty and can therefore only be affected as they develop.

The female reproductive system consists of:

- external genitalia
- internal genitalia.

EXTERNAL GENITALIA

The external genitalia, collectively known as the vulva, extend from the mons pubis anteriorly to the perineum posteriorly (Fig. 13.1). Laterally they extend to the outer aspects of the labia majora.

The *mons pubis* is a pad of fatty tissue that lies above the symphysis pubis of the pelvis. It has a covering of skin and after puberty is covered with hair. The mons pubis is not a structure of the reproductive system but functions as an overlying cushion to the bony pelvis below. The *perineum* is an area of strong muscle which supports the internal organs of the pelvic cavity.

The external genitalia consist of:

- two labia majora, which give protection to the internal genitalia
- two labia minora, which have a similar protective function
- the clitoris, which plays a role in promoting the pleasure of sexual intercourse
- the vaginal orifice, which allows access to the internal genitalia
- associated glands, which provide secretions to moisten and lubricate the external genitalia.

The labia majora

The *labia majora* are two folds of fatty tissue covered with skin, which extend from the mons pubis anteriorly to merge with the muscles of the perineum. The outer surface of the labia majora is covered with hair after puberty and the inner surface is smooth and contains sweat and sebaceous glands. The function of the labia majora is to protect the vagina: they enclose the vaginal orifice and the fatty tissue acts as a cushion.

The labia minora

The *labia minora* are two thin folds of skin lying within the labia majora. They are smooth, with no covering of hair, and contain a few sweat and sebaceous glands. Anteriorly, the labia minora each divide into two folds of skin and join to form the prepuce in front of the clitoris, and the frenulum behind it. Posteriorly they meet at the fourchette, a thin fold of skin at the rear of the vaginal orifice. The inner surfaces of the labia minora are normally in contact with each other and so also protect the vagina.

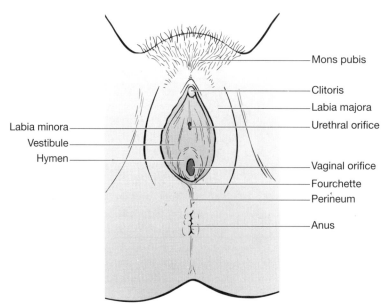

Figure 13.1 External genitalia.

The clitoris

The *clitoris* is a small projection of erectile tissue, about 25 mm long, richly supplied with blood vessels and nerve fibres. In response to stimulation, the clitoris becomes erect and filled with blood in a manner similar to the male penis. Its function is to enhance the pleasurable experience of sexual intercourse (Box 13.1).

The vaginal orifice

The *vaginal orifice*, or introitus, is situated between the two pairs of labia in an area commonly known as the vestibule. It lies behind the urethral orifice, which leads to the renal system. The vaginal orifice is covered internally by a membrane of skin called the hymen, which serves as protec-

---

Box 13.1   Female circumcision

Female circumcision is a traditional practice common in some African states, particularly Nigeria, Ethiopia, the Sudan and Egypt (Verralls 1993). As midwives are increasingly working with women from countries such as these, it is important for them to understand the procedure and its consequences, so they can give the women appropriate care.

There are several types of female circumcision, including (Wright 1996):

- excision of the prepuce of the clitoris, and suturing of the labia majora
- removal of the clitoris
- infibulation, which involves excision of the clitoris, labia minora and the majority of the labia majora. The remains of the labia majora are then sutured together leaving a small orifice for the passage of urine and menstruation.

These procedures are generally carried out on small girls, without the use of anaesthetics and in unhygienic conditions, leading to high morbidity and mortality rates (Morris 1996).

Female circumcision, also called female genital mutilation, has become a human rights issue for many, who are campaigning for it to be abolished. In the UK and many other western countries it is already illegal. However, changing attitudes in the countries where it is traditionally practised is difficult. Although carried out predominantly by Muslims, female circumcision is a cultural, not a religious custom.

Women who have been circumcised may experience considerable difficulties in labour (McConville 1998). They commonly require anterior episiotomy at delivery, because of the presence of extensive scar tissue around the external genitalia.

---

tion for the vagina and the other internal organs of the reproductive system. The *hymen* is ruptured on the occasion of first sexual intercourse, though it may previously have been damaged by physical activities (e.g. horse riding), or the use of tampons. The remnants of the hymen can usually still be seen as small tags of tissue, the *carunculae myrtiformes*.

At the entrance to the vaginal orifice lie the ducts of a pair of glands, *Bartholin's glands*. These open outside the vagina and secrete mucus to moisten the external genitalia. In the vestibule itself, on either side of the urethral orifice, are another pair of glands, *Skene's glands*, which also secrete mucus for the same purpose.

Blood, nerves and lymph

The external genitalia receive their blood supply from pudendal arteries, and corresponding veins drain blood away. The vulva is highly vascular and so tends to bleed heavily when damaged, but also to heal quickly.

Nerve supply is mainly from the pudendal nerves, which are branches of the sacral plexus. Lymph drainage is into the inguinal and external iliac glands.

INTERNAL GENITALIA

The internal genitalia consist of (Fig. 13.2):

- the vagina, where spermatozoa can be deposited, and the fetus can exit the body
- the uterus, where the embryo and fetus can be nurtured
- two uterine tubes, that provide a passageway through which the ova can reach the uterus
- two ovaries, which produce hormones and ova.

The vagina

The *vagina* is an elastic, fibromuscular canal that extends upwards and backwards from the vulva to the uterus, parallel to the plane of the pelvic brim. The walls of the vagina are usually in close contact, except at the upper end where the cervix projects into the vagina. Because of the position

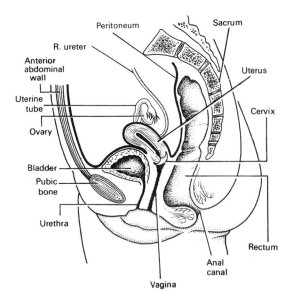

Figure 13.2 Sagittal section showing the organs of the pelvis. (Reproduced with permission from Wilson K J W, Waugh A 1996 Ross and Wilson Anatomy and Physiology in Health and Illness, 8th edn. Churchill Livingstone, Edinburgh)

of the cervix, the anterior wall of the mature vagina measures approximately 75 mm, and the posterior wall about 90 mm. Where the cervix projects into the vagina, four recesses or *fornices* (singular fornix) are formed. These are the anterior, posterior and lateral fornices (Fig. 13.3).

The functions of the vagina are:

● to allow the deposit and passage of spermatozoa during sexual intercourse

● to provide an outlet for the fetus and other products of conception
● to provide an outlet for the menstrual flow
● to act as a barrier to ascending infections.

The vaginal walls are composed of four layers:

1. an inner layer of *squamous epithelium* forming folds or rugae which allow the vagina to expand enormously to allow the passage of a fetus
2. a layer of *connective tissue* containing blood vessels
3. a *muscle layer* consisting of an outer layer of longitudinal muscle and an inner layer of circular muscle
4. an outer layer of *connective tissue*, continuous with that of other organs of the pelvis, containing blood and lymphatic vessels, and nerve fibres.

The vaginal walls contain no glands, but are kept moist by secretions from cervical glands and by seepage of fluid from blood capillaries. This fluid has an acid pH of 3.8–4.5, maintained by the presence of commensals in the vagina called *Döderleins bacilli*. These feed on glycogen, present in the vaginal walls, and convert it to lactic acid, which protects the vagina and other internal genitalia from infection. As the levels of glycogen in the vagina vary with the levels of ovarian hormones, this acid balance can be disturbed, most commonly during pregnancy, before

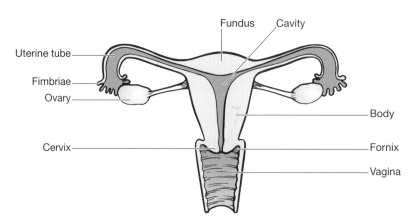

Figure 13.3 The internal genitalia.

puberty and during and after menopause. In such instances, pathogenic microorganisms can multiply readily, leading to an increased likelihood of vaginal infection (Box 13.2).

In front of the vagina lie the bladder and the urethra. Behind the vagina, at the point where the uterus enters, is a hollow in the peritoneum, called the *pouch of Douglas*. Running closely adjacent to the posterior wall of the vagina is the rectum. The perineal body, which supports the pelvic organs, is situated behind the vagina at the introitus.

Blood, nerves and lymph

The blood supply to the vagina comes from the vaginal, uterine and middle haemorrhoidal arteries, which are branches of the internal iliac arteries. Venous drainage is into the internal iliac veins.

Nerve supply is through the sacral plexus and the pudendal nerve. Lymphatic drainage is into the inguinal and iliac lymph nodes.

The uterus

The *uterus* is a hollow, pear-shaped muscular organ situated in the pelvic cavity between the bladder and the rectum. It is anteverted (tilted forwards) and anteflexed (curved forwards) (Fig. 13.2). The mature uterus measures approximately 75 mm long, 50 mm wide at the broadest point, and 25 mm thick, and weighs about 60 g.

The functions of the uterus are:

- to prepare to receive, protect and nourish a fetus
- to assist in the expulsion of the fetus, placenta and membranes at delivery
- to control blood loss from the placental site.

Macrostructure

The uterus consists of two main parts:

1. the corpus, or body
2. the cervix, or neck (Fig. 13.3).

The cervix is inserted into the vagina; the body lies in the pelvic cavity and at its upper aspect is joined to the two uterine tubes.

The corpus. The corpus or *body* of the uterus consists of the upper two-thirds of the uterus, so is approximately 50 mm long. Within the body lies the *cavity*, which is triangular, its apex pointing towards the cervix (Box 13.3). The anterior and posterior walls of the cavity are usually in close apposition. The upper rounded part of the body of the uterus is the *fundus*; the sections adjacent to the tubes are the *cornua*. The *isthmus* is a slightly constricted area at the junction of the body of the uterus and the cervix, measuring approximately 7 mm.

The cervix. The *cervix* is cylindrical, its lower portion projecting into the vagina. Running through the cervix is the *cervical canal* with, at its

---

Box 13.2 Vaginal infection

During pregnancy there are dramatic changes in the amounts and proportions of hormones released, and these affect the environment of the vagina. The body's resistance to infection is reduced at this time too (see Ch. 7). These factors combine to make pregnant women particularly susceptible to vaginal infections. By giving good advice on hygiene and diet, however, the midwife can assist women to keep vaginal infections to a minimum.

In early pregnancy, certain *vaginal infections* may infect the fetus, causing fetal abnormality, or even death. If contracted later in pregnancy, they may result in an infected neonate at birth (Wang & Smail 1989). It is important, therefore, for the midwife to watch out for any indications of infection, which should be treated swiftly.

It is common for vaginal discharge (leucorrhoea) to increase during pregnancy (Jamieson 1993). This must be distinguished from signs of vaginal infections, such as Candida albicans (*thrush*), a fungal infection which is especially likely to occur when taking antibiotics (Freeman 1995). Vaginal thrush at delivery is a common cause of oral thrush in the newborn.

Other organisms that can cause vaginal infection are the parasites *Trichomonas vaginalis*, which can cause a severe vaginitis, and *Chlamydia trachoma*, associated with widespread infection of the female reproductive system (Silverton 1993).

Bacteria are another type of infectious agent. They include the spirochaete *Treponema pallidum* that causes syphilis, *group B streptococcus* and *Neisseria gonorrhoeae*.

All of these microorganisms can be spread by sexual intercourse and many cause neonatal complications (Kelnar et al 1995).

Box 13.3 Anatomical anomalies

The uterus and other parts of the reproductive tract may not develop correctly during embryonic life. This can result in a variety of malformations. The uterus, uterine tubes and vagina all develop from embryonic structures known as Müller's ducts. During their development these ducts fuse at one end to produce the uterus and vagina. The other ends of the ducts remain open and become the uterine tubes. Incomplete fusion of Müller's ducts may occur (Matthew 1993). This will result in the presence of a *septum* down the centre of the uterus and possibly into the cervix and vagina. A less severe disruption of the developmental process may leave an indentation in the fundus of the uterus, a *bicornuate uterus*. Very rarely no fusion occurs, and the female infant has *two separate reproductive tracts*.

These malformations often remain undiagnosed until the woman becomes pregnant. The midwife may observe a *malpresentation*, which is found on scan to be due to a bicornuate uterus. This must be considered as one possible reason for a breech presentation. Any abnormality such as these may lead to a higher incidence of spontaneous abortion or intrauterine death. Because of the close relationship between the development of the reproductive and renal systems, any investigation into one must include investigations of the other.

top end, an opening into the uterus – the *internal os* – and at the other end, an opening into the vagina – the *external os*.

Microstructure

The uterus and cervix are made up of three layers of tissue:

1. an inner epithelium, the endometrium
2. a middle muscular layer, the myometrium
3. an outer layer of connective tissue, the perimetrium.

The endometrium. The inner epithelium lines the uterus and cervix and is called the *endometrium*. In the uterus, this consists of two layers:

1. the functional layer
2. the basal layer.

The *functional layer* is composed of highly glandular epithelial tissue that, after puberty, is built up and shed during each menstrual cycle under the influence of hormones. This layer is highly vascular, with spiral arterioles providing nour-

ishment for the constant proliferation of cells during the reproductive cycle. When a fertilised ovum becomes embedded, this layer provides the nourishment required for the growth and development of the embryo throughout pregnancy.

The *basal layer* is a permanent layer, which gives rise to the functional layer after each menstruation. This layer is also well supplied with blood in the form of straight arterioles that supply the necessary materials for the functional layer to be formed.

The cervix is lined with *columnar epithelium*, which secretes mucus to form a protective plug in the cervical canal to protect the internal genitalia from infection. Some epithelial cells are ciliated to assist the passage of spermatozoa. The arrangement of the strands of mucus alters throughout the menstrual cycle to either prevent penetration by spermatozoa, or to encourage their passage. The endometrium of the cervix is also arranged in folds similar to the vagina, called the *arbor vitae*, which allow dilatation during labour. The endometrial layer of the cervix is not shed during the menstrual cycle.

The myometrium. The middle layer of the uterine wall, the *myometrium*, is composed of three layers of muscle:

1. an inner circular layer
2. a middle oblique layer
3. an outer longitudinal layer.

The layers of muscle are thickest in the fundus of the uterus and thinnest in the cervix. Although it is possible to identify the individual layers, they are not distinct, the muscle fibres being intermingled with each other and with blood and lymph vessels, and nerve fibres. The myometrium plays a vital role during the process of pregnancy and childbirth.

The myometrium of the cervix contains some longitudinal smooth muscle that extends from the uterus, but the majority of muscle cells there are circular.

The perimetrium. The outer layer of the uterus and cervix, the *perimetrium*, is made up of a layer of peritoneum, which is draped over the uterus and the uterine tubes. At the lateral surfaces of the uterus there is a double fold of perimetrium that extends to the side walls of the pelvic cavity, forming the supporting broad ligament. There are two cavities in the peritoneum: the *pouch of Douglas* between the uterus and rectum, and the *uterovesicular pouch* between the uterus and bladder.

Blood, nerves and lymph

Blood supply to the uterus and cervix is from the uterine and ovarian arteries, which branch from the iliac artery and aorta. Branches of the uterine arteries – the radial arteries – penetrate deep into the myometrium, where they divide again into straight arterioles which supply the basal layer, and spiral arteries which nourish the functional layer. Venous drainage is into corresponding veins.

Nerve supply is from the sacral plexus. Lymphatic drainage is into internal iliac and inguinal lymph nodes.

Supporting structures

The uterus and cervix are held in place in the pelvis by ligaments. These are (Fig. 13.4):

- the *cardinal ligaments*, which run from the lateral surfaces of the cervix and vagina to the lateral walls of the pelvic cavity

- two *pubocervical ligaments*, which run from the cervix, under the bladder, forward to the pubic bones
- two *uterosacral ligaments*, which pass from the cervix in an upward and backward direction to the periosteum of the sacrum, encircling the rectum
- the *broad ligament*, attached to the lateral walls of the uterus, which it supports
- *round ligaments*, bands of fibrous tissue between the two folds of the broad ligament, extending from the cornua down to the tissues of the labia majora, which maintain the uterus in a position of anteversion and anteflexion.

The uterine tubes

The *uterine tubes*, also called the Fallopian tubes, extend laterally from each side of the uterus at the cornua (Fig. 13.3), between the folds of the broad ligament. The distal portions of the tubes bend backwards and downwards through the posterior wall of the broad ligament towards the ovaries, which lie behind the ligament.

The functions of the uterine tubes are:

- to propel the ovum towards the uterus
- to provide a passage for the spermatozoa to meet the ovum for fertilisation.

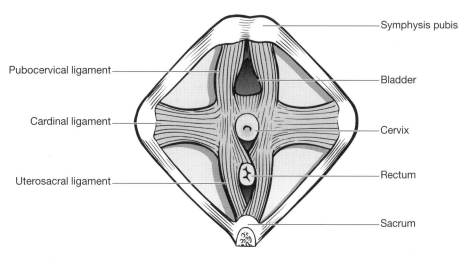

Figure 13.4   Supporting structures of the reproductive organs.

The uterine tubes are approximately 100 mm long and consist of:

- a narrow *isthmus* close to the cornua of the uterus, measuring approximately 25 mm
- the wider *ampulla*, approximately 50 mm
- the *infundibulum*, approximately 25 mm, which widens into finger-like projections called *fimbriae*.

The fimbriae lie over the ovaries and waft in the pelvic cavity, moving closer to the ovary at the time of ovulation. The lumen of the uterine tubes is open to the pelvic cavity at the fimbriae. When an ovum is released at ovulation, it is swept into the uterine tubes by currents set up by the fimbriae, and begins its journey towards the uterus.

The uterine tubes are very narrow and lined with *ciliated epithelium* arranged in folds. Once an ovum enters the uterine tube, it is wafted along the lumen by the cilia, the folds slowing down this process so that the ovum remains in the tube for as long as possible, to maximum its chances of being fertilised in the ampulla. Once fertilised, the ovum is propelled, in the same manner, to the uterus (Box 13.4). This also happens slowly, giving the ovum time to become sufficiently mature to embed in the endometrium of the uterus. This journey is thought to take several days if fertilisation has not taken place. The ovum is shed in the menstrual flow.

Surrounding the epithelium are two layers of *muscle*, an inner circular layer and an outer longitudinal layer. These muscular layers assist the propulsion of the ovum along the uterine tube by producing waves of peristalsis. Covering the uterine tubes is *peritoneum*, which forms the broad ligament.

Blood, nerves and lymph

The uterine and ovarian arteries and veins provide blood. Nerve supply is provided through the ovarian plexus, and lymphatic drainage is into the lumbar nodes.

Supporting structures

The uterine tubes are supported by the infundi-

> **Box 13.4** Ectopic pregnancy
>
> In rare instances after fertilisation, movement of the ovum along the uterine tube is delayed. The blastocyst embeds outside the uterus, usually in the wall of the tube. However, in 5% of such cases, the fertilised ovum embeds in the abdomen, on the ovary or in the cervix. Any pregnancy where a fetus develops outside the uterus is termed *ectopic pregnancy*. Tubal pregnancies are the most common type of ectopic pregnancy, occuring in 1 in 150 pregnancies. They are a major cause of maternal mortality in the UK (Griffiths 1998).
>
> A *tubal pregnancy* occurs usually as a result of narrowing or damage to the uterine tube caused by pathological changes or infection. Some factors that appear to increase the likelihood of a tubal pregnancy are increasing age, the use of intrauterine contraceptive devices, and previous abdominal surgery (Sweet 1997). *Signs of pregnancy* are apparent initially, but as the embryo increases in size the uterine tube becomes distended and the woman will complain of *abdominal pain*, possibly with a small amount of *vaginal bleeding* (Symonds & Symonds 1998). If diagnosis is delayed, the tube will rupture causing severe intra-abdominal haemorrhage with abdominal pain and *shock*. This is a surgical emergency and requires prompt treatment, which may include removal of, or surgery to, the uterine tube. Both of these interventions will reduce the woman's subsequent fertility (Gould 1997). However, if the condition is diagnosed early, medical treatment is possible that minimises the risks of surgery (Maiolates & Peddicord 1996).

---

bulopelvic ligaments. These are folds of the broad ligament, extending from the infundibulum to the lateral walls of the pelvis.

The ovaries

The *ovaries* are the female *gonads* or sex organs. They lie in the peritoneal cavity, in a small depression in the posterior wall of the broad ligament, one on each side of the uterus, close to the fimbriated ends of the uterine tubes.

The functions of the ovaries are:

- to produce ova regularly during the fertile years
- to produce the hormones oestrogen and progesterone.

The ovaries are dull white and almond shaped, with an irregular surface. After puberty they measure approximately 30 mm in length, 20 mm in width and are 10 mm thick. They weigh 5–8 g each.

Microscopically, the ovaries are covered by a layer of peritoneum, the *germinal epithelium*, enclosing a tough fibrous membrane, the *tunica albuginea* (Fig. 13.5). The ovary consists of an inner medulla and an outer cortex. The *medulla* contains blood and lymphatic vessels supported by connective tissue. The *cortex* contains ovarian follicles in various stages of development, embedded in fibrous tissue.

In the female fetus, *primordial* (primitive) *follicles* are formed by the 6th month of pregnancy. It is thought that approximately 5 million are present at this time. Most of these degenerate during the remaining pregnancy, leaving around 2 million at birth. Many more of these degenerate before puberty, and only 400–500 will eventually develop for ovulation and possible fertilisation. Any damage to the primordial follicles will affect the fertility of the woman, as no more are produced after the 6th month of pregnancy (Box 13.5).

Ovarian follicles undergo several stages of development during the 28 days of an average reproductive cycle. From about day five of the cycle, several primordial follicles start to mature under the influence of follicle-stimulating hormone from the pituitary gland. These are *secondary follicles*, and are composed of an outer covering of cells enclosing fluid, with an inner lining of granulosa cells surrounding an ovum.

Box 13.5 Infertility

In the UK 1 in 10 couples has difficulty conceiving (Llewellyn-Jones 1994). Fertility problems are often complex, and include female and male disorders (see Box 12.1). In women, *damage to the ovaries* at any time will have a profound effect on fertility, because all ova are present in a primitive form from early in the development of the female fetus. No regeneration is possible after birth.

The main types of female infertility relate to ovulation or damage to the uterine tubes. Hormonal disorders preventing regular *ovulation* can be treated relatively successfully (Taylor et al 1995). Damage to the uterine tubes, however, usually caused by *infection* or *endometriosis*, requires surgery, which is less successful. In such cases alternative forms of treatment, such as in-vitro fertilisation, carry a higher success rate (Prossar 1997). If the ovaries or any other part of the female reproductive system have been badly damaged or malformed (Box 13.3), there is likely to be no treatment (Quinn & Lowdermilk 1995).

Once follicle matures, into a Graafian follicle, it migrates through the cortex of the ovary towards the surface. Increasing amounts of oestrogen are also released from the maturing Graafian follicle. More and more fluid is secreted into it, raising the tension internally, making the covering increasingly thin, until finally it ruptures, releasing the ovum into the peritoneal cavity close to the fimbriae of the uterine tube. This is called *ovulation*, and is thought to be induced by hormonal changes. It is commonly accompanied by pelvic pain, known as *Mittelschmerz* or ovulation pain.

Ovulation occurs approximately once a month, from alternative ovaries. Occasionally more than

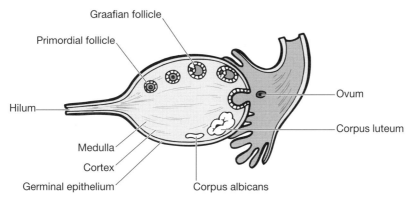

Figure 13.5 Microstructure of the ovary showing follicles in all stages of development.

one ovum is released, resulting in the possibility of a multiple pregnancy.

The ruptured Graafian follicle bleeds into the cavity vacated by the ovum. The granulosa cells multiply rapidly to produce a dense mass. The follicle becomes a *corpus luteum*, functioning as an endocrine gland producing oestrogen and progesterone for 14 days, after which it degenerates if fertilisation has not taken place. After degeneration, a white scar is left in the ovary, the *corpus albicans*.

Blood, nerves and lymph

Blood supply to the ovaries is from the ovarian arteries and into ovarian veins. Nerve supply is from the ovarian plexus. Lymph drainage is into the posterior abdominal nodes.

Supporting structures

The ovaries are attached to the *broad ligament* that weakly supports them. Further support is provided by the *ovarian ligaments*, which are attached to the cornua of the uterus. Laterally the ovaries are supported by the *infundibulopelvic ligaments*, that attach them to the lateral walls of the pelvic cavity.

HORMONAL CONTROL

The female reproductive system is fully functional from menarche to menopause. Menarche is the time of the first menstruation; menopause is the time when the reproductive (or menstrual) cycle ceases, usually around the age of 45–55. The reproductive cycle usually lasts about 4 weeks, and prior to the menopause will be interrupted only by pregnancy or breast-feeding.

The menarche

No hormonal activity relating to reproduction occurs in girls until the age of about 7, when pituitary hormones are released in response to stimuli from the hypothalamus. Ovarian follicles begin to produce small quantities of oestrogen, which increase gradually until, generally between the age of 10 and 16, the hormonal control of reproduction becomes mature and ovulation begins, followed by the first menstruation, the *menarche*.

Increasing levels of oestrogen during the period termed *puberty* produce many changes to the female body, principally:

- the deposition of fat to give the mature female shape
- growth of hair in the axilla and pubic area
- growth and development of the uterus, vagina and breasts
- the onset of menstruation.

The menopause

The *menopause*, also referred to as the climacteric or 'the change of life', is the period of time during which the reproductive cycle declines and then ceases altogether. It generally starts between the ages of 45 and 55, though it can begin in women as young as 35. This natural physiological process can take between 6 months and 3 years to complete.

In the early stages, the follicles remaining in the ovaries gradually produce less and less oestrogen. The reproductive cycles become irregular and, increasingly, ovulation does not take place. Once ovulation and oestrogen production have ceased, the woman is said to be post-menopausal.

It is the reduced oestrogen levels that cause many of the symptoms experienced by some menopausal and post-menopausal women, such as hot flushes, night sweats, emotional and sexual problems, and loss of bone density.

The reproductive cycle

The *reproductive cycle* is the result of the interactions of hormones from the hypothalamus, anterior pituitary gland and ovary. The outcomes of this hormonal interplay are:

1. the release of an ovum from the ovary
2. the preparation of the uterus to receive a fertilised ovum (Fig. 13.6).

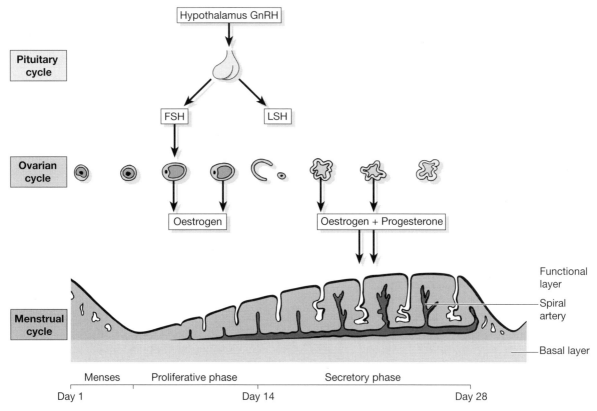

Figure 13.6 Summary of the reproductive cycle.

Each of these processes can be examined separately, as the ovarian and the menstrual cycles. However, they are both interdependent and occur concurrently. Together they make up the reproductive cycle which, in most women, lasts 28–30 days, though it can vary from 21–42 days, or more. Conventionally, the onset of menstruation is considered to be the first day of the cycle. At this time oestrogen and progesterone are at their lowest levels.

The ovarian cycle

The hypothalamus in the brain is the initiator of the reproductive cycle, although it releases its hormones in response to hormone levels in the bloodstream. The hypothalamus produces *gonadotrophin-releasing hormone (GnRH)* in response to low levels of oestrogen and progesterone. The

rising levels of GnRH stimulate the anterior lobe of the pituitary gland to secrete *follicle-stimulating hormone (FSH)*. This controls the growth and maturation of secondary follicles in the ovary, which also begin to secrete *oestrogen*. Eventually one secondary follicle matures more rapidly than the others, which degenerate. The remaining follicle matures into a Graafian follicle. This stage continues for an average of 14 days.

High oestrogen levels inhibit the release of FSH by the anterior pituitary gland. Instead, it releases *luteinising hormone (LH)* initially with a small, sudden increase that is thought to initiate ovulation. The Graafian follicle ruptures to release the ovum and cells proliferate to form the corpus luteum. The corpus luteum secretes *progesterone* as well as *oestrogen*. This continues for about 12 days, unless fertilisation of an ovum takes place. If the ovum is not fertilised, the corpus luteum degenerates, releasing decreasing amounts of oestrogen and progesterone. The reproductive cycle then begins again.

The menstrual cycle

The varying levels of oestrogen and later progesterone during the ovarian cycle also affect the endometrium of the uterus. The *endometrium* is composed of a basal layer capable of producing many cells to produce a thick temporary layer, the functional layer. The proliferation and shedding of the functional layer is referred to as the uterine or *menstrual cycle*.

The thickened glandular endometrium is well supplied with blood vessels and provides nourishment for the fertilised ovum. If no fertilised ovum is present, it is shed as the menstrual flow. The functional layer is composed of columnar epithelium interspersed with glands, supported by connective tissue, and containing many blood capillaries.

The development of the endometrium goes through three distinct phases:

1. menstruation, days 1–5
2. the proliferative phase, days 6–15
3. the secretory phase, days 16–28.

Menstruation. The endometrium is shed down to the basal layer. This is initiated when the spiral arteries of the endometrium go into spasm, leading to the withdrawal of the blood supply. As a result, the cells of the endometrium die (necrosis). Muscular contractions expel the dead tissue through the cervix. Blood and tissue loss is on average 50–150 ml in total.

The proliferative phase. The endometrium thickens and the glands lengthen under the influence of oestrogen from the Graafian follicle.

The secretory phase. The glands in the endometrium become coiled and produce nutritive secretions, such as glycogen, under the influence of both oestrogen and progesterone from the corpus luteum. The lining of the endometrium becomes more vascular and extra tissue fluid collects there. These conditions are optimal 7 days after ovulation, the time when a fertilised ovum is most likely to enter the uterus for embedding.

Each menstrual cycle indicates that the body is being prepared for pregnancy. Many women have irregular cycles. However, whatever the length of the cycle, the interval between ovulation and menstruation remains fairly constant. This interval is commonly 14 days – which means that in a 42-day cycle, ovulation occurs on day 28, and in a 21-day cycle, ovulation occurs on day 7. In other words, the length of a woman's secretory phase remains constant. It is her proliferative phase that varies, making her cycles longer or shorter. This can cause difficulties for a woman who experiences irregular cycles to plan or avoid a pregnancy if she is unable to use a mechanical or hormonal method of contraception (Box 13.6).

OOGENESIS

Oogenesis is the process by which mature ova are formed. It starts in the ovaries of the female fetus, where specialised cells begin a series of divisions and developmental changes, which are not completed until a mature ovum is released during each reproductive cycle, from the menarche to the menopause.

During early fetal life, primitive or *primordial germ cells* migrate from the yolk sac to the ovaries, where they develop into oogonia. *Oogonia* contain 46 chromosomes in 23 homologous (similar) pairs, as do all other cells in the fetus. During the 3rd month of fetal life, oogonia divide by *mitosis* to form larger primary oocytes, also containing 46 chromosomes.

After the 5th month of fetal life, the *primary oocytes* begin the early stages of the reduction division of *meiosis*. This division is not completed until each oocyte is ovulated, from puberty. The primary oocytes are each surrounded by a single layer of cells forming a primitive or *primordial follicle*.

From puberty, and at the start of each reproductive cycle, several primitive follicles respond to rising levels of FSH, by enlarging and maturing. During each cycle, only one continues this process of maturation, whilst the remainder degenerate. The primitive ovum completes the reduction division of meiosis, resulting in two cells. Each of these cells contains 23 chromo-

---

Box 13.6   Contraception

Many different *contraceptive methods* have been developed that allow women to choose not to become pregnant following sexual intercourse. Hormonal methods, such as the *contraceptive pill*, have proved very effective. These inhibit ovulation by supplying progesterone and/or oestrogen to interrupt the normal reproductive cycle. Hormonal *implants* such as Norplant, developed in the 90s, provide a constant supply of progesterone, and so avoid the problem of compliance associated with the pill and other methods. Though effective and convenient, hormonal contraceptives do produce side-effects in some women.

Barrier methods such as the male and female *condoms* and the *diaphragm* are another option. These have the advantage of not interfering with normal body functioning. The diaphragm works by lying diagonally across the cervix, preventing sperm from passing. Condoms have the additional benefit of protecting the users from sexually transmitted diseases. The male condom is the most popular method of contraception for both purposes (Silverstone 1997).

The *intrauterine device* (the coil), is another effective choice for some women. It works by preventing implantation of the fertilised ovum into the endometrium of the uterus.

For permanent infertility, *sterilisation* by ligation of the uterine tubes may be the method of choice.

Physiological methods can also be used if other forms of contraception are not acceptable. Collectively these methods are termed 'natural family planning'. Their effectiveness depends on which particular method is used, and how proficient the user is (Urwin 1997). Knowledge of the reproductive cycle enables a woman to calculate the 'safe periods' before and after ovulation, when fertilisation is impossible. Recognition of the cyclical changes to cervical secretions allows these times to be more accurately pinpointed. This is the basis of the *Billing's method* of contraception (Trent & Clark 1997). When combined with temperature readings, this method is known as the sympto-thermal method.

The most effective forms of contraception are male or female sterilisation, followed by hormonal methods. *Withdrawal* of the penis before ejaculation gives little protection against pregnancy, and is not recommended as a method of contraception.

---

somes (including an X sex chromosome), one from each homologous pair.

The *first polar body* is the smaller of the two cells, and it plays no further role in reproduction. The second cell contains the majority of the cytoplasm from the cell division, and it becomes the *secondary oocyte* that will subsequently become the mature ovum. The follicle itself becomes the *secondary follicle*. The secondary oocyte now enters the second division of meiosis, but this is not completed until fertilisation has occurred.

At ovulation both the secondary oocyte and the first polar body are discharged from the ovary. The secondary oocyte is wafted into the uterine tube and awaits fertilisation. Should a spermatozoon penetrate the ovum, the second meiotic division is immediately completed. This creates two cells, each containing 23 chromosomes, one once again being smaller than the other. The smaller cell is the *second polar body* and it subsequently disintegrates, as does the first polar body. The larger cell is now the fertilised *ovum*.

REFERENCES

Freeman S B 1995 Common genitourinary infections. Journal of Obstetric, Gynecologic and Neonatal Nursing 24(8):735–742

Gould D 1997 Ectopic pregnancy: causes and outcomes. Nursing Times 93(14):53–55

Griffiths J 1998 How to save eight lives a year. Nursing Standard 12(25):18

Jamieson L 1993 Preparing for parenthood: daily life in pregnancy. In: Bennett V R, Brown L K (eds) Myles textbook for midwives, 12th edn. Churchill Livingstone, Edinburgh, p 120

Kelnar C J H, Harvey D, Simpson C 1995 The sick newborn baby, 3rd edn. Baillière Tindall, London, p 346–348

Llewellyn-Jones D 1994 Fundamentals of obstetrics and gynaecology, 6th edn. Mosby, London, p 239

McConville B 1998 Female circumcision. Nursing Times 94(3):34–36

Maiolates C R, Peddicord K 1996 Methotrxate for nonsurgical treatment of ectopic pregnancy. Nursing implications. Journal of Obstetric, Gynecologic and Neonatal Nursing 25(3):205–208

Matthew J 1993 Structural abnormalities affecting pregnancy. In: Bennett V R, Brown L K (eds) Myles textbook for midwives, 12th edn. Churchill Livingstone, Edinburgh, p 377–378

Morris R 1996 The culture of female circumcision. Advances in Nursing Science 19(2):43–45

Prossar C 1997 Methods of in vitro fertilisation. Nursing Times 93(49):48–50

Quinn E B, Lowdermilk D L 1995 Common reproductive

concerns. In: Bobak I M, Lowdermilk D L, Jenson M D (eds) Maternity nursing, 4th edn. Mosby, St Louis, p 864–871

Silverstone T 1997 Condoms still the most popular contraceptive. Professional Care of the Mother and Child 7(4):108–110

Silverton L 1993 The art and science of midwifery. Prentice Hall, New York, p 235–350

Sweet B R (ed) 1997 Mayes' midwifery. A textbook for midwives, 12th edn. Baillière Tindall, London, p 520–522

Symonds E M, Symonds I M 1998 Essential obstetrics and gynaecology, 3rd edn. Churchill Livingstone, New York, p 89–94

Taylor A, Soubra A, Braude P 1995 Investigation and treatment. In: Meerbeau L, Denton J (eds) Infertility: nursing and caring. Scutari Press, London, p 71–75

Trent A J, Clark K 1997 What nurses should know about natural family planning. Journal of Obstetric, Gynecologic and Neonatal Nursing 26(6):643–648

Urwin J 1997 Current issues in contraception. Nursing Standard 11(19):39–45

Verralls S 1993 Anatomy and physiology applied to obstetrics. Churchill Livingstone, Edinburgh, p 87–90

Wang E, Smail F 1989 Infections in pregnancy. In: Chalmers I, Enkin E, Keirse M J N C (eds) Effective care in pregnancy and childbirth. Oxford University Press, Oxford, p 534–564

Wright J 1996 Female genital mutilation. Journal of Advanced Nursing 24(2):251–259

14

Fertilisation, the embryo and the fetus

Fertilisation occurs when a spermatozoon from the male unites with an ovum from the female. Approximately 265 days later, a newborn baby is delivered, capable of living independently of his mother.

During sexual intercourse, around 200–500 million spermatozoa are ejaculated in seminal fluid into the posterior fornix of the vagina. The majority either die in the harsh environment there or leak out. The remainder proceed on the long journey through the cervix, then the body of the uterus, along the uterine tube to the ampulla, where fertilisation usually occurs. This is a journey of approximately 200 mm, a vast distance for a microscopic cell.

During the fertile days of the female reproductive cycle, the cervical mucus becomes thin, stretchy and alkaline, providing favourable conditions for sperm survival. This mucus contains microscopic channels, that guide the spermatozoa towards the ovum.

Immediately after arrival in the vagina, the spermatozoa move into the cervix by rapid sideways movement of their head and flagellum (tail). As they pass through the cervix, and later the uterus and uterine tubes, they receive nourishment from the cells lining these structures.

Of the 200–500 million spermatozoa present in the original ejaculate, approximately 1 million reach the uterus, a few thousand reach the uterine tubes, and fewer than 100 are thought to meet the ovum, usually in the ampulla of the tube. This journey takes a few hours to complete. En route, the spermatozoa go through their final maturation process of *capacitation*, in which the protective covering on their head is removed to allow the activation of the enzymes carried in the acrosome.

At ovulation, the ovum is expelled forcibly from the ovary and is wafted into the uterine tube by the fimbriae. The ovum itself has no powers of movement, but is propelled along the uterine tube by the ciliated epithelium lining the tubes. Peristaltic waves in the uterine walls assist the process. If the spermatozoa reach the fimbriae of the uterine tube before the arrival of the ovum, they can wait for it there for up to 3 days – in some cases longer. Once the ovum is present, fertilisation by a spermatozoon will be attempted.

FERTILISATION

Although *fertilisation* usually takes place in the ampulla of the uterine tube, it can take place anywhere along its length. Spermatozoa home in on any egg-shaped mass they encounter, and very few actually reach the ovum itself. Those that do come into contact with the ovum butt against the corona radiata and zona pellucida that surround the cell membrane, releasing enzymes, including hyaluronidase, which are packaged in the acrosome in the head of the spermatozoon (Fig. 14.1). The enzymes from many spermatozoa break down the corona radiata and zona pellu-

---

Box 14.1 Multiple pregnancies

Occasionally, more than one developing fetus is detected during pregnancy. This is a multiple pregnancy. Around 1 in 100 pregnancies involve two fetuses, and 1 in 8000–9000 involve three fetuses. It is very rare for there to be more than three fetuses (Grant 1993), although quadruplets, quintuplets, sextuplets do occur naturally. Their incidence has increased as a result of certain types of infertility treatment (Ellings et al 1998). The risks, both during pregnancy and at delivery, of multiple pregnancies with more than three fetuses, are considerable (Silverton 1993).

A natural multiple pregnancy can come about in one of two ways. The first is when two or more ova are released at ovulation, each of which is fertilised. The resulting twins (termed binovular), triplets etc. are non-identical, and resemble each other as much or as little as any brothers or sisters. Alternatively, early in development, the embryo can split into two or more separate embryos. The resulting children are identical, and are referred to as monozygous, or uniovular.

In multiple pregnancies, there is a greatly increased risk of fetal abnormality, and therefore of abortion (Symonds & Symonds 1998). Occasionally one twin dies in utero, while the second develops normally. This lost twin may be aborted or may be retained in utero. A rare occurrence is that of a twin who has died in early pregnancy appearing at delivery as a flattened paper-thin fetus, a condition known as fetus papyraceous (Grant 1993).

Delivery of any multiple pregnancy carries an increased risk of complications and women expecting twins, triplets, etc. require close monitoring and are advised to plan delivery in an obstetric unit (Silverton 1993).

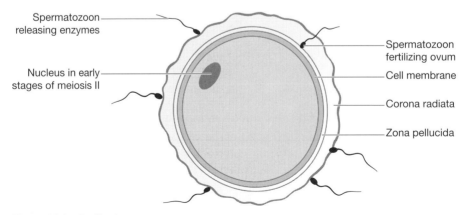

Figure 14.1 Fertilisation.

cida to allow access to the ovum. Only one spermatozoon will eventually penetrate the ovum. Once the spermatozoon has penetrated the cell membrane, the membrane alters its configuration to prevent any other spermatozoa entering (Box 14.1).

Spermatozoa can live for a maximum of 3–4 days. An ovum lives for maximum of 48 hours. Fertilisation is most likely to occur, therefore, when intercourse takes place not more than 48 hours before or 24 hours after ovulation.

Only the head of the spermatozoon is taken into the ovum, the tail having been shed. The DNA in the nucleus of the spermatozoon is then released, triggering the final meiotic division by the female chromosomes. Two sets of female chromosomes are formed, one being discarded as a second polar body and the other set joining with the male chromosomes to give the full complement of 46 chromosomes. As a result, all the information required to determine the development of a unique individual, combining both maternal and paternal characteristics, is present in the fertilised ovum, which is now called a *zygote*.

The zygote continues to move along the uterine tube for 3–5 days. During this time, mitotic cell division takes place, producing first 2, then 4, 8, 16, and then 32 cells, and so on, doubling the number of cells (Fig. 14.2) every 12–15 hours –

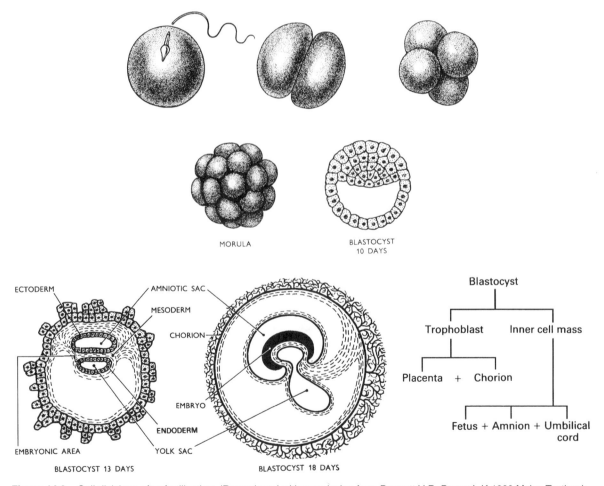

Figure 14.2 Cell divisions after fertilisation. (Reproduced with permission from Bennett V R, Brown L K 1999 Myles Textbook for Midwives, 13th edn. Churchill Livingstone, Edinburgh)

although the zygote does not increase in overall size. The cells remain inside the zona pellucida, preventing the zygote from adhering to the mucosa of the uterine tubes and from being recognised and rejected by the maternal immune system. Eventually a cluster of undifferentiated cells resembling a berry is formed in the zona pellucida. This is termed a *morula* (Latin for little mulberry).

As the cells continue to divide, the undifferentiated mass becomes organised into a fluid-filled cavity. This is the *blastocyst*. The outer layer of blastocyst cells is the *trophoblast*, and the remaining cells are clumped together at one end, forming the *inner cell mass*. The trophoblast will subsequently develop into the placenta and chorion, and the inner cell mass becomes the fetus, cord and amnion. Cell specialisation begins.

IMPLANTATION

The ovum, now developed into the blastocyst, reaches the uterus about 5 days after fertilisation. In the uterus the blastocyst lies close to the endometrium for a day or two more, to allow the trophoblast to secrete an enzyme which breaks down the endometrium surface. The blastocyst then embeds deep into the endometrium, where it can be nourished and continue to develop. A small implantation bleed from the vagina may be observed at this time, and may be mistaken as menstruation.

Small finger-like projections develop around the entire blastocyst from the trophoblast, aiding the process of *implantation* and anchoring the blastocyst firmly into the endometrium. These projections are called the primitive *chorionic villi*. Some of them will continue developing into the mature placenta, whilst the remainder will atrophy to form the chorionic membrane which lines the uterus. Implantation, or nidation, is normally complete by the 11th day after fertilisation.

Once the blastocyst becomes embedded, the endometrium is known as the *decidua*. Under the influence of the rising levels of oestrogen and progesterone of pregnancy, the decidua becomes several times thicker than the non-pregnant endometrium, and nourishes the fertilised ovum throughout pregnancy. The area where the blastocyst has burrowed into the decidua rapidly heals and covers over. That portion beneath the embedded blastocyst becomes the *decidua basalis*, and the portion covering the blastocyst, the *decidua capsularis*. The chorionic villi situated beneath the decidua capsularis subsequently atrophy, due to the lack of nutrients in this area.

THE EMBRYO

Once the blastocyst has become embedded in the decidua, it is known as the embryo (Fig. 14.3).

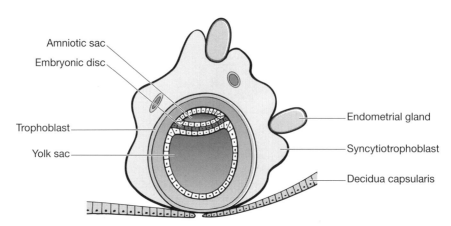

Amniotic sac
Embryonic disc
Trophoblast
Yolk sac
Endometrial gland
Syncytiotrophoblast
Decidua capsularis

Figure 14.3 The early embryo, day 12.

Embryo is the term given to the developing mass of cells from implantation until 8 weeks' gestation. It is during this time that all the body systems and organs are laid down in a rudimentary form. For the remaining 30 weeks, they have simply to grow and mature.

The embryo undergoes rapid development from this time. The first stage is the formation of two enclosed cavities lying in close proximity to each other: the amniotic and yolk sacs. The embryo develops from an area between these two sacs, the *embryonic disc*. Three layers of cells develop in this region:

1. the layer closest to the amniotic sac is the *ectoderm*, and it will form the skin and much of the central nervous system of the embryo
2. the central layer, the *mesoderm*, will form the bones, muscles, heart and blood vessels, and certain internal organs such as the kidneys and reproductive organs
3. the *endoderm* lies close to the yolk sac and will form much of the digestive and respiratory organs, as well as the glands and mucous membranes.

The amniotic sac is filled with fluid and will eventually enclose the embryo. The yolk sac provides nourishment for the trophoblast until the chorionic villi are sufficiently mature to take over this role.

Rapid development in the form of *organogenesis*, organ formation, takes place until the 8th week of gestation. The main stages of embryonic development are listed below.

- Day 13: Chorionic villi begin to secrete *human chorionic gonadotrophin* (hCG), which stimulates the corpus luteum in the ovary to continue producing the hormones necessary to maintain the pregnancy until the placenta is mature enough to take over this role (Box 14.2).
- Day 15: A thick band of cells, *the primitive streak*, appears in the midline of the dorsal surface of the embryo. Blood vessels begin to form. Cell specialisation begins.
- Days 18–21: The primitive nervous system begins to fold into position. The heart begins to twitch. Primitive eyes and ears begin differentiation. Red blood cells begin development.

Box 14.2   Diagnosis of pregnancy

Many women quickly suspect they are pregnant, because of the early symptoms they experience, such as amenorrhoea, nausea and tender breasts, caused by the different and rising levels of hormones in their body.

It is unusual nowadays to confirm pregnancy by vaginal examination. Instead, one of the simplest methods of diagnosing pregnancy is by examining urine for human chorionic gonadotrophin (hCG). This hormone is secreted from the trophoblast of the developing embryo from implantation, to maintain the corpus luteum until the placenta can take over hormonal control of the pregnancy. Sufficient hCG is present in maternal blood for adequate amounts to be excreted and show up in the urine by the 28th day of pregnancy (Alexander et al 1989). Sensitive blood tests can pick up hCG earlier, soon after implantation (Klopper 1991). By 8 weeks, the pregnancy can be confirmed by ultrasound.

- Weeks 3–4: The heart begins to pump blood, and the brain divides into forebrain, midbrain and hindbrain. Outlines of the eyes can be seen above the mouth. Lungs begin to form. Features of the gastrointestinal system can be identified. Somites – future vertebrae and muscles – appear to either side of the midline.
- Week 5: Rapid brain growth continues. Limb buds appear. The umbilical cord is formed. The heart chamber is divided by septa.
- Week 6: The liver begins to function. Rudimentary kidneys and genitalia form. Eyes migrate to the front of the face (Fig. 14.4). Cartilage begins to form the skeleton. Muscle differentiation begins.
- Week 7: Eyelids form, as well as the gallbladder, palate and tongue. The neck becomes visible. The diaphragm develops to separate the abdominal and thoracic cavities. Bone cells begin to replace cartilage. Arms and legs begin movement.
- Week 8: Hands and feet are now well formed. The heart has four chambers and beats at 40–60 beats per minute. Major blood vessels form, and circulation begins through the umbilical cord. External genitalia can be distinguished as male or female.

By the end of week 8, all the body systems and organs are formed, and the embryo becomes known as the fetus (Fig. 14.5). The mother has only missed two menstrual cycles, and the uterus is still in the pelvic cavity.

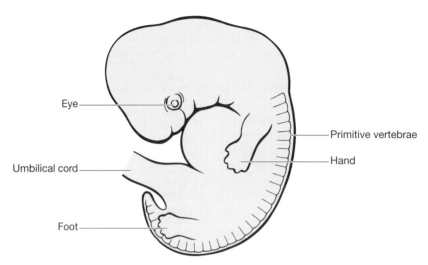

Figure 14.4 Embryo, week 6.

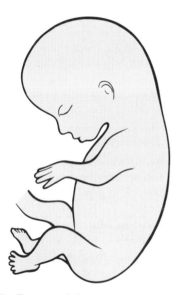

Figure 14.5 Fetus, week 8.

The uterus is an ideal environment for the development of the embryo, and yet many embryos develop major defects, due to either environmental or genetic factors, or a combination of both. Many of these grossly abnormal embryos are aborted spontaneously during the first 5 or 6 weeks of pregnancy. Often the mother does not even realise she was pregnant, thinking her period merely late. Whilst genetic defects are usually unavoidable, environmental damage can be minimised if, from before conception, the pregnant woman considers carefully her diet and environment, and avoids noxious substances such as cigarettes and drugs (Box 14.3).

For the first 14 days after conception, the embryo is largely protected from harm by the zona pellucida. It is not until after implantation that the embryo is exposed to teratogens circulating in the fluids of the mother's body. A *teratogen* is any substance, process or agent that produces a malformation in the embryo or fetus. Common teratogens are drugs, chemicals, infectious agents and radiation. The degree of damage to the embryo depends very much on the stage of development of each system or organ. Each system has *critical periods* of development (Moore 1989). During the fetal period, teratogens will not cause major structural defects as all the organs have already been formed. Minor structural defects may occur but fetal damage tends to result in mild to serious functional abnormalities, such as mental retardation or blindness.

FETAL DEVELOPMENT

The fetal period extends from the 8th week of gestation until delivery, which happens, on average, at 38 weeks. Most systems have been formed before the onset of fetal life, but their functioning has yet to be fully developed. Some

Box 14.3   Preconception care

Approximately 2% of babies born at or near term have some form of defect (Kelnar et al 1995). Many of these are caused by environmental factors, which could be avoided by ensuring good health before the pregnancy occurs (Lumley & Astbury 1989).

Preconception care aims to enable both partners to be in optimum health before conception. Any health problems are detected and treated, where possible, before a pregnancy is attempted. Factors examined include:

- physical health, weight and age
- reproductive health, taking into consideration the intervals between births, and the type(s) of contraception used
- exercise, to improve overall health, especially of the heart and lungs
- previous medical history, looking at conditions such as epilepsy and diabetes, the presence of infections in the vagina, and immunity to rubella
- abuse of substances such as alcohol, cigarettes, illegal or over-the-counter drugs
- relatives' medical history, to highlight any genetic defects that could be passed on
- environmental risks at work, such as exposure to anaesthetic gases, and at home, such as catching toxoplasmosis from cleaning out cat litter trays
- diet – a well-balanced diet being basic to the health of both parents and especially to the health of a subsequent fetus.

Taking the first letter of each of these factors enables couples who are planning a pregnancy to be adequately PREPARED for their future pregnancy, with advice from health professionals (Dickerson 1995). This will minimise the risks to the unborn child of environmental hazards (Paul 1997).

further differentiation of body organs continues until the 20th week. The main stages of fetal development are listed below.

- Weeks 8–12: The head constitutes half the fetal length. Teeth form in the gums and fingernails can be seen. The intestines become established in the abdominal cavity and the fetus begins to swallow amniotic fluid and pass urine. Blood begins to form. The external genitalia differentiate and can be identified.
- Weeks 13–16: The fetus grows rapidly, almost doubling in length. Facial features migrate to their correct position and the face is identifiable as human. Both muscle and bone develop rapidly, enabling plenty of fetal movement to occur. Meconium begins to form in the gut.
- Weeks 17–24: The fetal heart can be heard by

fetal stethoscope, and the mother begins to feel movement. Vernix is formed, indicating functioning sebaceous glands. The lungs are well formed, and capillaries are developing around the alveoli. Hair develops on the head, eyebrows and eyelids. The eyes are structurally complete.

- Weeks 25–28: Subcutaneous fat is laid down and the eyes open. Lung physiology is sufficiently developed to enable gas exchange to begin (Box 14.4). The nervous system can control temperature and breathing movements.
- Week 29: The fetus is fully formed and the organs are able to function to some extent.

For the remainder of pregnancy, organ physiology matures and the fetus continues to lay down fat and muscle. The nervous system continues myelinisation beyond term.

Box 14.4   The preterm infant

The problems that preterm babies have depend on how premature they are, and how well developed their body systems are. Common problems in babies born well before term include temperature regulation, respiration, feeding, jaundice and infection (Thomson 1993).

In the preterm infant the heat-regulating centre in the hypothalamus is immature (Param 1995). Additionally, stores of brown fat and subcutaneous fat have not been laid down and there is reduced muscular activity. Care must be taken therefore to use warmed or heated equipment for the preterm infant, and to keep him covered if at all possible.

To sustain respiration, ventilator support may be needed and expert care is required to ensure adequate oxygenation. Apnoea is common in babies less than 34 weeks' gestation, and so the necessary equipment must be available.

Adequate feeding is essential to provide sufficient glucose for the metabolic needs of the infant. As many of the primitive reflexes required for taking milk feeds are absent or poorly developed, nutrition may need to be provided intravenously or via a nasogastric tube. Breast milk is best, although some supplements may be required (Jones 1994).

Jaundice is more likely in the preterm infant, because his liver will be particularly immature. Treatment must be initiated quickly if bilirubin levels rise to a toxic level.

Preterm infants have a reduced ability to fight infection, as they have had insufficient time in utero to acquire maternal immunoglobulins, and their own ability to produce antibodies will be immature.

Delivery of a fetus before term should therefore ideally be carried out in a specialist unit that has the necessary neonatal services.

REFERENCES

Alexander S, Stanwell-Smith R, Buekins P, Keirse M J N C 1989 Biochemical assessment of fetal well-being. In: Chalmers I, Enkin E, Keirse M J N C (eds) Effective care in pregnancy and childbirth. Oxford University Press, Oxford, p 455–476

Dickerson J 1995 Good preconception care starts at school. Modern Midwife 5(11):15–18

Ellings J M, Newman R B, Bowers N A 1998 Prenatal care and multiple pregnancy. Journal of Obstetric, Gynecologic and Neonatal Nursing 27(4):457–465

Grant B 1993 Multiple pregnancy. In: Bennett V R, Brown L K (eds) Myles textbook for midwives, 12th edn. Churchill Livingstone, Edinburgh, p 365–376

Jones E 1994 Breast feeding in the preterm infant. Modern Midwife 4(1):22–26

Kelnar C J H, Harvey D, Simpson C 1995 The sick newborn baby, 3rd edn. Baillière Tindall, London, p 197

Klopper A 1991 Placental metabolism. In: Hytten F, Chamberlain G (eds) Clinical physiology in obstetrics, 2nd edn. Blackwell Scientific, Oxford, p 397–400

Lumley J, Astbury J 1989 Advice for pregnancy. In: Chalmers I, Enkin E, Keirse M J N C (eds) Effective care in pregnancy and childbirth. Oxford University Press, Oxford, p 237–254

Moore K L 1989 Before we are born: basic embryology and birth defects, 3rd edn. W B Saunders, Philadelphia

Param L 1995 Specific problems of the newborn at risk. In: Bobak I M, Lowdermilk D L, Jenson M D (eds) Maternity nursing, 4th edn. Mosby, St Louis, p 777–781

Paul M 1997 Occupational reproductive hazards. Lancet 349: 1385–1388

Silverton L 1993 The art and science of midwifery. Prentice Hall, New York, p 224–234

Sweet B R (ed) 1997 Mayes' midwifery. A textbook for midwives, 12th edn. Baillière Tindall, London, p 177

Symonds E M, Symonds I M 1998 Essential obstetrics and gynaecology, 3rd edn. Churchill Livingstone, New York, p 125

Thomson E 1993 Small and large babies. In: Bennett V R, Brown L K (eds) Myles textbook for midwives, 12th edn. Churchill Livingstone, Edinburgh, p 559–571

15

The pregnant uterus

The uterus undergoes immense changes in size and shape during pregnancy. These have a considerable impact on the body as a whole, altering the functioning of other organs and systems. Many of these alterations are necessary to maintain the pregnancy; others are merely side-effects, but often cause discomfort to the pregnant woman.

Labour depends entirely on efficient contraction and retraction of uterine muscle. The anatomy of the vagina allows the passage of the fetus into the outside world. On completion of labour and delivery, the uterus is ideally structured to prevent haemorrhage, and to revert to its non-pregnant state.

THE PREGNANT UTERUS

The size of the uterus increases dramatically during pregnancy. The *non-pregnant* uterus measures 75 mm in length, 50 mm in width and 25 mm in depth (Fig. 15.1). *At term*, it measures an average of 300 mm by 230 mm by 200 mm. The non-pregnant uterus weighs approximately 60 g, increasing to 900 g at 40 weeks of pregnancy. These remarkable increases in size and weight are controlled by oestrogen, which acts on the myometrium to increase the size of individual muscle cells (*hypertrophy*), and the number of muscle cells (*hyperplasia*). These two processes account for the growth which occurs up to 20 weeks' gestation; for the second half of pregnancy, growth is mainly due to the uterus stretching to accommodate the fetus.

Following implantation, the endometrium of

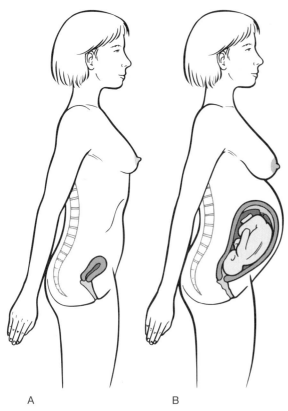

Figure 15.1 Change in the size of the uterus during pregnancy. A: non pregnant; B: pregnant.

the uterus becomes thicker and increasingly vascular, under the influence of oestrogen and progesterone from the corpus luteum. During pregnancy, the endometrium is known as the decidua. The *decidua* is thickest and most vascular in the fundus and upper body of the uterus, and it is here that the blastocyst most frequently embeds. Oestrogen stimulates the development of many new blood vessels in the uterine walls to provide sufficient oxygen and nutrients for these considerable changes to take place. The decidua provides all the nourishment for the blastocyst until the chorionic villi of the placenta are sufficiently developed to take over.

Growth of the uterus can be measured through the abdominal wall throughout pregnancy. Adequate growth of the uterus gives a good indication of the health and growth of the fetus. It also gives some indication of fetal size. Regular

palpation of the uterus reveals landmarks from which the gestation of the fetus can be estimated:

- At 12 weeks the fundus can be palpated just above the symphysis pubis
- At 20–22 weeks the fundus will normally be at the level of the umbilicus
- At 36 weeks the fundus will normally have reached the xiphisternum.

As the uterus grows, it also changes shape and position. The narrow *isthmus*, situated at the junction of the uterus and cervix measures only 7 mm in the non-pregnant uterus. It becomes elongated from implantation until around 10 weeks, by which time it measures 25 mm (Fig. 15.2). The uterus as a whole takes on a globular shape, sitting on an elongated stalk formed from the lengthened isthmus. At 12 weeks the uterus is in an upright position, having risen out of the pelvis, although it is usually inclined slightly to the right, due the position of the colon. This is referred to as *right obliquity of the uterus*. The fetus now takes up most of the cavity of the uterus, which takes on a more globular shape overall.

By the 30th week of pregnancy, the uterus can be seen to consist of two main parts. What was originally the isthmus has become the *lower uterine segment*, the walls of which contain circular and longitudinal smooth muscle layers. The walls of the remaining portion of the uterus,

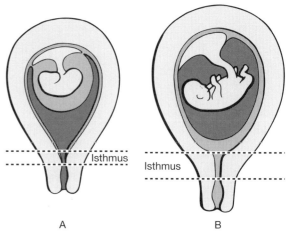

Figure 15.2 The enlarging isthmus during the early weeks of pregnancy. A: 6 weeks; B: 10 weeks.

the upper uterine segment, are thicker, as they contain these muscles plus a layer of oblique muscle.

By the 36th week of pregnancy, the lower uterine segment is well formed, measuring 80–100 mm long. Due to good muscle tone and softening of pelvic muscles and ligaments, the presenting part of the fetus moves into the lower uterine segment, giving the appearance of a decrease in fundal height. The movement may be into the true pelvis (engagement), particularly in the primigravida (a woman having her first baby). *Engagement* has occurred when the widest diameter of the presenting part, for example the head, has passed through the pelvic brim. Engagement in multiparous women often only occurs once labour begins, because abdominal muscles are more relaxed.

From around the 16th week of pregnancy, the uterine muscle undergoes intermittent gentle contractions that maintain muscle tone. These are known as Braxton Hicks contractions, and are felt by many women from early pregnancy. However, some women do not feel these contractions until they become stronger towards the end of pregnancy, and they may misinterpret them as labour.

The cervix

The cervix plays a vital role during pregnancy, acting as a barrier against infection. From early in pregnancy, progesterone influences the endocervical cells to secrete a plug of mucus to occlude the cervical canal, preventing passage of any microorganisms. This *operculum* remains in the cervical canal until labour begins, when dilatation of the cervix loosens it and it is shed as the '*show*' through the vagina, often accompanied by a small amount of blood (Box 15.1).

The vagina

Throughout pregnancy, the vagina is affected by the high levels of circulating hormones, particularly oestrogen. The muscle of the vaginal walls increases in thickness and the walls themselves become more elastic. An increase in the fluids

---

> **Box 15.1**   Incompetent cervix
>
> In 20% of recurrent abortions, particularly those which occur in the second trimester, the cervix is found to be dilating (without painful contractions) early in pregnancy (Grant 1989a). This condition is due to *cervical incompetence*. The cervix will usually have been damaged previously by dilatation and curettage (D and C), traumatic birth or uterine abnormality (Poole 1995).
>
> Treatment is designed to prevent premature dilatation of the cervix. Cervical cerclage is performed, a surgical procedure in which a nonabsorbable ribbon or suture is placed around the cervix. The suture is removed when labour begins, or 7 days before term. Treatment is very successful, with 80% of women delivering after the 36th week of pregnancy.

---

produced by the cells lining the vagina cause the discharge to be more profuse (*leucorrhoea*). The normal equilibrium of the vagina is disturbed by the increased hormones: the environment becomes more acid, preventing invasion by many bacteria, although some vaginal infections, particularly thrush, are more likely (Wang & Smail 1989).

Other structures

The ovaries cease functioning during pregnancy, due to the high levels of oestrogen and progesterone. The uterine tubes become stretched by the growing uterus and are pulled into an almost vertical position towards the end of pregnancy. The external genitalia receive an increased blood supply during pregnancy, also due to increased hormonal activity.

FIRST STAGE OF LABOUR

Labour is the physiological process during which the fetus, placenta and membranes are expelled through the birth canal after the 24th week of pregnancy. The initiation of labour is fully described in Chapter 3, and is thought to be the result of increased sensitivity of the myometrium to the effects of hormones, particularly oestrogen.

The first stage of labour begins with regular painful uterine contractions and ends when full dilatation of the cervix is achieved. It takes on average 12–14 hours in the primigravida, and 6–10 hours in the multiparous woman. However, the length of the first stage varies considerably between individuals and is influenced by both physiological and psychological factors (Crowther et al 1989).

The two processes involved in the first stage – uterine contraction and cervical dilatation – are described below.

Uterine contraction

Three factors govern *uterine contraction*:

1. fundal dominance
2. polarity
3. contraction and retraction.

Fundal dominance describes the initiation of each uterine contraction in the fundus of the uterus close to one of the cornua (Fig. 15.3). It is from this point that the contraction spreads across the fundus and down though the main body of the uterus to the cervix. This effect can be felt abdominally. Once the contraction has spread across the uterus, it fades from all areas simultaneously. The contraction lasts longest and is at its strongest at the fundus.

The result of fundal dominance is that the upper segment of the uterus contracts powerfully, whilst the lower uterine segment contracts less strongly and dilates. *Polarity* is the term which describes this neuromuscular harmony between the upper and lower segments, or poles,

of the uterus. In the absence of highly organised and coordinated muscular contractions (polarity) uterine function would be ineffective (Box 15.2).

The third factor involved in efficient uterine contraction is *contraction* and *retraction* of uterine muscle cells. After each contraction, the muscle cells never fully relax, but maintain a small degree of contraction. With each successive contraction, therefore, the muscle cells become shorter. This is what is meant by the term retraction. The result is that the upper segment of the uterus becomes gradually smaller and thicker, and its cavity becomes smaller, so the fetus is pushed down into the pelvis.

Cervical dilatation

Late in pregnancy, the internal os begins to dilate as a result of strengthening Braxton Hicks contractions. This is termed *effacement* of the cervix (Fig. 15.4). Once labour begins, uterine muscle fibres become shorter throughout the body of the uterus, so the internal os becomes part of the lower uterine segment. The cervix is fully effaced once the full length of the cervical canal has become one with the lower uterine segment. In the primigravida this process is usually well established before labour begins, whereas in the multigravida, effacement may take place along with cervical dilatation.

With the onset of labour, the external os of the cervix begins to dilate (Fig. 15.4D). As the uterine contractions grow stronger, so the muscle cells

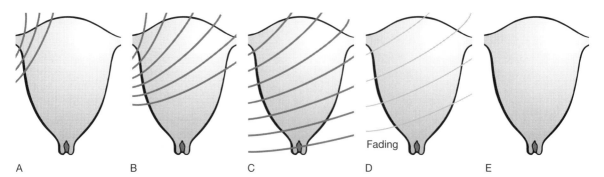

A   B   C   D Fading   E

Figure 15.3 Fundal dominance of uterine contractions. A: Contraction begins at the cornu. B: Contraction spreads over the fundus. C: Contraction involves the entire uterus. D: Contraction fades from all parts together. E: Contraction complete.

Box 15.2   Abnormal uterine action

Neuromuscular harmony is essential in the process of cervical dilatation: without coordinated contraction and retraction of uterine muscle, the cervix may not dilate. In some women the process of labour is slow and ineffective, either because the contractions are too weak or because they are incoordinate. In such cases it may be necessary to augment labour by administering synthetic oxytocin, syntocinon, to increase the efficiency of uterine contractions. In other women, labour is extremely rapid. Several types of abnormal uterine action have been identified, and are described below.

Hypotonic uterine action may occur at the onset of, or during, labour. Contractions are weak and infrequent. The cervix dilates slowly or not at all. Hypotonic contractions may be due to a long latent phase, in which case the pregnant woman can be encouraged to be active until true labour begins. In the primigravida, hypotonic uterine contractions may occur early in labour, with no known cause. In any labouring woman, hypotonic contractions may develop due to cephalopelvic disproportion (CPD) or malpresentation.

Incoordinate uterine action describes the situation where there is no neuromuscular harmony. Uterine contractions are frequent and painful, but the cervix is slow to dilate. This condition occurs in 4–6% of primigravida women (Llewellyn-Jones 1994). The cause is not always apparent, but may be due to malposition or mild CPD. Treatment involves correcting any dehydration or ketoacidosis and augmenting labour. In rare instances, the cervix ceases to dilate due to cervical dystocia, a condition caused by a scarred cervix or an anatomical abnormality (Silverton 1993).

In a *precipitate labour*, excessive uterine contractions occur, with strong and painful contractions from early in labour and rapid dilatation of the cervix. The labouring woman is often unprepared for this and so the baby may be delivered in an inappropriate environment. During a precipitate labour, the fetus may become distressed, because of the lack of time between contractions for the placenta to become perfused with oxygen and nutrients. Alternatively, the uterus may be overstimulated by the administration of syntocinon, and *hypertonic contractions* result (Keirse & Chalmers 1989). Part of the midwife's role is to observe induced or augmented labour to ensure that contractions do not occur too frequently.

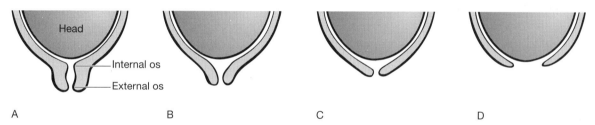

Figure 15.4   Effacement of the cervix. A: Cervix is closed. B: Cervix is partially effaced. C: Cervix is fully effaced. D: Cervix begins to dilate.

undergo increased contraction and retraction. Assessment of *cervical dilatation* is a good indication of the progress of labour. To allow the full-term fetus to pass through the cervix, a dilatation of 10 cm is required.

The regular painful uterine contractions that bring about cervical dilatation usually begin at 15–20 minute intervals, and last 30–40 seconds. The intervals shorten and the contractions become more intense, until at the height of labour, contractions occur every 2–3 minutes, each lasting for a full minute. During each contraction the placenta is compressed and blood flow is reduced. The fetus who has been healthy throughout preg-

nancy can accommodate this. However, contractions that come more frequently or last for more than one minute will starve the fetus of oxygen and may lead to fetal distress.

Other physiological changes

There are other important physiological changes which take place during the first stage of labour. These are described below:

● A *retraction ring* forms between the upper and lower uterine segments during labour. This is a ridge that may be palpable through the abdominal wall. It is formed at the junction where the thickened wall of the upper uterine segment meets the much thinned and distended wall of the lower segment. As labour progresses, the retraction ring may be felt to rise up the abdominal wall as the cavity becomes smaller and the fetus descends into the pelvis.

- The intensity of contractions increases as labour progresses, causing an *increase in intra-uterine pressure*, which can be measured using an internal transducer. However, this is an invasive procedure and so intrauterine pressure will normally be assessed externally, either by the midwife palpating the uterus during contractions, or by using an external transducer connected to a cardiotocograph (Box 15.3).
- The uterus is never fully relaxed during labour and the extent of the residual pressure can be felt by palpating the uterus. This is known as assessing the *resting tone* of the uterus. A low resting tone is essential between contractions to allow the placenta to become perfused with fresh blood for the respiration and nutrition of the fetus.
- Effacement and dilatation of the cervix lead to

Box 15.3 Cardiotocography

A *cardiotocograph* (CTG) can be used to monitor the condition of the fetus during pregnancy and labour. An ultrasound transducer is strapped to the abdomen of the woman where the fetal heart is clearly audible. This allows the fetal heart rate and variability (a sign of fetal wellbeing), to be monitored over time, and can be used as part of a biophysical profile to determine fetal health. During labour, an external pressure transducer can also be positioned on the fundus of the uterus to monitor uterine contractions. These two monitors allow the fetus's response to uterine contractions to be observed.

The use of a CTG in labour is the subject of much debate. In low-risk women, CTG monitoring has been found to be no better than intermittent auscultation with a Pinard stethoscope or hand-held Doppler ultrasound (Grant 1989b). Often, interpretation of the tracing is open to debate, leading at times to unnecessary intervention (Dover & Gauge 1995, Neilson 1993). In many obstetric units, therefore, use of a CTG is discouraged in low-risk women, although it can be of great value in those with complicated labours (Gibb 1997). In the face of increased litigation, however, the temptation to have proof on paper of the condition of the fetus – however low the degree of risk – remains (Symon 1997).

---

the chorion becoming detached from the decidua of the uterus. This allows a small quantity of amniotic fluid to protrude into the cervix, and the presenting part of the fetus separates this from the remaining amniotic fluid. The small bag of fluid in front of the presenting part is called the *forewaters*, whilst the fluid behind the fetus is the *hindwaters*. As labour progresses, the presence of amniotic fluid around the fetus, and particularly in front of the presenting part, equalises pressure and provides partial protection to the fetus from the direct effect of the contracting uterine walls.

- *Rupture of the membranes* surrounding the fetus occurs as a result of increasing pressure in the uterus. This usually occurs spontaneously towards the end of labour and can be considered as a vaginal douche in preparation for delivery.
- With each contraction of the uterus the force of the fundal contraction travels along the axis of the fetus down to the presenting part and then to the cervix, where it plays an important role in cervical dilatation. This is called *fetal axis pressure*.

SECOND STAGE OF LABOUR

The second stage of labour begins once the cervix is fully dilated, and lasts until the fetus is delivered. This is commonly 1–2 hours in the primigravida, and 30–60 minutes in the multiparous woman (Watson 1994). Uterine contractions become *expulsive* and force the fetus through the birth canal. Often this is accompanied by rupture of the membranes. The mother feels compelled to aid this process by active pushing (Peterson 1997). The pressure of the contractions along the fetal axis encourages the presenting part – usually the head – to become increasingly flexed, presenting the smaller diameters of the fetal skull to distend the birth canal (Fig. 15.5).

As the fetal head moves through the birth canal, the soft tissues in the pelvic cavity are displaced. The bladder is pushed up into the abdomen, stretching the urethra. This may cause the woman to experience some difficulty passing urine. The rectum becomes flattened into the sacrum. The deep pelvic floor muscles (the levator ani), are thinned and displaced laterally. The superficial

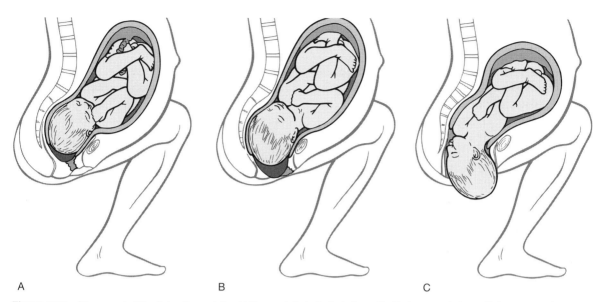

Figure 15.5   Movement of the fetus through the birth canal. A: Late first stage. B: Early second stage. C: Late second stage.

muscles become thinned and stretched. As the fetus is delivered, the introitus is distended dramatically, but recoils immediately once the delivery is complete.

THIRD STAGE OF LABOUR

Once the baby is delivered, the mother becomes involved in the new life that has emerged from her body and often pays little or no attention to the third stage of labour. Yet in many ways this is the most hazardous stage for the mother: the placenta must be expelled from the uterus, leaving a open wound through which 500 ml of blood pass per minute.

Placental separation begins when the fetus is expelled from the uterine cavity. The placental site becomes halved in size, the placenta being peeled off the uterine wall. At the same time the placenta itself becomes squeezed by uterine contraction, so blood in the intervillous spaces is forced into the veins in the spongy layer of the decidua. Venous return from the uterus is greatly reduced, causing blood vessels in the decidua to become congested. These burst, aiding – along with a subsequent contraction – the process of placental separation from the uterine wall. The placenta is expelled into the lower uterine segment, stripping the membranes from the decidua, and with the next contraction, both the placenta and membranes are delivered.

The separation of the placenta can occur in one of two ways (Fig. 15.6):

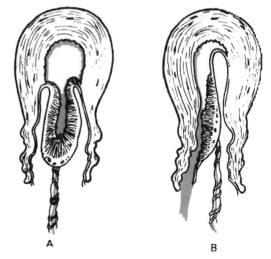

Figure 15.6   Delivery of the placenta. A: Schultze method of delivery. B: Matthews Duncan method of delivery. (Reproduced with permission from Bennett V R, Brown L K 1999 Myles Textbook for Midwives, 13th edn. Churchill Livingstone, Edinburgh)

1. In the *Schultze* method of separation, that most commonly seen, the placenta is forced away from the uterine wall by a collection of blood, called a retroplacental clot. This process begins at the centre and the placenta therefore falls to the lower uterine segment with the fetal surface facing the cervix. This means that as the placenta is delivered, the amnion is enclosing the chorionic surface and any blood lost. Blood loss is minimal with this method.

2. In the *Matthews Duncan* method the placenta separates from its border, slipping down the uterine wall. The maternal surface is delivered first and blood loss appears slightly increased.

Once the placenta has separated, the bleeding must be stopped, i.e. haemostasis must begin. The site where the placenta has been attached is open to the maternal circulation. Three factors prevent torrential blood loss:

1. uterine *contraction and retraction* brings the walls of the uterus into close apposition, exerting pressure on the placental site (Fig. 15.7)

2. the uterine blood vessels become clamped by the *'living ligatures'* of the oblique muscle fibres of the myometrium, through which they are woven

3. *clots* are rapidly formed in the vessels of the placental site.

The third stage of labour may be *actively managed* by the midwife, by the use of oxytocic drugs given with the delivery of the fetus. Such intervention reduces the risks of increased blood loss during this stage (Prendiville & Elbourne 1989). An actively managed third stage will last only 5–10 minutes, whereas unaided, the physiological process may take from 20 minutes to 1 hour.

Once delivered, the placenta and membranes must be examined by the midwife to ensure that they are complete. Evidence of a placental abnormality, such as a missing umbilical vessel, may suggest a fetal abnormality. If the placenta or membranes are not complete, the newly delivered mother will be closely observed for haemorrhage or infection.

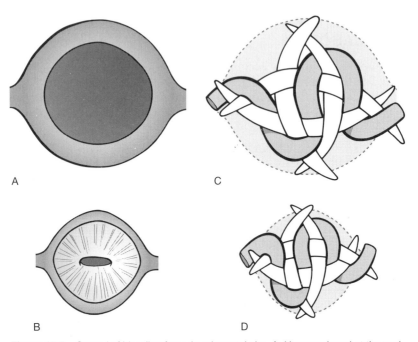

A

C

B

D

Figure 15.7 Control of bleeding from the placental site. A: Uterus relaxed at the end of the second stage. B: Uterus contracted and retracted at completion of the third stage. C: Anatomy of the oblique muscle fibres. D: Contraction of the 'living ligatures'.

THE PUERPERIUM

The puerperium is the period of up to 6 weeks after delivery, during which the uterus and other structures of the reproductive system return to their prepregnancy state. The return of the uterus to its normal size, tone and position is called *involution*. At the end of labour, the uterus weighs approximately 1 kg. This is reduced to 60 g by the end of the puerperium.

Three processes are involved in involution:

1. autolysis, in which muscles are broken down
2. ischaemia, which is a reduction in blood flow to the decidua
3. continued contraction and retraction of muscle cells.

Autolysis

The muscles of the uterus increase during pregnancy to ten times their normal length, and five times their normal thickness. *Autolysis* involves the release of proteolytic enzymes that digest these muscle cells, returning them to their prepregnancy size. Phagocytes remove the debris produced by autolysis. This process is incomplete, because some elastic tissue remains within the myometrium, preventing the uterus from totally regaining its original structure.

Ischaemia

Ischaemia is the result of the constriction of uterine blood vessels by the contraction of the uterus. This is to prevent blood loss from the placental site, but it also restricts blood flow to the decidua as a whole. As a result, the decidua dies and is shed as lochia. A new endometrium begins to form from the 10th day postpartum and is usually complete by 6 weeks.

Contraction and retraction

Contraction and retraction of muscle fibres occurs under the influence of oxytocin, and continues the process of involution. Some women feel these contractions as *afterpains*, particularly those women who have had previous pregnancies. Breast-feeding encourages oxytocin release, and so aids the process of involution. Involution of the uterus results in a reduction in the size of the placental site, which becomes covered in granular tissue and subsequently by the new endometrium.

Lochia

Lochia is the term given to the materials discharged from the uterus from the completion of the third stage until 3–4 weeks postnatally. The appearance of lochia pass through three principal stages as involution progresses:

1. *Lochia rubra* are discharged for 3–4 days, and are red due to the presence of blood from the placental site. Shreds of decidua, vernix and amniotic fluid are passed with this lochia.
2. *Lochia serosa* are passed for 5–9 days, during which time they change from pink to brown. They contain less blood and more serum with leucocytes and organisms.
3. *Lochia alba* last from 10–28 days and are yellowish-white. They contain leucocytes, cervical mucus and debris.

Close observation of the lochia by the midwife will confirm the normal process of involution. The quantity, colour and odour must be noted. Persistent lochia rubra may indicate that the uterus has retained products of conception. Scanty or offensive lochia may indicate the presence of infection, especially if they are accompanied by pyrexia.

Palpation of the fundus of the uterus gives an indication of the rate of involution: within 24 hours of delivery the fundus should be at the level of the umbilicus. It should then decrease in size, until by day 10 it has usually returned into the pelvis and can no longer be palpated. As it returns to the pelvic cavity, the uterus usually regains its anteverted and anteflexed position.

The cervix

The cervix is soft and vascular after delivery. This vascularity reverses rapidly during the puerperium, and the cervix regains a hard consistency within 3–4 days of delivery. By day 10 of the puerperium, the cervical canal has reformed with an internal and external os. The external os closes to a 10 mm slit, never regaining the narrow circular os present before the first delivery.

Other organs

The remaining organs of the reproductive system also return to their previous structure and position during the puerperium. The ovaries and uterine tubes become pelvic organs. The vagina regains its elastic shape. All the supporting structures of the reproductive organs are stretched during pregnancy, but should regain their tone with normal activity.

REFERENCES

Crowther C, Enkin M, Keirse M J N C, Brown I 1989 Monitoring the progress of labour. In: Chalmers I, Enkin E, Keirse M J N C (eds) Effective care in pregnancy and childbirth. Oxford University Press, Oxford, p 833–845

Dover S, Gauge M 1995 Fetal monitoring – midwifery attitudes. Midwifery 11(1):18–27

Gibb D 1997 Really understanding the cardiotocograph. Professional Care of the Mother and Child 7(5):125–128

Grant A 1989a Cervical cerclage to prolong pregnancy. In: Chalmers I, Enkin E, Keirse M J N C (eds) Effective care in pregnancy and childbirth. Oxford University Press, Oxford, p 633–646

Grant A 1989b Monitoring the fetus during labour. In: Chalmers I, Enkin E, Keirse M J N C (eds) Effective care in pregnancy and childbirth. Oxford University Press, Oxford, p 877–878

Keirse M J N C, Chalmers I 1989 Methods for inducing labour. In: Chalmers I, Enkin E, Keirse M J N C (eds) Effective care in pregnancy and childbirth. Oxford University Press, Oxford, p 1065–1066

Llewellyn-Jones D 1994 Fundamentals of obstetrics and gynaecology. Mosby, St Louis, p 168–172

Neilson J P 1993 Cardiotocography during labour. British Medical Journal 306:347–348

Peterson L 1997 Pushing techniques during labour: Issues and controversies. Journal of Obstetric, Gynecologic and Neonatal Nursing 26(6):719–726

Poole J H 1995 Hypertension, hemorrhage and maternal infections. In: Bobak I M, Lowdermilk D L, Jenson M D (eds) Maternity nursing. Mosby, St Louis, p 575–576

Prendiville W, Elbourne D 1989 Care during the third stage of labour. In: Chalmers I, Enkin E, Keirse M J N C (eds) Effective care in pregnancy and childbirth. Oxford University Press, Oxford, p 1145–1169

Silverton L 1993 The art and the science of midwifery Prentice Hall, New York, p 347

Symon A 1997 The importance of cardiotocographs. British Journal of Midwifery 5(4):192–194

Wang E, Smail F 1989 Infections in pregnancy. In: Chalmers I, Enkin E, Keirse M J N C (eds) Effective care in pregnancy and childbirth. Oxford University Press, Oxford, p 534–564

Watson V 1994 The duration of the second stage of labour. Modern Midwife 4(6):21–22

16

The placenta, cord and membranes

The fetus develops and grows rapidly throughout pregnancy, and so requires nutrients and gases in abundance. It is unable to acquire these substances from the bloodstream at the necessary speed or to manufacture the complex substances it needs for its development. Instead, the placenta performs these functions, metabolising the substances required, removing wastes and producing the necessary hormones.

The fetal circulation develops separately from the mother's circulation and includes vessels in the umbilical cord, a temporary structure which enables fetal blood to pass through the placenta. A double layer of membrane develops around the fetus enclosing amniotic fluid that maintains a stable environment and cushions the fetus from external forces.

THE PLACENTA

Functions

The placenta is the organ which attaches the embryo to the uterus wall. It is very complex, and carries out many of the functions that the immature fetus is unable to perform for itself. The placenta has five principal functions:

1. *Respiration* – fetal lungs are immature until late in pregnancy, and do not begin to function until after delivery. The placenta absorbs oxygen and excretes carbon dioxide for fetal metabolism.

2. *Nutrition* – the placenta absorbs the nutrients the fetus needs, and breaks them down with enzymes into simpler molecules for use in fetal

cells. Some nutrients are stored by the placenta, to be used as the need arises. Glucose, for example, is stored by the placenta as glycogen.

3. *Excretion* – wastes produced by the fetus are removed from fetal blood and excreted by maternal organs.

4. *Protection* – the placental barrier is limited, but it does prevent the passage of most bacteria. Small microorganisms, such as viruses, however, can pass through, and may affect the developing fetus. Some protective antibodies, such as the immunoglobulin IgG, transfer from maternal to fetal blood late in pregnancy and serve to protect the fetus from harmful organisms for several months after birth. Most drugs also pass through the placenta, and may damage the fetus.

5. *Hormone production* – the placenta acts as a complex endocrine gland, producing many different hormones. Human chorionic gonadotrophin (hCG) is produced by the early villi in large amounts to maintain the corpus luteum – and hence the pregnancy – until the placenta has developed sufficiently to take over. hCG levels later fall. Other essential hormones produced by the placenta are progesterone and oestrogen (manufactured in conjunction with the fetal adrenal glands), both of which are required to develop relevant maternal organs for the pregnancy. Human placental lactogen is also produced, for glucose metabolism, as are corticosteroids, adrenocorticotrophic hormone (ACTH) and thyroid-stimulating hormone.

Development of the placenta

During the implantation process, the blastocyst begins to develop finger-like projections from the trophoblast over its entire surface (Fig. 16.1). These are the developing *chorionic villi*. Once implantation is complete, those villi with the most abundant blood supply (in the decidua basalis), proliferate, whilst the remainder degenerate and form the chorionic membrane (Fig. 16.2). By the 10th week of pregnancy, the placenta has formed from these closely packed villi.

As the chorionic villi penetrate the decidua, they erode the walls of maternal blood vessels, allowing pools of blood to form, called *sinuses*.

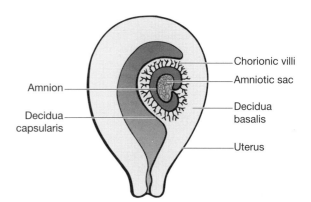

Figure 16.1 Early embryo, showing proliferation of chorionic villi.

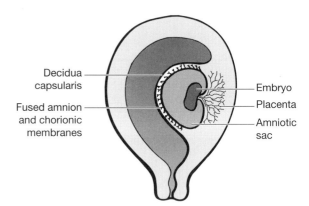

Figure 16.2 Early development of the placenta.

Some villi burrow deeply into the decidua to serve as anchorage for the placenta. The remaining villi float in maternal blood sinuses, where the exchange of nutrients and gases can take place between maternal and fetal blood (Fig. 16.3). There is no direct contact between fetal and maternal blood. Maternal blood returns to the general circulation, where wastes can be removed and nutrients absorbed by maternal organs. Fetal blood is passed along the blood vessels in the umbilical cord, which has developed from a central point in the placenta, to the fetal circulation.

The *placenta* is fully formed by 10 weeks, but is a relatively loose structure, becoming more compact as it matures. Between 12 and 20 weeks' gestation, the placenta weighs more than the fetus, and carries out all metabolic functions for

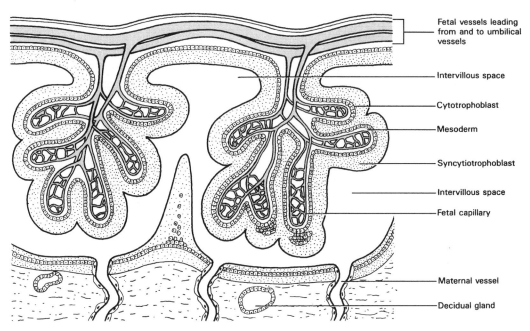

Fetal vessels leading from and to umbilical vessels

Intervillous space

Cytotrophoblast

Mesoderm

Syncytiotrophoblast

Intervillous space

Fetal capillary

Maternal vessel

Decidual gland

Figure 16.3 Chorionic villi lying in maternal blood sinuses. (Reproduced with permission from Bennett V R, Brown L K 1999 Myles Textbook for Midwives, 13th edn. Churchill Livingstone, Edinburgh)

the fetus. As fetal organs develop, so placental function alters accordingly.

The placenta at term

The placenta is flat, and round or oval in shape. At term it is approximately 200 mm in diameter, and 25 mm thick at its central point, tapering towards the edges. It weighs on average 600 g, although this varies with the weight of the fetus. The placenta is expected to weigh approximately 1/6 the weight of the fetus.

Implantation of the placenta usually occurs near to the fundus of the uterus, on either the anterior or posterior surface, where the decidua is at its thickest.

The placenta is commonly described with reference to:

- the maternal surface
- the fetal surface.

The maternal surface

The *maternal surface* of the placenta is attached to the decidua, and so has a deep-red, bloody appearance. This surface is arranged into 15–20 irregular lobes, called *cotyledons*, that are divided by deep grooves called *sulci* (Fig. 16.4A). Each cotyledon is divided into numerous lobules, which each contain one chorionic villus. These resemble the roots of a tree plunging deep into the substance of the placenta from the fetal surface, dividing many times to lie in maternal blood sinuses. In this way, a *large surface area* is formed, through which nutrients and gases can be exchanged (Box 16.1).

Each villus contains fetal blood cells and plasma, covered by a single layer of *cytotrophoblast cells* and the *syncytiotrophoblast*. Four layers of cells therefore divide fetal blood from maternal blood, but all necessary nutrients and gases can pass through these layers by passive or active transport.

The fetal surface

The *fetal surface* of the placenta lies next to the fetus (Fig. 16.4B). It is covered by the amniotic membrane, which gives it a white glistening appearance. The *umbilical cord* arises from the

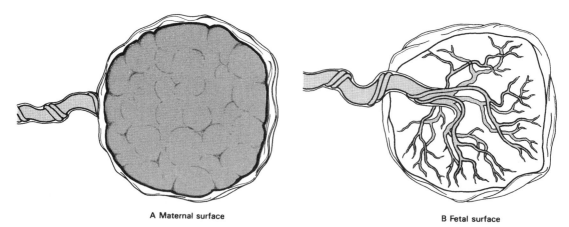

A Maternal surface   B Fetal surface

Figure 16.4   Macrostructure of the placenta. A: Maternal surface. B: Fetal surface. (Reproduced with permission from Bennett V R, Brown L K 1999 Myles Textbook for Midwives, 13th edn. Churchill Livingstone, Edinburgh)

Box 16.1   Haemorrhage

The placenta embeds over a large area of the decidua of the uterus. Chorionic villi burrow into the decidua, opening maternal blood vessels to form sinuses. These sinuses are continuous with the maternal circulation. At term, 500–700 ml of blood pass through the placental site every minute (Sleep 1993). Should the placenta separate, partially or completely, without the uterus contracting to tie off (or ligate) the exposed blood vessels, blood loss will be very rapid.

During the prenatal period, partial separation of the placenta may occur as a consequence of pathological conditions associated with the pregnancy, such as pregnancy-induced hypertension, essential hypertension or trauma (Blackburn & Loper 1992). Maternal smoking and illegal drug abuse have also been implicated. Partial separation of the placenta prenatally is termed a placental abruption or *abruptio placenta*. Another cause of haemorrhage from the placental site prenatally, is an abnormally situated placenta, as is the case in *placenta praevia* (Box 16.5).

Partial separation of the placenta can also occur during labour and delivery, leading to *intrapartum haemorrhage*. In many cases no direct cause for this is found, though it is sometimes due to a short cord, or the placenta partially separating after the delivery of a first twin, when the uterine cavity becomes smaller.

A major haemorrhage from the placental site after delivery of the baby is still a significant cause of maternal mortality and morbidity in the UK, and is a major cause of death in the developing world (Kwast 1991). The term *postpartum haemorrhage (PPH)* is applied when blood lost is greater than 500 ml, or sufficient to cause shock. There are two types of PPH:

1. a primary PPH
2. a secondary PPH.

A *primary PPH* occurs within 24 hours of delivery, and may occur before the placenta has been delivered or after the third stage has been completed. The direct cause of a primary PPH is the failure of the uterus to contract and retract adequately. There are many possible reasons for this to occur, including:

* prolonged labour, where the uterine muscle has become exhausted
* conditions where the uterus has been overdistended, as is the case in multiple births or polyhydramnios
* the placenta being retained in the uterus (Llewellyn-Jones 1994).

Often, however, no cause can be identified. Treatment is to remove the placenta, if still in the uterus, to 'rub up' a contraction and administer an oxytocic drug.

A *secondary PPH* commonly occurs 7–10 days after delivery. The two main causes of this condition are *infection*, and *retained products* in the uterus. The latter case can arise if a small section of the placenta, or a blood clot, is retained in the uterus after delivery, preventing complete contraction and retraction of the uterus. Treatment for a secondary PPH is as above, with removal of the retained products or treatment of the infection.

placenta on this surface, usually centrally, and is covered with a continuation of the amnion. Blood vessels can be seen radiating out from the cord under the layer of amnion, with each cotyledon receiving its own branch of the umbilical artery and vein.

THE UMBILICAL CORD

The *umbilical cord* develops to connect the placenta to the fetus at the fetal umbilicus. At term, the cord is on average 500 mm long (although this can vary considerably), and 20 mm thick. Enclosed within the cord, and protected by it, are *two umbilical arteries* and *one umbilical vein*, continuous with the fetal circulation. The cord itself is composed of *Wharton's jelly*, a form of connective tissue. Covering the cord is a layer of *amnion* continuous with that surrounding the fetal sac. The umbilical cord has a spiral twist, which gives it added strength.

After delivery, the umbilical cord has no further function. It is ligated close to the fetal abdomen, interrupting the circulation. The blood remaining within it clots, the tissue atrophies and the cord separates from the umbilicus around the 5th day of life.

FETAL MEMBRANES

On examination of the placenta, two membranes can be identified:

1. the chorion
2. the amnion.

The *chorion* is the outer membrane lining the cavity of the uterus. It develops from the trophoblast of the early embryo, and is thick and friable, with an opaque appearance. It is continuous with the edges of the placenta.

The *amnion* is the membrane closest to the fetus, and it secretes amniotic fluid. It is smooth and transparent, and stronger than the chorion. The amnion also covers the fetal surface of the placenta and the umbilical cord.

Amniotic fluid

Amniotic fluid (also called *liquor*), is produced

Box 16.2 Amniocentesis

Examination of the amniotic fluid (liquor) can reveal information about the condition of the fetus. Cells shed from the fetus's skin carry its DNA, and so can be used for chromosome analysis. In this way, *genetic abnormalities* can be determined early in pregnancy, and a decision made about the continuation of the pregnancy. If, later in pregnancy, a decision has to made about the risks to a fetus of continuing a compromised pregnancy, the maturity of the lungs can be assessed by sampling the liquor and measuring the *lecithin:sphingomyelin* ratio present (Mattson 1995).

The process of sampling amniotic fluid is termed *amniocentesis*. The placental site and position of the fetus are determined by ultrasound, and a needle is inserted into a pool of liquor through the abdominal wall. This procedure does carry a risk of spontaneous abortion or preterm labour (CEMAT 1998, Green & Statham 1993), and this must be considered when making the decision to perform amniocentesis.

Blood tests carried out in early pregnancy will determine the likely risk of carrying a fetus with Down's syndrome or neural tube defect. If the risk is high, amniocentesis can be offered to the mother to provide a firm diagnosis (Wright 1994).

---

continuously by the amnion. It is recycled constantly by fetal swallowing, and fetal urine and lung fluids add to its composition (Box 16.2). It cushions the fetus from the pressure of the uterine walls, from the noises of other body systems, and during labour, from the pressure of the presenting part on the dilating cervix. The amount of amniotic fluid at term is approximately 1000 ml (Box 16.3).

ANOMALIES OF THE PLACENTA, CORD AND MEMBRANES

Occasionally, the placenta develops in such a way that its structure at term is not as described above (Box 16.4). Often this will not affect the birth process, but in rare instances the anomaly will cause difficulties during the delivery of the fetus or the placenta.

One such anomaly is called a *succenturiate lobe* (Fig. 16.5A). This is a small extra lobe of placenta which develops alongside the main placenta. Blood vessels will run through the membranes to

---

Box 16.3 Abnormal quantity of amniotic fluid

The amount of liquor present in the uterine cavity at term is, on average, 1000 ml. It is normal for the amount to vary between individuals, and according to the stage of pregnancy. However, if the quantity varies to a dramatic extent, it can cause clinical difficulties. Excessive amniotic fluid is termed polyhydramnios; insufficient fluid, oligohydramnios.

Polyhydramnios describes the situation where the volume of liquor exceeds 1500 ml. Often the quantity is 3000 ml before it becomes clinically apparent. Polyhydramnios occurs in 1 in 250 pregnancies, and is usually associated with a congenital defect in the fetus, such as oesophageal atresia or an open neural tube defect, or can be the result of maternal diabetes or a multiple pregnancy (Rankin 1993). The discomfort to the mother is considerable, aggravating minor disorders of pregnancy such as breathlessness, heartburn and constipation. Because of the enlarged uterus, the fetus may frequently change position – termed an unstable lie (Hofmeyr 1989) – necessitating close observation during the final weeks of pregnancy.

Care must also be taken during labour, as the sudden decompression of the uterus when the membranes rupture may cause *placental abruption* or a *prolapsed umbilical cord*. A malpresentation of the fetus may result. Often a *controlled artificial rupture of membranes (ARM)* is carried out before term in theatre, where an immediate Caesarean section can be carried out if necessary. After delivery, the baby must be examined for abnormalities and the mother closely observed for postpartum haemorrhage.

In *oligohydramnios*, there is less than 500 ml of liquor present. This condition is also associated with fetal abnormality, such as an absence of kidneys, a condition known as renal agenesis, or Potter's syndrome (Jonquil 1997). For the fetus, life is very uncomfortable, with lack of space preventing movement and lack of liquor drying out the skin. Labour will proceed without complication from this condition, although it may be induced early if there is a possibility of placental insufficiency. The baby should be examined soon after birth to identify any abnormalities (Skovgaard & Silvonek 1993). Commonly the neonate has compression deformities, such as a squashed face and talipes (club-foot).

Box 16.4 Hydatidiform mole

A *hydatidiform mole* is a rare condition in which placental growth is grossly abnormal. Chorionic villi proliferate over the entire trophoblast, becoming filled with fluid, which replaces blood vessels, and the entire structure comes to resemble a bunch of grapes (Poole 1995). The fetus is starved of nutrients and essential gases, so dies and is absorbed. However, the uterus continues to enlarge, usually much more rapidly than normally expected. The chorionic villi continue to secrete many hormones, giving a strongly positive result to any pregnancy test, and later exacerbating the minor disorders of pregnancy such as *nausea and vomiting* (Mace 1995). Early pregnancy-induced hypertension may also develop (Jonquil 1996). Diagnosis may be suspected because of the increased uterine size, but often the first clinical signs are vaginal bleeding. Ultrasound will confirm the diagnosis.

After removing the contents of the uterus, the woman will be closely monitored to ensure that a rare complication of this condition, *choriocarcinoma*, does not occur. This condition develops in 3% of women who have had a hydatidiform mole, usually within 1 year of its occurrence (Sweet 1997).

---

causing *infection* or *secondary haemorrhage* during the puerperium.

The midwife will examine the placenta and membranes after delivery, and if a small hole is seen in the membrane, it may indicate the retention of a succenturiate lobe of the placenta.

Another anomaly occurs when the cord is inserted into the membranes some distance from the placenta (Fig. 16.5B). This unusual placement is called a *velamentous insertion* of the cord. In this case too, the blood vessels will run through the membranes, and if they lie over the cervical os they may rupture and cause a severe *haemorrhage* directly from the fetus. The situation where blood

this lobe, and its presence may result in one of two rare difficulties:

1. an *intrapartum bleed* may be caused if the membranes lie over the cervical os, and they and the vessels running through them either intentionally or spontaneously rupture

2. alternatively, on delivery of the placenta, this extra lobe may be retained in the body,

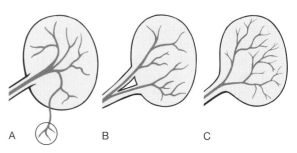

Figure 16.5 Placental anomalies. A: Succenturiate lobe. B: Velamentous insertion of the cord. C: Battledore insertion of the cord.

Box 16.5 Placenta praevia

The placenta may embed in any position in the decidua of the uterus. If it embeds abnormally low down in the uterine cavity, it may cover the cervical os, either before, or once it begins, to dilate. This condition is known as a *placenta praevia*, and the placenta will encroach on the lower uterine segment as it develops during pregnancy. During the later months of pregnancy, the lower uterine segment stretches and the placenta becomes detached from the decidua, resulting in vaginal blood loss.

The cause of the abnormal implantation of the embryo is not known, but factors that may be associated with this condition are a scarred uterus, maternal smoking, a larger than usual placenta, such as occurs with a multiple pregnancy, and multiparity, as the uterine cavity will have been enlarged with each pregnancy (Fraser & Watson 1989).

Placenta praevia is classified according to its position in relation to the cervical os (Rankin 1993). *Types I* and *II* may be safely delivered vaginally, although the labour must be closely monitored. *Types III* and *IV*, however, cannot be delivered by vagina, as massive haemorrhage will result, with probable fetal death and possible maternal death. It is essential, therefore, to identify the presence of a placenta praevia during pregnancy, and determine its grade before labour commences. Often a non-engaged presenting part near term leads the midwife to suspect this condition. Ultrasound is a valuable method of confirming the diagnosis.

It is hard to predict the probable outcome of a placenta praevia (Love & Wallace 1996). For this reason, once it has been diagnosed, the woman may be advised to remain in the obstetric unit, in case she haemorrhages. This can be very frustrating for her, as she will feel well and may have family commitments that she believes she is neglecting. Flexible visiting arrangements and assistance with childcare and finance may be required.

vessels lie over the cervical os is termed a *vasa praevia* (Box 16.5). A less serious complication of this condition is that, during active delivery of the placenta, the cord may break away, or separate, from the placenta.

A *placenta accreta* is an anomaly which occurs as a result of anchoring chorionic villi burrowing too deeply into the decidua, and reaching the uterine muscle. In such cases, separation of the placenta after delivery is difficult or impossible to achieve. *Manual removal* will be attempted, but if this is not successful, the placenta may need to be left in the uterus to be reabsorbed. This will greatly increase the risk of *infection* and *postpartum haemorrhage*.

Other anomalies that may occasionally occur, but which have no clinical significance, include:

- a *circumvallate placenta*, in which the membranes are doubled back at the edges, appearing to be joined near the centre of the placenta
- a *battledore insertion*, in which the cord may be attached at the very edge of the placenta (Fig. 16.5C), and so may separate as a result of controlled cord traction
- *bipartite* or *tripartite placentae* occur when two or three separate large lobes make up the placenta, each with a branch of the umbilical cord leaving the lobe and joining a short way from the lobes to make one cord.

The maternal surface of the placenta may also have anomalies. *Infarcts* may be present, which are areas of dead placental tissue caused by an interruption of blood flow. These will remain red initially, but later become white and fibrosed. Placental infarcts may occur in any placenta, but may be especially numerous if the mother has suffered from pregnancy-induced hypertension. Other common features are small gritty deposits, which are composed of mineral salts. This *calcification* is of no clinical significance.

Anomalies of the cord include those associated with the placenta described above. Other variations are in the cord's length or thickness. A *short cord* may cause *delay in the descent* of the fetus during delivery. The fetus can become entangled in a *long cord*, resulting in a *true knot* in the cord

Box 16.6 Exomphalus

In rare cases, a defect can develop in the abdominal wall of the fetus, allowing its abdominal organs to protrude into the base of the cord. This is a congenital umbilical hernia or *exomphalus*, and often occurs along with other fetal abnormalities (Kelnar et al 1995). As soon as the baby is born, the exomphalus is immediately covered with wet gauze, to prevent fluid loss, infection or damage, until surgery can be arranged.

A similar condition involving the herniation of abdominal contents through a defect elsewhere in the abdominal wall is *gastroschisis*. In cases of gastroschisis, there is an even more urgent need to protect the neonate's protruding abdominal organs which, unlike an exomphalus, are not covered with the amniotic membrane.

or in *loops of cord* around a limb or the neck. A *thin cord* may easily *separate* whilst undertaking controlled cord traction. Often an irregularity in the amount of Wharton's jelly present in one section of the cord will suggest a knot in the cord which, on examination, will be seen to be a *'false' knot*. In rare cases, the intestines will *herniate* into the base of the umbilical cord (Box 16.6).

REFERENCES

Blackburn S T, Loper D L 1992 Maternal, fetal and neonatal physiology. A clinical perspective. WB Saunders, Philadelphia, p 93

CEMAT 1998 Randomised trial to assess safety and fetal outcome of early and midtrimester amniocentesis. Lancet 351:242–247

Fraser R, Watson R 1989 Bleeding during the latter half of pregnancy. In: Chalmers I, Enkin E, Keirse M J N C (eds) Effective care in pregnancy and childbirth. Oxford University Press, Oxford, p 600–608

Green J, Statham H 1993 Testing for fetal abnormality in routine antenatal care. Midwifery 9(3):124–135

Hofmeyr G J 1989 Breech presentation and abnormal lie in late pregnancy. In: Chalmers I, Enkin E, Keirse M J N C (eds) Effective care in pregnancy and childbirth. Oxford University Press, Oxford, p 651–663

Jonquil S G 1996 Molar pregnancy: a case study and review. Midwifery Today 39:35–38

Jonquil S G 1997 The flow of waters. Midwifery Today 41:15–16

Kelnar C J H, Harvey D, Simpson C 1995 The sick newborn baby, 3rd edn. Baillière Tindall, London, p 219–221

Kwast B A 1991 Postpartum haemorrhage: its contribution to maternal mortality. Midwifery 7:64–70

Llewellyn-Jones D 1994 Fundamentals of obstetrics and gynaecology. Mosby, St. Louis, p 33

Love C O B, Wallace E M 1996 Pregnancies complicated by placenta praevia. What is appropriate management? British Journal of Obstetrics and Gynaecology 103(9):864–867

Mace K 1995 Hidden misery of hydatidiform mole. Modern Midwife 5(10):15–17

Mattson S 1995 Assessment for risk factors. In: Bobak I M, Lowdermilk D L, Jenson M D (eds) Maternity nursing, 4th edn. Mosby, St Louis, p 544–548

Poole J H 1995 Hypertension, haemorrhage and maternal infections. In: Bobak I M, Lowdermilk D L, Jenson M D (eds) Maternity nursing, 4th edn. Mosby, St Louis, p 578–581

Rankin S 1993 Disorders of the pregnancy. In: Bennett V R, Brown L K (eds) Myles textbook for midwives, 12th edn. Churchill Livingstone, Edinburgh, p 320–334

Skovgaard R L, Silvonek A L 1993 Oligohydramnios. Literature review and case study. Journal of Nurse-Midwifery 38(4):208–215

Sleep J 1993 Physiology and management of the third stage of labour. In: Bennett V R, Brown L K (eds) Myles textbook for midwives, 12th edn. Churchill Livingstone, Edinburgh, p 219

Sweet B E (ed) 1997 Mayes' midwifery, 12th edn. Baillière Tindall, London, p 519–520

Symonds E M, Symonds I M 1998 Essential obstetrics and gynaecology, 3rd edn. Churchill Livingstone, New York, p 68

Wright L 1994 Prenatal diagnosis in the 1990s. Journal of Obstetric, Gynecologic and Neonatal Nursing 23(6):506–515

17

The fetus

The fetus has two anatomical adaptations which are essential to its intrauterine survival, and its subsequent successful delivery. These are:

1. fetal circulation to pass through the placenta, not the lungs
2. fetal skull bones which are not completely ossified at term.

The midwife requires a good knowledge of these adaptations to allow her to understand the process of delivery and fetal adaptation to extrauterine life.

During intrauterine life, the fetus relies on the placenta to meet its nutritional, respiratory and excretory needs. Fetal circulation is adapted to bypass the lungs and direct blood to and from the placenta, through temporary structures in the circulatory pathways. Immediately after birth, these structures stop working, and the neonate is capable of carrying out all vital functions independently of the mother.

The incomplete ossification of fetal skull bones permits some flexibility during the process of delivery. Whatever the presentation of the fetus during labour, the fetal skull is the largest part to deliver. Knowledge of the shape and diameters of the skull (and those of the mother's pelvis), enables the midwife to assist in the delivery process and identify difficulties if they occur.

FETAL CIRCULATION

Four temporary structures are located in the fetal circulation, which redirect blood through the umbilical cord to the placenta, where they pick up oxygen and necessary nutrients, and away from the lungs, which are not functional during intrauterine life. These structures are (Fig. 17.1):

1. the ductus venosus, through which oxygenated blood is directed from the umbilical vein directly to the inferior vena cava

2. the foramen ovale, situated between the atria, through which blood flows to bypass the pulmonary circulation

3. the ductus arteriosus, between the pulmonary arteries and the aorta, which further prevents blood flow into the pulmonary circulation

4. two hypogastric arteries that direct deoxygenated blood from the lower extremities back through the umbilical arteries to the placenta.

Fetal circulation before birth

Oxygen diffuses from maternal blood through four layers of cells in the chorionic villi into branches of the *umbilical vein* in the placenta (Fig. 17.1). It is this vein which carries the oxygenated blood to the fetus, through the umbilical cord, towards the inferior vena cava in the fetal abdomen. Here, the first temporary structure, the *ductus venosus*, diverts the majority of the blood directly into the inferior vena cava. The remaining blood travels along the portal vein to the liver, where it provides essential nutrients and oxygen. From the liver, deoxygenated blood travels along the hepatic artery to the vena cava. Oxygenated blood from the ductus venosus mixes with deoxygenated blood from the lower limbs and the liver, and all other organs therefore receive mixed oxygenated and deoxygenated blood.

From the venae cavae, blood enters the right atrium of the heart. The majority of this blood is immediately directed through the oval window – the *foramen ovale*, an opening in the septum between the two atria – into the left atrium. Blood then travels from the left atrium to the left

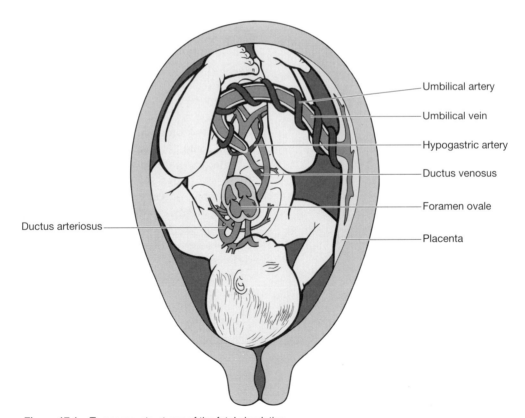

Figure 17.1 Temporary structures of the fetal circulation.

ventricle and into the aorta, so bypassing the pulmonary circulation and the non-functioning lungs. In this way the brain directly receives a good supply of oxygenated blood.

Some blood, however, does pass into the right ventricle of the heart and out into the pulmonary arteries. To prevent the majority of this blood reaching the lungs, the third temporary structure – the *ductus arteriosus* – directs most of the blood into the aorta and so into the systemic circulation. Blood flow continues through the aorta to the body. This is mixed oxygenated and deoxygenated blood.

Branching from each iliac artery is a *hypogastric artery*. It is through these temporary structures that the majority of the blood is returned, through the umbilical arteries, to the placenta. Some, however, flows to the lower limbs.

Fetal blood

Using the placenta for respiration is not as efficient as using mature lungs, and fetal blood is there-fore modified to ensure adequate oxygenation. *Red blood cells* are more plentiful and larger than those required soon after birth. They also have a *shorter lifespan* – 90 days, compared with the 120-day life of adult cells. *Fetal haemoglobin* (HbF) is slightly different to adult haemoglobin (HbA), enabling it to carry oxygen at lower pressures (Kelnar et al 1995). Towards the end of pregnancy HbF begins to be replaced with HbA.

Fetal circulation after birth

Soon after birth, the newborn infant takes his first breath and expands his lungs. This is brought about by several stimuli:

- a slight *hypoxia* (oxygen deficiency), due to the depression of placental circulation during uterine contractions
- *compression* and *decompression* of the chest wall and fetal skull during delivery through the restricted space of the birth canal
- *changes in sensory input*, from the muted confines of the uterus to the loud, bright, cold (relatively) place of birth.

Box 17.1   The Apgar score

Immediately after birth, the neonate is physically examined to ensure that the necessary physiological changes have taken place to enable him to live independently of the mother. One of the most common methods of assessing the infant's condition is by using the Apgar score, a system based on five specific signs that can be quickly checked:

1. heart rate
2. respiratory effort
3. muscle tone
4. response to stimuli
5. colour.

The Apgar score is deduced at 1 minute after birth, and at 5 and 10 minutes if required. It is calculated by giving a mark of 0, 1 or 2 for each of the signs. The ideal score is 10. A score of 8 shows that the neonate is in good condition, one of 4–7 indicates the need for some resuscitative measures, whereas a baby scoring 1–3 will require urgent resuscitation (Letko 1996).

The infant takes a deep breath, to inflate the lungs and respiration commences (Box 17.1). This begins the process of altering the fetal circulation to that required in extrauterine life. With the inflation of the lungs, blood flows into the net-work of capillaries surrounding the alveoli of the lungs, *lowering pressure in the right atrium*. Pulmonary blood is then returned to the *left atrium, raising the pressure* there. The difference in pressure between the right and left atria causes a flap of tissue on the left side of the foramen ovale to close over this structure. Over the next few months this becomes permanently fused. Blood is no longer able to divert through the septum, and passes instead into the right ventricle and into the pulmonary circulation.

The ductus arteriosus is also bypassed in this process, and subsequently blood pressure in the pulmonary artery falls, whilst systemic blood pressure rises. The direction of fetal blood flow is reversed. Higher oxygen levels cause the ductus arteriosus to constrict over the next few days, eventually closing to form one of the ligaments of the heart.

The birth of the baby has resulted in the sepa-ration of the umbilical cord. A decrease in blood flow returning from the placenta further lowers the pressure in the right atrium, aiding the process described above. Blood is no longer able to pass along the hypogastric arteries, umbilical arteries and vein, and ductus venosus. Each of these structures gradually changes function, forming ligaments.

THE FETAL SKULL

The bony skull of the fetus protects the delicate brain within it. Unlike in the adult, the fetal skull is made up of separate bones, which are able to move independently of each other, and to some extent overlap, so that the skull can more easily accommodate to the diameters of the maternal pelvis during labour and delivery. During early fetal life these bones are composed of membrane, which is gradually replaced by bone from central points of ossification. This process continues into adulthood, to allow development and growth of the brain throughout the early years of life.

The regions of the fetal skull important in understanding the delivery process are:

- the bones covering the cerebral hemispheres
- the sutures dividing these bones
- the two fontanelles.

The fetal skull is made up of the vault, face and base. The *vault* consists of:

- *two frontal* bones
- *two parietal* bones
- *two temporal* bones, of little significance in the birth process
- *one occipital bone.*

These bones are named after the regions of the cerebrum they cover (Fig. 17.2). The central points of ossification can be identified on the vault, and are called the *frontal bosses, parietal eminences* and *occipital protuberance.* The bones of the *face* and *base* of the skull are fused at term and so allow little movement, but they need to be considered when assessing the diameters of the skull (see below).

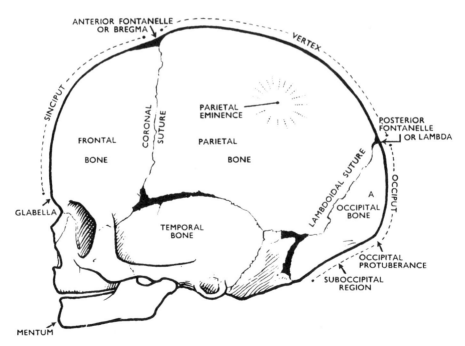

Figure 17.2 The bones of the fetal skull. (Reproduced with permission from Bennett V R, Brown L K 1999 Myles Textbook for Midwives, 13th edn. Churchill Livingstone, Edinburgh)

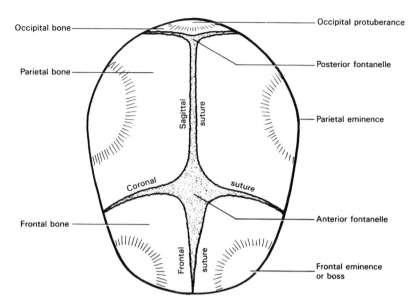

Figure 17.3 The sutures and fontanelles of the fetal skull. (Reproduced with permission from Bennett V R, Brown L K 1999 Myles Textbook for Midwives, 13th edn. Churchill Livingstone, Edinburgh)

The significant landmarks of the fetal skull are (Figs 17.2 and 17.3):

- the *sinciput* – the forehead
- the *mentum* – the chin
- the *bregma* – the anterior fontanelle
- the *lambda* – the posterior fontanelle
- the *vertex* – the highest point on the fetal skull, midway between the parietal eminences
- the *occiput* – the area over the occipital bone
- the *glabella* – the bridge of the nose.

The bones of the fetal skull are attached to each other by *sutures* composed of soft fibrous tissue, which make movement and overlapping possible. Four sutures in particular are relevant to the identification of fetal position (Fig. 17.3):

- the *frontal suture*, which joins the frontal bones
- the *sagittal suture*, which unites the two parietal bones
- the *coronal suture*, which joins the frontal bones to the parietal bones
- the *lambdoidal suture*, which unites the posterior margins of the parietal bones to the occipital bone.

Where three or more sutures meet, enlarged areas of soft fibrous tissue are formed. These are the *fontanelles*. There are two fontanelles:

1. the bregma
2. the lambda.

The anterior fontanelle, the *bregma*, is located where the two frontal and two parietal bones meet, i.e. where four sutures meet. The bregma is kite-shaped, and measures 20–25 mm wide by 25–30 mm long. This area does not ossify until the infant is 18 months old.

The posterior fontanelle, the *lambda*, is situated where the parietal bones meet the occipital bone i.e. where three sutures meet. This fontanelle closes soon after birth. The fontanelles allow further overlapping of the fetal skull bones (moulding) and are also useful indicators to the midwife when identifying the position of the fetal head during labour (Box 17.2).

Diameters of the fetal skull

Knowing the diameters of both the mother's pelvis and the fetal skull allows the midwife to understand the practical implications of the

---

Box 17.2 Vaginal examination

One method of determining the progress of labour is to carry out a *vaginal examination* (Cassidy 1993) to investigate:

- the consistency, dilatation and effacement of the cervix
- the presence of amniotic membranes
- the presentation and position of the presenting part of the fetus
- how well the presenting part is applied to the dilating cervix.

Other factors that may affect the progress of labour can also be determined, such as:

- the presence of cord or placenta
- the degree of moulding
- the presence of stools in the rectum
- the degree of relaxation of the woman.

The *position of the fetal head* can be determined by identifying the sutures and fontanelles presenting through the cervix. These can give an indication of the rotation and descent of the fetus as it moves through the pelvis. For example, a fetal head in which the sagittal suture is in the diagonal diameter of the pelvis, with the posterior fontanelle palpable, will indicate that this fetus is well flexed, with the suboccipital bregmatic diameter of 9.5 cm presenting. This is the ideal vertex presentation. If, however, the anterior fontanelle is palpated, this will suggest an erect fetus with the occipital frontal diameter of 11 cm presenting, i.e. the presenting part is 1.5 cm wider. This presentation is still likely to deliver vaginally, but there may be increased moulding, with possible injury to the internal structures of the fetal skull and more damage to the soft tissues of the perineum at delivery.

Box 17.3 Minor injuries to the fetal head

The fetal skull may be injured if labour is prolonged, delivery is instrumental or operative, or if the presentation or position of the fetus varies from the ideal vertex presentation. Any injuries must be recognised swiftly by the midwife, so that she can reassure the mother and guide her in caring for her newborn baby. The two most common injuries are caput succedaneum and cephalhaematoma (Sweet 1997).

A *caput succedaneum* is an oedematous swelling which forms on the presenting part of the fetal skull. It is caused by prolonged pressure on the cervix as it dilates. A caput often occurs in labours where the fetal head is in a posterior position in the pelvis. Although it may cause anxiety for the mother, a caput succedaneum is harmless to the baby and usually disappears within 36–48 hours.

A *cephalhaematoma* develops after birth. It is caused by rupture of small blood vessels under the periosteum of the bone of the skull, as a result of friction during delivery between the fetal head and the maternal pelvis. This commonly occurs in cases of mild cephalopelvic disproportion or rapid deliveries, where the fetus has little time to accommodate to the diameters of the pelvis. Like a caput succedaneum, this is a minor injury, but will not disappear completely for up to 6 weeks.

---

presentation and position of the fetus as it moves through the birth canal. Where space available is minimal – due to a large fetus, a small pelvis, or a combination of the two – it is essential to be aware of the position of the fetal skull in order to predict the feasibility of vaginal delivery of the fetus (Box 17.3).

Two types of fetal skull measurements are taken:

1. longitudinal measurements
2. transverse measurements.

There are 5 key *longitudinal measurements*, all diameters across specific parts of the fetal skull (Fig. 17.4). During delivery, the attitude of the fetal head determines which of these diameters is presenting. The term *attitude* refers to the degree of flexion of the fetal head with its body. Table

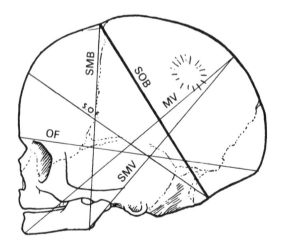

Figure 17.4 Possible presenting diameters of the fetal skull. (Reproduced with permission from Bennett V R, Brown L K 1999 Myles Textbook for Midwives, 13th edn. Churchill Livingstone, Edinburgh)

17.1 gives a complete inventory of which attitudes correspond to which presenting diameters. Given that, on average, the largest diameter of a woman's pelvic brim, cavity and outlet is 13 cm, it will be apparent which presentations may cause difficulty during delivery.

Table 17.1   Fetal head diameters presenting during labour

Attitude	Presentation	Presenting diameter	Average size
Well flexed	Vertex	Suboccipital bregmatic	9.5 cm
Partially flexed	Occipitoposterior	Suboccipital frontal	10 cm
Erect	Cephalic	Occipital frontal	11.5 cm
Partially extended	Brow	Mentovertical	13.5 cm
Partially extended	Face	Submentovertical	11 cm
Extended	Face	Submentobregmatic	9.5 cm

Two *transverse diameters* have significance in the process of delivery:

1. the biparietal diameter
2. the bitemporal diameter

The *biparietal diameter*, between the parietal eminences, measures an average of 9.5 cm. This is the widest transverse diameter, and *crowning of the head* occurs once this diameter has passed through the introitus. The *bitemporal diameter*, between the two extreme points of the coronal suture, measures about 8 cm. It has little significance normally.

Moulding

Moulding is the overlapping of fetal skull bones at the suture line. It occurs as the skull passes through the pelvis during delivery, and is a normal adaptation to the small diameters of the maternal pelvis. It results in a decrease in the diameters presenting during labour and an increase in the diameters at right angles to those presenting. At delivery, the skull shape appears distorted, which can be worrying for the parents.

The most common presentation at term is vertex, in which the suboccipital and biparietal diameters can be reduced by moulding by as much as 15 mm, whilst the mentovertical diameter is elongated. The full-term neonate delivered with a cephalic presentation will usually experience some degree of *moulding*.

In the preterm infant, the skull is less ossified and so moulding can be excessive. This puts a strain on the structures beneath including the folds of dura mater. The postmature infant, on the other hand, has slightly increased ossification of the skull bones, so there is less opportunity for them to move relative to each other. This does not normally cause a problem, unless there is a borderline disproportion between skull and pelvis.

Internal anatomy of the fetal skull

The fetal brain is delicate, and can be damaged by the process of birth, especially if the baby is preterm. The vault of the fetal skull protects the two cerebral hemispheres that make up the substance of the brain. Covering the brain are the meninges, which provide protection and blood to the cerebrum. Folds of the outermost layer of the meninges, the *dura mater*, dip in between the hemispheres of the cerebrum.

The fold of dura mater situated between the two cerebral hemispheres is the *falx cerebri* (Fig. 17.5). A second fold runs horizontal to this, between the cerebral hemispheres and the cerebellum. This is a crescent-shaped structure, called the *tentorium cerebelli*. Two *sinuses* containing blood run along the margins of both the falx cerebri and the tentorium cerebelli. The *superior sagittal sinus* runs along the upper aspect of the falx cerebri, and the *inferior sagittal sinus* runs along the lower aspect of the falx. The *straight sinus* runs along the margin of the falx cerebri and the tentorium cerebelli. Two *lateral sinuses* pass along the outer aspect of the tentorium cerebelli. The *great vein of Galen*, which is situated at the junction of the falx cerebri and the tentorium cerebelli, drains into the straight sinus.

If the fetal skull undergoes a greater degree of moulding than is usual, or if the moulding is in an abnormal direction, or occurs too rapidly, then the junction between the falx and the tentorium may tear. This usually occurs through the tentorium, and is termed a *tentorial tear*. It involves the sinuses and the great vein of Galen, and may lead to brain damage or death.

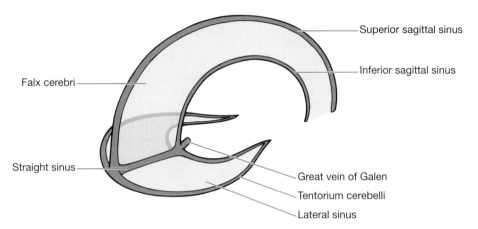

Superior sagittal sinus

Inferior sagittal sinus

Falx cerebri

Straight sinus

Great vein of Galen

Tentorium cerebelli

Lateral sinus

Figure 17.5 Internal structures of the fetal skull.

REFERENCES

Cassidy P 1993 The first stage of labour: physiology and early care. In: Bennett V R, Brown L K (eds) Myles textbook for midwives. Churchill Livingstone, Edinburgh, p 159–163

Kelnar C J H, Harvey D, Simpson C 1995 The sick newborn baby, 3rd edn. Baillière Tindall, London, p 255

Letko M D 1996 Understanding the Apgar score. Journal of Obstetric, Gynecologic and Neonatal Nursing 25(4):299–303

Sweet B (ed) 1997 Mayes' midwifery. A textbook for midwifery, 12th edn. Baillière Tindall, London, p 906–909

18

The female pelvis

Knowledge of the female pelvis and pelvic floor is essential to understanding the processes of labour. The pelvis and its landmarks aid identification of fetal position, and the muscles of the pelvic floor are involved in the rotation of the fetus as it moves through the birth canal.

THE PELVIS

In order to be born, the fetus must negotiate the one principal obstacle that prevents easy exit from the reproductive system: the maternal pelvis. The pelvic girdle is a strong bony structure, which articulates with the lumbar vertebrae superiorly and the heads of femur laterally. The pelvis is an essential part of the skeleton because it makes possible activities such as walking and running, sitting and kneeling. It also protects the pelvic organs, which include the reproductive organs, and to a lesser extent, some of the lower abdominal organs. Attached to the pelvis are the muscles of the pelvic floor, which in part support the position and physiology of the pelvic organs, particularly the bladder, vagina, uterus and rectum.

Although the female pelvis is adapted for childbearing, it is not ideal: the upright posture of the human animal has not included full evolution of the skeleton to this posture. The spinal column, for example, has four curves and the pelvis is tilted, producing a marked curve in its axis. This curve has to be negotiated by the fetus in the process of birth.

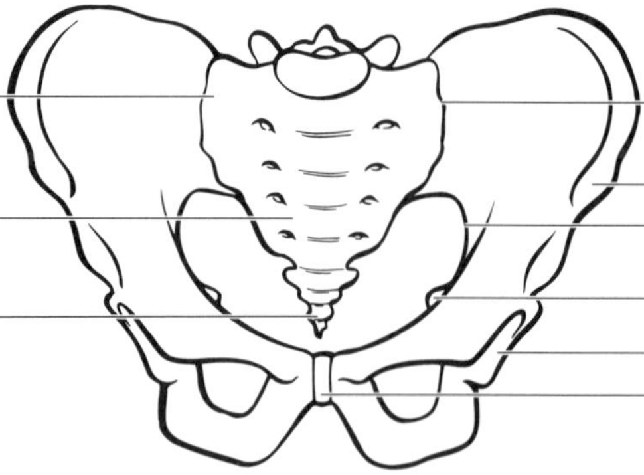

Sacral ala

Sacrum

Coccyx

Sacroiliac joint

Innominate bone

Iliopectineal line

Ischial spine

Acetabulum

Symphysis pubis

Figure 18.1 The bones of the pelvis.

The pelvis is composed of four bones (Fig. 18.1):

- two innominate bones, which form the side walls of the pelvis
- one sacrum, which forms the rear of the pelvis
- one coccyx, which forms the base of the spinal column and pelvis.

These bones articulate at four joints:

- two sacroiliac joints, which allow some movement
- the symphysis pubis, which allows some movement
- the sacrococcygeal joint, which allows free movement.

The innominate bones

The *innominate bones* are each composed of three parts or bones (Fig. 18.2):

1. the ilium
2. the ischium
3. the pubis.

These bones meet in the acetabulum, the fossa forming the socket for the hip joint. In childhood they are separate bones divided by cartilage. By the age of 20–25, however, they are fused together and are immovable.

The ilium

The *ilium* forms the upper flattened portion of the innominate bone. Its upper border forms the *iliac crest*, which is the area the hands rest on when placed on the hips. At its anterior point is the *superior iliac spine* and 25 mm below this is the *inferior iliac spine*. Its lower extremity is formed by the *posterior superior* and *inferior iliac spines*. Above the cleft of the buttocks there are two small dimples to either side of the spinal column,

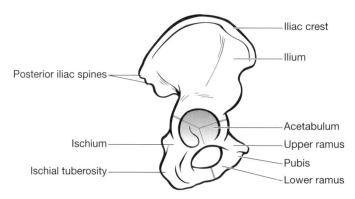

Iliac crest

Ilium

Posterior iliac spines

Acetabulum

Ischium

Upper ramus

Pubis

Ischial tuberosity

Lower ramus

Figure 18.2 Principal features of an innominate bone.

which mark the position of these spines. The upper two-fifths of the acetabulum is formed by the iliac bone. The outer surface of the ilium is rough and is an attachment for the gluteus muscles of the buttocks. The inner surface is smooth and concave, and is termed the iliac fossa. A ridge beneath the fossa is significant as a landmark to separate the false pelvis from the true pelvis in obstetric terms. This ridge is the *iliopectineal line*, and has a prominence, the *iliopectineal eminence*, where the ilium and pubis fuse.

The ischium

The *ischium* is a much smaller bone and is the inferior portion of the innominate bone. It comprises two-fifths of the acetabulum plus a large thickened area of bone, called the *ischial tuberosity*. The tuberosities can be felt through the buttocks and bear the weight of the body when sitting. On the inside of the ischium, posterior to the acetabulum, the *ischial spine* can be felt. This can be palpated vaginally and used to define the descent of the fetus (Box 18.1). If particularly prominent, the ischial spines may influence the space available in the pelvis for the passage of the fetus.

The pubis

The *pubis* is a small bone situated at the front of the pelvis. It is composed of a body and two rami. The *upper ramus* joins the ilium at the iliopecti-neal eminence and forms one-fifth of the acetab-ulum. The *lower ramus* fuses with the ramus of the ischium. The two lower rami of the two pubic bones form the *suprapubic arch*, the bodies of which meet at the *symphysis pubis*. The supra-pubic angle needs to be at least 90° to enable the passage of the fetus.

The sacrum

The *sacrum* is situated between the two ilia and forms the posterior wall of the pelvis. It is wedge-shaped, and is composed of five fused vertebrae. The first vertebra has a prominent upper margin, the *sacral promontory*, which if too pronounced, can obstruct the descent of the fetus into the pelvis. The internal surface of the sacrum has a deep curve, which if flattened, can also prevent the descent of the fetus into the pelvis. Widened wings of bone called *sacral alae* are situated to each side of the first sacral vertebrae. Four pairs of foramina (openings) are situated to each side of the midline in the sacrum, allowing the passage of nerves into and out of the spinal cord.

The coccyx

The *coccyx* is a small triangular-shaped bone situ-ated beneath, and articulating with, the sacrum. It is composed of four fused rudimentary vertebrae, which are evolutionary remnants of an ancestral tail. The coccyx is hinged with the sacrum, and moves backwards during the passage of the fetus.

Supporting structures

Because of its need for strength and stability, the pelvis is provided with powerful ligaments:

- *sacroiliac ligaments* run in front of and behind the sacroiliac joint
- *pubic ligaments* are present both in front of and behind the symphysis pubis
- *sacrotuberous ligaments* run from the ischial tuberosities to the sacrum
- *sacrospinous ligaments* run from the ischial spines to the sacrum.

Box 18.1   Stations in the pelvis

Knowledge of the landmarks of the pelvis can be useful in the assessment of progress in labour. During vaginal examination, for example, the midwife can identify the ischial spines and determine the level of the presenting part of the fetus in relationship to these spines (Cassidy 1993). To do this, she imagines a line drawn between the spines, and the distance of the leading edge of the presenting part is estimated in centimetres above or below this line. For example, if the fetus is found to be 1 cm below the imaginary line, the station of the presenting part is described as +1; 2 cm above the line will be –2. Other factors that can be used to assess progress include abdominal examination and monitoring of contractions.

Late in pregnancy, it may be observed that the head of the fetus has not engaged into the pelvis. If the woman is expecting her second or subsequent baby, this is not unusual. It may be, however, that during labour the fetal head still does not move into the pelvis. One possible reason for both these situations is that the fetus is too large to pass through the pelvis, a condition termed cephalopelvic disproportion (CPD). This may be because the fetus is larger than average, the pelvis is smaller than average, or a combination of the two (Olah & Neilson 1993). It could also be due to the pelvis having been damaged by trauma or malnutrition. CPD occurs in 5% of term pregnancies (Lowdermilk 1995). Delivery may only be possible by Caesarean section.

In cases where CPD is suspected, the obstetrician will examine the pregnant women vaginally and possibly by erect lateral X-ray of the pelvis to estimate whether vaginal delivery is possible. There is debate over the value of pelvic assessment, because the effect of fetal attitude and position cannot be predicted (Thubisi et al 1993). Therefore, where there is thought to be only a mild degree of CPD, the mother may be allowed a 'trial of labour', with close monitoring throughout. Abdominal examination will indicate whether there is movement into the pelvis, and vaginal examination will determine rotation and descent of the fetus. One good indication of the severity of CPD is the degree of moulding that is observed on the fetal skull (Vacca & Keirse 1989).

Pelvic joints and ligaments all relax during pregnancy, due to the increased levels of hormones in the body. This fractionally increases the pelvic size, which may be vitally important for a successful delivery if there is a degree of disproportion between the size of the fetus and the size of the pelvis (Box 18.2).

Physiological parameters of the pelvis

For obstetric purposes the pelvis can be considered to consist of the false pelvis above the iliopectineal line, and the true pelvis below this. The false pelvis plays no part in the process of childbirth.

The shape and diameters of the *true pelvis* are vitally important in allowing the passage of the fetus. The true pelvis consists of (Fig. 18.3):

- the brim
- the cavity
- the outlet.

The fetus rotates within these sections accommodating to the largest diameters.

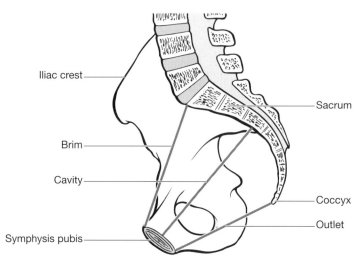

Figure 18.3 Relevant diameters of the true pelvis.

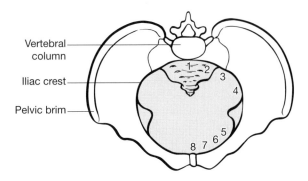

Figure 18.4 Landmarks of the pelvic brim.

The pelvic brim

The pelvic *brim* is roughly oval in shape, and its landmarks are shown on Figure 18.4. They are:

- the sacral promontory (1)
- the sacral alae (2)
- the sacroiliac joints (3)
- the iliopectineal lines (4)
- the iliopectineal eminences (5)
- the upper borders of the superior pubic rami (6)
- the upper borders of the bodies of the pubic bone (7)
- the upper border of the symphysis pubis (8).

The pelvic cavity

The pelvic *cavity* extends from the brim to the outlet. It contains no specific landmarks, but forms the *curve of Carus*, through which the fetus must pass (see pelvic inclination below, and Fig. 18.5).

The pelvic outlet

The pelvic *outlet* is ovoid or diamond shaped, and its perimeter is partly formed by ligaments. The landmarks of the pelvic outlet are shown on Figure 18.6. They are:

- the lower border of the symphysis pubis (1)
- the pubic arch, formed by the inferior pubic rami (2)
- the ischial spines (superior landmarks) and ischial tuberosities (inferior landmarks) (3)
- the sacrotuberous and sacrospinous ligaments (4)

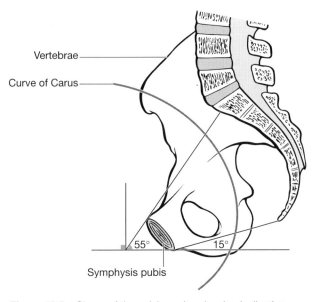

Figure 18.5 Shape of the pelvic cavity, showing inclination.

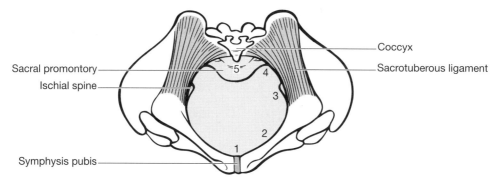

Figure 18.6 Landmarks of the pelvic outlet.

• the tip of the coccyx, then the lower aspect of the sacrum once the coccyx has hinged backwards (5).

Diameters of the pelvis

The *gynaecoid* pelvis (the most common type of female pelvis), is usually the correct shape and size to allow the fetus to pass, but if the fetus is larger than average or the pelvis smaller than average, or a combination of the two, labour may be prolonged or obstructed.

The brim, cavity and outlet are all shaped in such a way that their diameters can be estimated and used to identify the route taken by the fetus as it negotiates the pelvis. Combined with a knowledge of the presentation, position and attitude of the fetus, this information enables the midwife to:

• identify whether there is sufficient room for the passage of the fetus
• understand why the fetus rotates as it moves through the pelvis, accommodating to the spaces and prominent landmarks it encounters
• predict any difficulties that may develop.

The average diameters of the typical female pelvis are shown in Table 18.1.

Two other diameters are relevant to the passage of the fetal head through the pelvis, particularly if in a posterior position:

1. the *sacrocotyloid diameter*, which extends from the sacral promontory to the iliopectineal eminence on the same side, should be at least 90 mm long

Table 18.1 Average diameters (in cm) of the female pelvis.

Pelvic diameter sections	Antero-posterior diameter	Oblique diameter	Transverse diameter
Brim	11cm	12cm	13cm
Cavity	12cm	12cm	12cm
Outlet	13cm	12cm	11cm

2. the *diagonal conjugate*, the diameter from the apex of the pubic arch to the sacral promontory, should be at least 12.5 cm.

Pelvic inclination

Because of the curvature of the spine, the pelvis as a whole is inclined markedly from the horizontal. This means the fetus cannot travel straight downwards to be delivered, but has to follow a curve (Box 18.3). Using the pelvic brim as a landmark, the plane of the brim is at an angle of 55° to the horizontal, while the plane of the

Box 18.3   Positions in labour

The fundamental relationship between the pelvis and the fetus is altered by the position the woman adopts both during labour and delivery. In developed countries, the medicalisation of childbirth has restricted the mobility of women, yet those who are allowed to follow their instincts will often adopt an upright position (Kitzinger 1989). In this way, gravity assists the movement of the fetus through the pelvis. The attitude of the fetus becomes increasingly flexed as it moves through the pelvis. If the mother remains mobile, during delivery she will thrust her pelvis forward and this will move her spine and sacrum backwards allowing more room in the pelvis (Sutton 1996). Delivering in a recumbent position restricts the movement of the joints of the pelvis and thus reduces the diameters of the pelvis. Adopting different positions during labour has also been found to give greater comfort and pain relief (Watson 1994).

The modern delivery suite will normally provide a range of equipment to enable the labouring woman to adopt the position of her choice (Nelki & Bond 1995). Any procedures that are required to monitor the process of labour should adapt to these positions (Shermer & Raines 1997). Bean bags, pillows, wedges and floor mattresses can be of great value. Birthing chairs are less restricting on the pelvis than delivery beds. The midwife will be required to provide help and support to enable the woman to find a position of comfort.

outlet is just 15°. This is because of the differences in length of the anterior and posterior walls of the pelvis (4.5 cm and 12 cm respectively). An imaginary line drawn at right angles to these planes describes the path the fetus takes as it passes through the pelvis (Fig. 18.5). This is the *curve of Carus*.

Pelvic shape

As with all human characteristics, the shape

and size of the female pelvis vary between individuals. Most females have the gynaecoid pelvis described above, which varies in size to some extent, but has the optimal shape for childbirth. *Nutritional* and *traumatic* factors may alter the size or affect certain sections of the pelvis. *Hereditary* factors may result in a pelvis of a different shape, such as an android, anthropoid or platypelloid pelvis, or a combination of shapes (Fig. 18.7). Information that may point to an abnormal pelvis may be obtained from the history given by the woman at the beginning of pregnancy. This can be further assessed during the later stages of pregnancy, when monitoring the descent of the fetus into the pelvis once it engages into the pelvic brim, and when gauging the diameters of the pelvis during vaginal examination. However, the only true measurement of the pelvis is obtained by delivery itself.

PHYSIOLOGICAL CHANGES THROUGH THE CHILDBEARING YEAR

Pregnancy

During pregnancy the hormones *progesterone* and *relaxin* act on the ligaments of the body, including those in the pelvis, resulting in movement in the underlying joints and a slight enlargement of the diameters of the pelvis (Russell & Reynolds 1997). This will allow more room for the passage of the fetus, but will also give rise to movement of the joints. The pregnant woman may therefore complain of *lower back pain*, possibly with discomfort when walking.

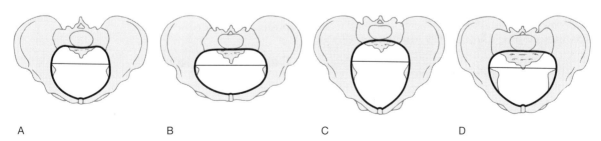

A   B   C   D

Figure 18.7   Types of pelvis. A: Gynaecoid. B: Platypelloid. C: Anthropoid. D: Android.

Labour

The diameters of the pelvis and the curve of Carus determine the passage of the fetus through the pelvis during labour. Knowledge of the diameters of the pelvic brim, cavity and outlet, and of the presenting diameters of the fetus allows the midwife to anticipate the correct descent of the fetus during labour, and be aware of any deviation from this.

The rotation of the presenting part of the fetus is commonly called the *mechanism of labour*. This process will be described below, for a labour in which the fetal head is presenting (cephalic presentation) in a well-flexed attitude.

The mechanism of labour

The most common position for a cephalic presentation is *left occipital anterior (LOA)*, in which the occiput of the fetal skull faces the left anterior surface of the mother's abdomen. The head of the fetus is flexed well onto the chest, so the diameter presenting into the pelvis is the *suboccipito-bregmatic diameter (SOB)*, which measures 9.5 cm (on average). As the fetal head descends into the brim of the pelvis, it adapts its largest diameter to the largest diameter of the pelvis. So the SOB diameter enters the pelvic brim in the transverse position (diameter 13 cm see Table 18.1).

The fetal head goes on to descend through the pelvic cavity, which has equal diameters in all directions. It is here that the head rotates through 90°, to the largest diameter of the pelvic outlet, which is the anteroposterior (AP) diameter (1.3 cm). This rotation is facilitated by the muscles of the pelvic floor. The lowest point of the fetal skull meets these muscles, which are hammock shaped and deflect the head into the AP position. In this way, the fetal head can be delivered accommodating the largest diameters of the pelvic outlet, inflicting the minimum damage to the soft tissues involved.

Once the fetal head has passed through the pelvis, the shoulders have to follow. These are usually smaller, and are at right angles to the largest diameter of the fetal head. They also rotate to accommodate to the diameters of the pelvis. The trunk of the fetus will rotate through 45° to position the shoulders in the AP diameter of the pelvic outlet, again to minimise trauma. The midwife must await this rotation before encouraging the mother to deliver the body of the fetus.

Postnatal

The hormonal influences on the musculoskeletal system, including the pelvis, are rapidly removed once the placenta has been delivered. The ligaments tighten again to restrict movement of the bones of the pelvis.

THE PELVIC FLOOR

Because humans walk upright, a strong structure is required to support the contents of the pelvic cavity. This structure is the *pelvic floor*, a thick band of tissue, principally muscle, which extends from the symphysis pubis to the sacrum, and between the lateral walls of the pelvis, across the pelvic outlet. The pelvic floor also plays an important role in micturition and defaecation, and in sexual intercourse.

During pregnancy, it is vital in supporting the vast increase in weight of the uterus and its contents, and during labour and delivery it directs the movement and rotation of the fetus.

The pelvic floor consists of muscles, ligaments and connective tissue that includes the pelvic peritoneum, the supporting ligaments of the uterus, and two layers of muscle. A deep layer of muscle directly supports the vagina and indirectly supports the uterus, whilst a superficial muscle layer provides support for the urethral, vaginal and anal sphincters, and overall strength to the pelvic floor. The layers of the pelvic floor form a hammock-shaped structure from the symphysis pubis to the sacrum.

Deep muscle layer

The *deep muscle layer* is the more important of the two muscle layers in terms of the normal physiology of the bladder, vagina, uterus and rectum. The deep muscles are collectively known as the *levator ani* muscles. They are attached anteriorly

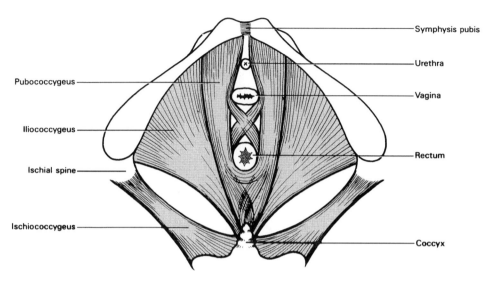

Figure 18.8 Deep muscle layer of pelvic floor. (Reproduced with permission from Bennett V R, Brown L K 1999 Myles Textbook for Midwives, 13th edn. Churchill Livingstone, Edinburgh)

to the pubic bone, laterally to the ischial spines and posteriorly to the coccyx and sacrum.

Three main muscle groups make up the levator ani muscles (Fig. 18.8):

1. The *pubococcygeus muscles*, as their name suggests, extend from the inner aspect of the pubic bone to the coccyx. Three main bands can be identified. The first surrounds the urethra, the second surrounds the vagina inserting into the vaginal walls and perineum, and the final band loops around the anus inserting into the walls of the anal canal, with some fibres crossing over in the perineum. This group can be considered to be the most vital of the deep muscles, as they surround and support the urethra, lower third of the vagina and rectum.

2. The *iliococcygeus muscles* extend from the inner aspect of the iliac bone, and fibres from each side meet in the midline in the perineum, before extending to the coccyx.

3. The *ischiococcygeus muscles* arise from the ischial spines and pass to the lower sacrum and upper coccyx. These muscles help support the sacroiliac and sacrococcygeal joints of the pelvis.

Blood, nerves and lymph

Blood is supplied to all these muscles from the pudendal arteries and veins. Nerve supply is provided by the third and fourth sacral nerves and lymph drains into the inguinal and external iliac glands.

Superficial muscle layer

The *superficial muscles* of the pelvic floor are much smaller than the levator ani, but are vitally important in maintaining the overall strength of the pelvic floor (Fig. 18.9). *Ischiocavernosus muscles* extend from each ischial tuberosity to the clitoris. The *bulbocavernosus muscles* arise in the perineum, pass around the vagina and embed in the clitoris. The *transverse perineal muscles* extend from the ischial tuberosities to the perineum, where they intermingle with muscles of the perineal body.

Other muscles

Two other sets of muscles in the pelvic floor play important roles in their own right: these are the external anal and urethral sphincters. The *external anal sphincter* surrounds the anal orifice, with some fibres extending back through the perineal body to attach to the coccyx. The *external sphincter of the urethra* arises and embeds in the pubic bone, having passed above and below the

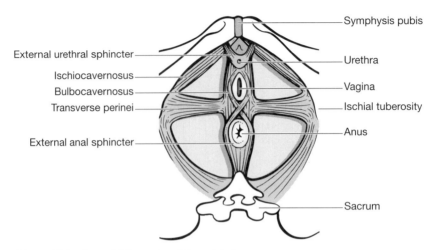

Figure 18.9 Superficial muscles of the pelvic floor.

urethra. These sphincters play a vital role in the control of defaecation and micturition respectively.

The remaining areas of the pelvic floor are filled with ligaments, connective tissue and fat. Blood, lymph and nerve supply come from the same sources that serve the deep muscle layer.

The perineal body

The *perineal body* is the name given to the muscles and connective tissue situated between the vaginal and rectal canals. It is the area most likely to be damaged during delivery. It is commonly described as being triangular, with the base being the skin lying between the vaginal and anal orifices, and the apex the point where the vagina and rectum are in close proximity. Each side of the triangle is 35–40 mm long.

The perineal body is a vital part of the pelvic floor, as it is the place where many of the muscles of the pelvic floor join. It consists of:

● the layer of skin at the base
● the bulbocavernosus and transverse perinei of the superficial muscles
● the pubococcygeus of the deep muscles.

The functions of the perineal body are to assist in the processes of birth and defaecation. It may become torn or incised during childbirth, and so may subsequently need suturing.

Effective functioning of the pelvic floor depends on the maintenance of good muscle tone. Regular activity and exercise will maintain tone, and pelvic floor exercises can be taught that will encourage tone, if carried out on a regular basis throughout life (Bishop et al 1992).

PHYSIOLOGICAL CHANGES THROUGH THE CHILDBEARING YEAR

Pregnancy

The muscles of the pelvic floor become *relaxed* during pregnancy, due to the effects of the hormones, particularly relaxin. Though aiding the process of birth, this softening may also lead to *stress incontinence*, particularly in the latter stages of pregnancy: on coughing, laughing or sneezing, a small quantity of urine may escape from the relaxed urethral sphincter (MacArthur et al 1991).

Labour

During labour, the muscles of the pelvic floor will aid the *expulsive action* of the birth canal, which pushes out the fetus. All the tissues around the birth canal will become greatly distended, with the rectum and posterior structures of the pelvic floor being pushed downwards and outwards. Anterior structures will be moved upwards and forwards, away from the birth canal. Immediately after delivery, all these structures will resume their correct position, but the pelvic floor muscles will need time to regain their tone.

Damage to the pelvic floor

However good the delivery technique, the perineum and surrounding structures, such as the vulva, can be damaged during childbirth (Lavin & Smith 1996). This damage can be accidental, e.g. a tear, or deliberate, as in the case of an episiotomy.

The degree of damage caused by a *tear* can be classified, to aid diagnosis and treatment:

- A *first degree* tear is one where there is minor damage involving the fourchette and perineal skin.
- A *second degree* tear involves both the fourchette and the muscles of the pelvic floor – either the superficial muscles only, or the deep muscles too.
- A *third degree* tear is considered very serious because it involves the external anal sphincter as well as the structures of a second degree tear. It may therefore have an impact on the subsequent continence of faecal matter.

Any of the above may be accompanied by tears or grazes to the labia or clitoris, or vaginal and cervical lacerations. *Labial* and *clitoral* tears can often be left to heal spontaneously, provided there is good vulval hygiene. However *vaginal* and *cervical* tears must be sutured quickly, as they are associated with high blood loss (Box 18.4).

Episiotomy

An *episiotomy* is a surgical incision into the perineum before delivery, intended to aid the birth of the fetus. Episiotomy was developed historically in the belief that a planned incision would maintain tone in the pelvic floor and prevent prolapse, and that it would heal better than a tear. However, these beliefs have been questioned in the light of recent evidence (Sleep et al 1989, Henrikson et al 1994). At present, episiotomy is carried out principally for instrumental delivery or because of fetal distress (Stamp 1998).

Box 18.4   Trauma

During delivery, trauma can occur to any part of the internal or external genitalia. It can range from bruising or grazing, to small tears that are left unsutured or large second or third degree tears or episiotomies (Ball 1993). Internally, any part of the genital tract can sustain damage, from the vagina through the cervix to the uterus itself.

The degree of pain felt by the mother varies considerably. The woman who has sustained slight damage may feel as much pain as the woman with a major degree of tissue damage. The woman who has had an epidural throughout labour may find postnatal pain particularly severe. Tears around the clitoral area are often particularly painful. The midwife should not assume she understands the amount of pain a woman is feeling, and she should give adequate analgesia to meet the individual woman's needs.

During the early hours after delivery, the midwife must investigate expressions of severe discomfort described by the mother.

One particularly painful condition that can occur unexpectedly is a *haematoma*. A ruptured blood vessel continues to bleed beneath the surface of the vulva, or indeed in any pelvic tissue, and causes a swelling of varying size. This is commonly associated with a sutured laceration in which the vessel has not been ligated during the repair process. If small, this can be left to dissipate, with analgesia and icepacks to relieve the pain. However, if large, the haematoma may require excision.

Episiotomy entails incision of the fourchette, the skin of the perineum, the posterior vaginal wall and the superficial muscles of the pelvic floor. As this is a deliberate surgical incision, it is essential that the woman give informed consent to the procedure.

There are two main types of incision (Fig. 18.10):

1. mediolateral
2. midline.

Midwives in the UK most commonly use the *mediolateral* incision. This involves an incision that commences at the fourchette and is then directed through a 45° angle between the anus and the ischial tuberosity. This incision avoids both Bartholins gland and the anal sphincter, but is considered to be more complex to repair than the midline incision. The *midline* episiotomy follows the midline from the fourchette towards the anus. It is associated with smaller blood loss and easier repair, but if it extends it is more likely

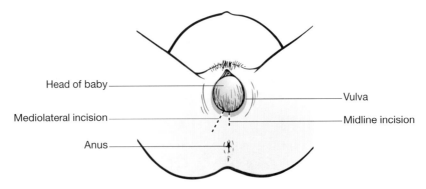

Figure 18.10 Types of episiotomy.

than the mediolateral incision to involve the anal sphincter (Helwig et al 1993).

Postnatal

The muscles of the perineum must stretch significantly during childbirth, but they regain their supporting function very quickly afterwards (Peschers et al 1997). Postnatal exercises and early ambulation can aid this process and prevent many long-term problems, such as urinary incontinence and prolapse (Parsons 1997). Increased blood flow to the genitalia (caused by raised progesterone levels during pregnancy) may lead to a degree of oedema and bruising in the early postpartum days. Damage to the perineum can also cause much *discomfort* and *pain* during the puerperium, and the midwife will be required to suggest both pharmacological and non-pharmacological methods of pain relief so the woman is better able to carry out her role as carer to the newborn baby.

REFERENCES

Ball J 1993 Complications of the puerperium. In: Bennett V R, Brown L K (eds) Myles textbook for midwives, 12th edn. Churchill Livingstone, Edinburgh, p 477–479

Bishop K R, Dougherty M, Mooney R, Gimotty P, Williams B 1992 Effects of age, parity, and adherence on pelvic floor response to exercise. Journal of Obstetric, Gynecologic and Neonatal Nursing 21(5):401–406

Cassidy P 1993 The first stage of labour: physiology and early care. In: Bennett V R, Brown L K (eds) Myles textbook for midwives, 12th edn. Churchill Livingstone, Edinburgh, p 161–162

Helwig J, Throp J, Bowes W 1993 Does midline episiotomy increase the risk of third and fourth degree lacerations in operative vaginal deliveries? Obstetrics and Gynaecology 82: 275–279

Henrikson T B, Bek K M, Hedegaard M, Secher N J 1994 Methods and consequences of changes in use of episiotomy. British Medical Journal 309:1255–1258

Kitzinger S 1989 Childbirth and society. In: Chalmers I, Enkin E, Keirse M J N C (eds) Effective care in pregnancy and childbirth. Oxford University Press, Oxford, p 102

Lavin J, Smith A R 1996 Pelvic floor damage. Modern Midwife 6(5):14–16

Lowdermilk D L 1995 Labor and birth at risk. In: Bobak I M, Lowdermilk D L, Jenson M D (eds) Maternity nursing, 4th edn. Mosby, St Louis, p 698

MacArthur C, Lewis M, Knox E G 1991 Health after childbirth. HMSO, London, p 253

Nelki J, Bond L 1995 Positions in labour: a plea for flexibility. Modern Midwife 5(2):19–24

Olah K S J, Neilson J P 1993 Failure to progress in the management of labour. British Journal of Obstetrics and Gynaecology 101(1):1–3

Parsons C 1997 The importance of a healthy pelvic floor. Modern Midwife 7(1):10–14

Peschers U M, Schaer G N, DeLancey J O 1997 Levator ani function before and after childbirth. British Journal of Obstetrics and Gynaecology 104(9):1004–1008

Russell R, Reynolds F 1997 Back pain, pregnancy, and childbirth. British Medical Journal 314:1062–1063

Shermer R H, Raines D A 1997 Positions during the second stage of labour: moving back to basics. Journal of Obstetric, Gynecologic and Neonatal Nursing 26(6):727–734

Sleep J, Roberts J, Chalmers I 1989 Care during the second stage of labour. In: Chalmers I, Enkin E, Keirse M J N C (eds) Effective care in pregnancy and childbirth. Oxford University Press, Oxford, p 1129–1144

Stamp P 1998 Care of the perineum in the second stage of labour: a study of views and practices of Australian midwives. Midwifery 13(2):100–104

Sutton J 1996 A midwife's observations of how the birth

process is influenced by the relationship of the maternal pelvis and the foetal head. Journal of the Association of Chartered Physiotherapists in Women's Health 79:31–33

Thubisi M, Ebrahim A, Moodley J, Shwini P M 1993 Vaginal delivery after previous caesarean section: is X-ray pelvimetry necessary? British Journal of Obstetrics and Gynaecology 82:421–425

Vacca A, Keirse M J N C 1989 Instrumental vaginal delivery. In: Chalmers I, Enkin E, Keirse M J N C (eds) Effective care in pregnancy and childbirth. Oxford University Press, Oxford, p 1216–1218

Watson V 1994 Maternal position in the second stage of labour. Modern Midwife 4(7):21–24

19

The female breast

The female breasts, or mammary glands, are accessory organs of reproduction. They are required to provide nourishment for the neonate after birth. However, they also play a significant role in the attraction of the adult male to the female, and in enhancing the act of sexual intercourse. The breasts are rudimentary until puberty, when the reproductive organs become sufficiently mature to enable reproduction to take place. During pregnancy, the breasts develop further, under the influence of hormones. Once the fetus has been delivered, sudden decrease in these hormones stimulates milk production.

Both male and female neonates have rudimentary breasts at birth. In the male, the breasts remain in this state throughout life. In the female, breast tissue is produced as a result of the release of oestrogen and progesterone during puberty.

The mature female breast consists of:

- one areola, which provides lubrication during lactation (milk secretion)
- one nipple, through which milk is excreted
- many alveoli, in which milk is produced
- tubules and ducts, through which milk passes from the alveoli to the nipple.

THE BREAST

External structure

The two mature female *breasts* are modified exocrine glands that are capable of secreting milk. One is situated on each side of the midline on the anterior chest wall (Fig. 19.1). They extend

217

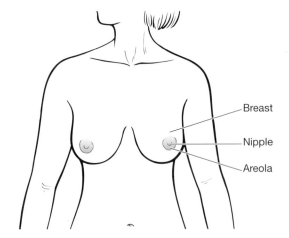

Figure 19.1 External structure of the breasts.

from the second to the sixth rib, and laterally from the sternum to the axilla, over the pectoralis muscles, to which they are attached by connective tissue. Strands of connective tissue run through the breasts giving them support. Each breast is hemispherical in shape, with an axillary tail extending towards the axilla. Breast size varies considerably between individuals, and throughout an individual's life.

At the midpoint on the exterior surface of the breast lies an area of pigmentation, the *areola*, measuring on average 25 mm in diameter. The degree of pigmentation varies between individuals. Opening into the areola are sebaceous glands, *Montgomery's tubercles*, which secrete a sebum-like substance to lubricate the nipple during pregnancy and breast-feeding. At the centre of the areola is the *nipple*, a highly sensitive erectile structure (Box 19.1). Within the nipple are plain muscle fibres that act like a sphincter to prevent the leakage of milk during pregnancy and lactation. Leading into the nipple are 16–20 openings from the lactiferous tubules. Both the areola and the nipple are pink in colour until pregnancy, when they darken.

Internal structure

Internally, the breast consists of 16–20 *lobes*, divided by bands of fibrous tissue (Box 19.2). Each lobe contains a *lactiferous duct* leading to an *ampulla*, or reservoir, just beneath the nipple (Fig. 19.2). It is here that milk is stored. Each lobe is divided into a number of *lobules*, each of which contain a lactiferous duct, along which milk is directed from the many alveoli where it is manu-

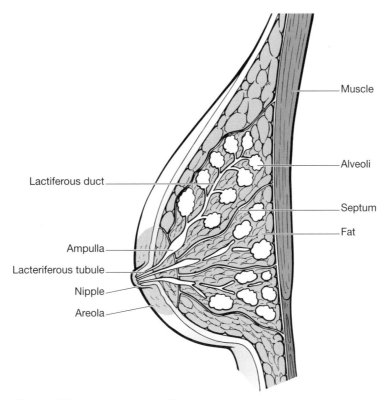

Muscle

Alveoli

Septum

Fat

Lactiferous duct

Ampulla

Lacteriferous tubule

Nipple

Areola

Figure 19.2   Internal structure of the breast.

factured. Between these structures is a variable amount of fatty tissue, that determines the size of the breast.

The *alveoli* are clustered around lactiferous ducts, like bunches of grapes. The alveoli are composed of milk-secreting cells, *acini*, which extract the nutrients necessary for milk production from the network of capillaries that surround each alveolus. Also enclosing each alveolus are *myoepithelial cells* (Fig. 19.3), which have the capacity to contract under the influence of oxytocin, squeezing the milk out of the alveolus and into the lactiferous ducts.

Blood, nerves and lymph

Blood is supplied to the breasts by the mammary arteries and upper intercostal arteries. Venous drainage is into mammary and axillary veins.

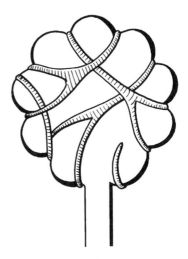

Figure 19.3   Microstructure of an alveolus. (Reproduced with permission from Bennett V R, Brown L K 1999 Myles Textbook for Midwives, 13th edn. Churchill Livingstone, Edinburgh)

Lymphatic drainage is extensive and is principally into the axillary glands, with some drainage into the mediastinal glands. The lymphatic systems of the two breasts are in direct communication.

There is little nerve supply to the breasts as they are largely controlled by hormones. However, the skin is supplied by branches of the thoracic nerves, and the nipple and areola are supplied by the autonomic nervous system.

PHYSIOLOGICAL CHANGES THROUGH THE CHILDBEARING YEAR

Pregnancy

From the 6th week of pregnancy, the breasts undergo considerable enlargement and development in response to the increasing levels of the hormones of pregnancy (Silverton 1993). Oestrogen is responsible for the growth of the lactiferous ducts and tubules. Progesterone, prolactin and human placental lactogen (HPL) results in the proliferation and enlargement of the alveoli. The pregnant woman may feel *tingling* in her breasts, and increased *sensitivity* to touch. Blood supply to the breasts increases, with *visible veins* appearing on their surface.

By the 12th week of pregnancy, the nipples and areola have become more *pigmented*. Montgomery's tubercles have become more pronounced and begin secreting lubricants. By the 16th week of pregnancy, *colostrum* has been formed under the influence of HPL and prolactin, although the high levels of oestrogen and progesterone prevent milk formation. By the 24th week of pregnancy, *secondary areola* have formed. These are areas of pigmentation around the areola. On average each breast enlarges by 50 mm and by 1500 g in weight during pregnancy.

Colostrum is the precursor of milk. It is highly nutritious and contains many immunoglobulins, which supplement the protection against infections the newborn has gained from the mother via the placenta throughout pregnancy. Because colostrum is formed from early in pregnancy, it is immediately available to the neonate after delivery.

Labour

Once the third stage of labour has been completed, the placenta, and the many hormones it secretes, are no longer in the body. The resulting dramatic decrease in the levels of oestrogen and progesterone in particular, initiate *lactation*.

Postnatal

As oestrogen and progesterone levels decrease, prolactin levels increase, stimulating the production of *milk* (lactation). Colostrum continues to be produced for the first day or two after delivery, and this gradually changes in composition to milk. This is encouraged by suckling the neonate from birth, but if the mother chooses not to breast-feed, milk will still be produced to some degree. However, lack of stimulation of the breasts will result in the cessation of milk production.

Two main hormones are involved in lactation (Fig. 19.4):

1. *prolactin* from the anterior lobe of the pituitary gland influences the *production of milk*
2. *oxytocin* from the posterior lobe controls the *ejection of milk*.

Whenever the baby suckles, the production of prolactin is stimulated. Frequent breast-feeding, including night feeds, will maintain good prolactin levels. Milk ejection is a *neuroendocrine* response. Stimulation, created either by the baby suckling, by the sound of the baby crying, or simply by thinking of the baby, will result in the release of oxytocin from the posterior lobe of the pituitary gland. This acts on the myoepithelial cells surrounding the alveoli, which contract and expel milk from the alveoli and through the lactiferous ducts. This *milk ejection reflex* or 'let down' of milk can be very forceful: the milk enters the baby's mouth with little help from his tongue and jaw action.

For the mother who is breast-feeding, the early postnatal days see many changes in breast function. Initially the breasts are soft and the baby suckles frequently, taking small amounts of colostrum. By the 3rd or 4th day, the breasts

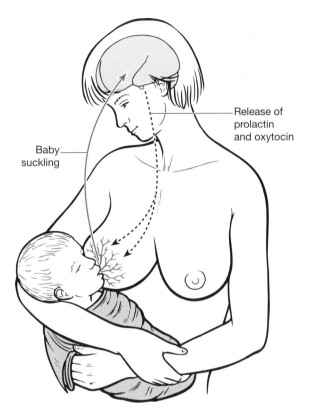

Baby
suckling

Release of
prolactin
and oxytocin

Figure 19.4 Hormonal control of lactation.

become full and colostrum changes to milk. At this time the breasts may become *sore* (Duffy et al 1998) and *engorged*, and the baby may have difficulty latching on (Woolridge 1986). This commonly comes at a time when the mother's spirits are low. However, much help and encouragement from the midwife will help her through this uncomfortable period enabling breast-feeding to settle into a pleasant experience.

The composition of colostrum and breast milk is very complex. Colostrum is a transparent yellow colour, and has a higher protein content than breast milk (Fisher 1993). The proteins contain a high proportion of immunoglobulins, giving the neonate extra protection against infection in the early days after birth. Carbohydrate and fat levels are lower than in breast milk. Although the amount of colostrum taken by

the neonate is small, it is very nutritious and protective.

Breast milk varies in composition and amount throughout the day, and as the infant grows. It meets the nutritional requirements of the full-term neonate perfectly. It is a complete food and drink for the baby, requiring no supplements in the form of formula feeds or water. Constituents of breast milk include the following (Sweet 1997):

- *Protein*, in smaller proportions than in formula feeds. This is easily and completely digested and leaves little waste. The principal protein found in breast milk is *lactalbumin*, with *caseinogen* present in smaller quantities. These proteins contain amino acids, including two – *cystine* and *taurine* – which are not present in formula milk. These are important as they are involved in growth and in the development of the brain.
- *Fat*, which is rapidly broken down by lipase, also present in breast milk, and activated in the intestines.
- *Lactose*, a specific form of sugar which is quickly absorbed. It plays an important role in the absorption of calcium and in the growth of protective commensals in the gut.
- *Vitamins A, B complex, C, D, E and K*, in sufficient quantities to meet the baby's needs.
- *Iron* and *zinc*, both essential ingredients in human diets.
- Minerals such as *sodium, potassium, calcium* and *phosphorus*, all at lower levels than in formula milk, to prevent dehydration (Sachdev et al 1991).
- Immune factors such as *macrophages, immunoglobulins, lysozyme, lactoferrin* and the *bifidus factor*, which protect the infant from infection.

The neonate

The rudimentary breasts both male and female infants have can be somewhat *enlarged* at birth. This occurs in response to the high levels of maternal hormones crossing the placenta during fetal development. This enlargement is transient and rapidly resolves within 3–4 weeks.

REFERENCES

Dahlen H 1993 Lactation mastitis. Nursing Times 89(36):38–40

Duffy E P, Percival P, Kershaw E 1998 Postnatal effects of an antenatal group teaching session on postnatal nipple pain, nipple trauma and breast feeding rates. Midwifery 13(4):189–196

Fisher C 1993 Feeding. In: Bennett V R, Brown L K (eds) Myles textbook for midwives, 12th edn. Churchill Livingstone, Edinburgh, p 521–522

MAIN Trial Collaborative Group 1994 Preparing for breast feeding: treatment of inverted and non-protractile nipples in pregnancy. Midwifery 10(12):200–214

Renfrew M, Fisher C, Arms S 1990 Bestfeeding: getting breastfeeding right for you. Celestial Arts, Berkley, p 124–126

Sachdev H P S, Krishna J, Puri R K 1991 Water supplementation in exclusively breast fed infants during the summer in the tropics. Lancet 337:929–933

Scott A, Forsyth S 1996 Breast feeding and antibiotics. Modern Midwife 6(7):14–16

Silverton L 1993 The art and science of midwifery. Prentice Hall, New York, p 526–528

Smale M 1992 The National Childbirth Trust book of breastfeeding. Vermillion, London, p 100

Sweet B (ed) 1997 Mayes' midwifery, 12th edn. Baillière Tindall, London, p 802–804

Woolridge M W 1986 Aetiology of sore nipples. Midwifery 2:172–176

Glossary

Glossary

Abortion Spontaneous miscarriage before the fetus is viable (i.e. before the 24th week of pregnancy); or, the deliberate termination of a pregnancy

Abruptio placenta The partial or complete separation of the placenta from its site after the 24th week of pregnancy

Acid aspiration syndrome Mendelson's syndrome – in which stomach acid is inhaled during general anaesthesia, causing pulmonary irritation and oedema

Acid base balance The normal ratio of acid and alkaline ions required to maintain the pH of the blood and body fluids

Acidosis A condition in which the pH of the blood is less than 7.35

Acquired immunity Specific immunity

Acrosome A package containing enzymes in the head of a spermatozoon

Acute A term applied to symptoms that occur suddenly and for a short period of time

Adaptation (Sensory): a process by which neurones transmit fewer impulses despite the stimulus remaining the same

Aerobic (Of a metabolic process): requiring oxygen

Aetiology The cause of a disease

Afterpains Pain felt due to uterine contraction in the post-natal period

Agglutination Cells clumping together

Agglutinogen An antigen located on the surface of erythrocytes that determines blood group and Rhesus factor

Alkalosis A condition in which the pH of the blood is greater than 7.45

Allergen A substance which provokes an allergic reaction

Alpha fetoprotein A plasma protein excreted into amniotic fluid by the fetus

Amenorrhoea The absence of menstruation

Amniocentesis The removal of amniotic fluid from the uterus through the abdominal wall

Amniotic fluid see Liquor amnii

Amniotomy The rupture of the membranes surrounding the fetus

Ampulla (of uterine tube) The longest and widest portion of the uterine tube, between the infundibulum and the isthmus of the tube

Anaemia deficiency of red blood cells

Anaerobic (Of a metabolic process): occurs in the absence of oxygen

Anaesthesia Loss of sensation

Analgesia Insensitivity to pain

Anencephaly The congenital absence of the cranium including partial or total absence of the cerebral hemispheres

Anomaly A variation from the norm

Anteflexion The bending forwards of the uterus

Antenatal Relating to pregnancy

Anteversion The tilting of the uterus to the front

Anti-D immunoglobulin An antibody against the Rhesus factor

Antibody A protein produced by lymphatic tissue in response to antigens, which circulates in the plasma to attack antigens and render them harmless

Antigen Any substance which stimulates the production of antibodies

Antipyretic A substance that reduces fever

Apex The pointed end of an organ such as the cone-shaped heart

Apgar score A system devised to apply a numerical score to the condition of a neonate immediately after birth

Apnoea Cessation of breathing

Arbor vitae Branch-like ridges in the endothelium of the cervix

Areola Pigmented area around the nipple of the breast

Association area (Cerebral cortex): an area of the cerebral cortex which integrates with other areas controlling the same function

Asthma Respiratory condition in which there is wheeze and difficulty in expiration

Atrial septal defect Malformation of the septum between the atria of the heart

Atrophy The wasting of an organ or tissue

Attenuation A process by which pathogenic microorganisms are made less virulent

Attitude The degree of flexion of the fetal body

Augment (Uterine contractions): increase intensity of uterine contractions

Autoimmunity A disordered immune response against constituents of the body's own tissues

Autolysis The breakdown of tissue after the death of its cells; self destruction

Autoregulation (Blood): the local regulation of blood flow to an organ

Baby blues Mood swings associated with the early days of the postnatal period

Basal ganglia Areas of grey matter in the cerebrum

Bilirubin Bile pigment formed by the breakdown of haemoglobin

Binovular twins (also called Dizygotic twins) Non-identical twins, derived from two separate ova

Biophysical profile A method of examining the health of the fetus

Biorhythms Inherent cyclical rhythms of body systems

Blastocyst An early stage of embryonic development, consisting of the trophoblast and an inner cell mass

Blood–brain barrier The barrier formed by astrocytes around the blood vessels of the brain

Bonding Mother–infant interaction

Brain stem The collective name for the midbrain, medulla oblongata and pons Varolii

Bregma Anterior fontanelle

Broad ligament A double layer of peritoneum attaching the uterus to the lateral walls of the pelvis

Brown fat A specialised type of fat present in the newborn that can be metabolised for heat production

Caesarean section A surgical procedure in which the fetus is delivered through an incision in the lower uterine segment

Calcification The laying down of calcium salts in tissue

Capacitation The process by which the enzymes present in the acrosome of the spermatozoon are exposed for the process of fertilisation

Capillary bed The term applied collectively to all capillaries

Caput succedaneum Oedematous swelling of the fetal head due to prolonged pressure

Cardiac sphincter The upper narrowed portion of the stomach where the oesophagus enters

Cardinal ligament The ligament attaching the uterus to the lateral walls of the pelvis

Cardiotocograph An electrical device which monitors fetal heart rate and rhythm, and the strength and frequency of uterine contractions

Carpel tunnel syndrome A tingling and numbness of the hand resulting from pressure on the median nerve as it passes through the carpel tunnel of the wrist

Carunculae myrtiformes Remnants of the hymen

Catheterisation The insertion of a catheter into the urethra, usually to release urine

Cell division Process by which cells reproduce

Cell-mediated immunity A type of immunity in which T-lymphocytes attach to antigens to destroy them

Cephalhaematoma A swelling of blood under the periosteum of the fetal scalp due to shearing forces

Cerebral cortex The outer layer of the cerebral hemispheres containing the cell bodies of neurones, within which nerve impulses are interpreted and acted on

Cerebrospinal fluid Fluid contained within the ventricles and subarachnoid space of the nervous system

Cervical Relating to the neck or the cervix

Cervix The lower third of the uterus

Chemotaxin A chemical released to attract phagocytes

Childbearing year The period which spans pregnancy, labour and the puerperium

Chloasma An area of pigmentation on the face, which develops during pregnancy

Cholestasis Cessation of the flow of bile

Chorionic villus A minute projection extending into the decidua

Choroid plexus Blood vessels in the roof of the ventricles of the brain which produce cerebrospinal fluid

Chromosome A linear sequence of genes in the nucleus of a cell, composed mostly of DNA, which transmits genetic information

Chronic Prolonged

Cilia Hair-like processes projecting from cell membranes

Circumcision The removal of the foreskin of the penis

Cleft palate An opening in the hard palate, caused by incomplete fusion

Coccygeal Relating to the coccyx

Coitus Sexual intercourse

Collagen A protein contained in connective tissue

Colostrum The first secretions of the breasts, from the 16th week of pregnancy until full production of breast milk

Commensal A microorganism which causes no harm to the host

Complement A complex series of proteins circulating in the blood that are activated during the non-specific immune response

Compliance Ability of lung tissue to expand

Congenital Present at, and existing from the time of birth

Conjugated Joined together, e.g. bilirubin and water to allow excretion

Constipation Infrequent, difficult passage of hard stools

Continence The ability to control micturition

Contraception The prevention of conception or of the implantation of a fertilised egg

Contractility The ability of cells to shorten

Contraction The shortening of muscle fibres, or narrowing of a diameter of the pelvis

Convulsion A violent, involuntary contraction of muscles

Cornua The junctions of the uterus and uterine tubes

Corona radiata Layers of cells surrounding the ovum

Corpus Body

Corpus albicans Literally 'white body', the scar tissue that replaces the degenerated follicle in the ovary

Corpus luteum The yellow glandular body formed in the ovary after ovulation, secreting oestrogen and progesterone

Cortex The outer layer of an organ

Cot death Sudden infant death from unknown cause

Cramp Painful spasmodic muscular contraction

Craving Intense desire

Cretinism Severe mental retardation caused by hypothyroidism

Cricoid cartilage Cartilage covering the trachea that can be used to occlude the oesophagus

Critical period The interval in which embryonic systems/organs undergo their greatest development

Curettage A surgical procedure involving scraping the endometrium of the uterus

Cyanosis A bluish discoloration of skin or mucous membranes due to lack of oxygen in underlying blood vessels

Cystitis Inflammation of the bladder

Decidua The endometrium in pregnancy

Defaecation Evacuation of the rectum

Degeneration Deterioration in the structure of tissue, preventing its full function

Dehydration Loss of water

Denaturation The breakdown of the structure of a protein

Deoxyribonucleic acid The nucleic acid in all cell nuclei, that form the basic structure of genes

Depression Lowering of mental mood

Dermatome An area of the body served by one spinal nerve

Diabetes mellitus A disorder of carbohydrate metabolism caused by a deficiency or absence of insulin from the islets of Langerhans, required to control blood glucose levels

Diarrhoea Loose watery stools

Diastole Relaxation of the heart between contractions

Differential diagnosis The diagnosis of a disease whose symptoms are the same as several other diseases

Differentiation (Embryology): the process in embryonic development whereby unspecialised cells or tissues become specialised for particular functions

Diploid Containing two of each chromosome. All cells in the body are diploid, except gametes

Dislocation The displacement of a bone from its joint

Diuresis The passage of copious amounts of urine

Dizygotic twins See Binovular twins

Döderleins bacilli Commensals of the vagina that maintain an acidic environment

Dysmenorrhoea Painful menstruation

Dyspnoea Difficulty breathing

Eclampsia Condition progressing from preeclampsia in which convulsions occur

Ectoderm Outer layer of embryonic tissue

Ectopic pregnancy Pregnancy in which the fertilised egg embeds outside the uterus

Effacement (also called Ripening) Shortening of the cervix, resulting in the loss of the cervical canal

Ejaculation Expulsion of semen from the penis

Elasticity The ability of a structure to regain its original shape after having been stretched

Elimination The removal of waste

Embolism A clot that travels in the bloodstream

Embryo The product of conception from implantation until 8 weeks' gestation

Embryonic disc A collection of cells in the blastocyst from which the embryo is formed

Endocrine gland A ductless gland where hormones are manufactured then absorbed directly into the bloodstream

Endometriosis The presence of tissue resembling endometrium outside the uterus, which undergoes cyclical change in response to reproductive hormones

Endometrium The lining of the uterus

Endorphin A neuropeptide that acts as an analgesic

Engagement Movement of the widest presenting part of the fetus through the pelvic brim

Engorgement The accumulation of tissue fluids and/or milk in the breasts

Enzyme A biological catalyst which brings about a chemical reaction

Epidural anaesthesia The introduction of a local anaesthetic into the epidural space to block selected spinal nerves

Epidural space The potential space between the dura mater and the vertebral column

Epilepsy A disease of the nervous system in which convulsions occur

Episiotomy Surgical incision of the perineum during delivery

Erythrocyte Red blood cell

Extrauterine Outside the uterus

Fallopian tube Uterine tube that conducts ova from the ovary to the uterus

Falx cerebri A double fold of dura mater separating the two cerebral hemispheres

Fenestration Opening in a vessel wall

Fertilisation The union of a spermatozoon and an ovum

Fetus The product of conception from its 8th week of gestation until delivery

Fissure A cleft e.g. in an organ

Fistula An abnormal opening between two organs

Flagellum A tail-like projection from a cell membrane

Fluid balance The maintenance of a balance of fluids in the body, as a result of measured ingested and excreted fluids

Folic acid One of the B vitamins required for the normal development of red blood cells

Follicle A small vesicle containing an ovum

Fontanelle An area of membrane between the bones of the fetal skull

Forewaters The bag of amniotic fluid formed in front of the presenting part of the fetus

Fornix One of four recesses formed by the protrusion of the cervix into the vagina

Fossa A hollow

Fourchette The fold of skin where the labia minora join posteriorly

Functional layer The layer of endometrium which is affected by the reproductive hormones

Fundus The base of a hollow organ situated furthest from the opening

Gamete A reproductive cell such as the ovum or spermatozoon

Ganglion A collection of nerve fibres

Gene The basic unit of genetic material, consisting of a section of DNA

Genetics The study of inheritance

Genitalia The organs of reproduction

Gestation The normal period of time required for the fetus to mature sufficiently to live independently of the mother

Glabella The bridge of the nose

Globin A protein used in the manufacture of haemoglobin

Glucagon A hormone that stimulates the production of glucose from glycogen

Glycogen The form in which carbohydrates are stored in the liver and muscle

Glycosuria The presence of glucose in urine

Gonad A hormone-secreting reproductive gland in both males and females that produces gametes

Gonadotrophin A hormone that acts on the gonads

Gonorrhoea A sexually-transmitted disease

Graafian follicle A fluid-filled vesicle containing an ovum

Gravid Pregnant

Grey matter The area of the cerebrum containing cell bodies and unmyelinated neurones

Guthrie test A test carried out on neonates on the sixth or seventh day after delivery to screen for phenylketonuria and other metabolic disorders

Gynaecoid (Pelvis): the type of pelvis most suited to childbirth

Haematoma An accumulation of blood, usually clotted, in tissue, or an organ or a space

Haemoglobin The molecule found in red blood cells responsible for the transportation of oxygen

Haemolysis The breakdown of red blood cells

Haemolytic disease of the newborn An anaemia caused by the destruction of fetal red blood cells by maternal antibodies – usually the result of rhesus incompatibility

Haemorrhage Excessive blood loss

Haemorrhagic disease A bleeding disorder caused by a lack of clotting factors

Haemorrhoids (piles) Varicose veins in the anal region

Haemostasis The cessation of bleeding

Haploid Containing a single set of unpaired chromosomes, half the normal complement of chromosomes i.e. gametes are haploid

hCG Human chorionic gonadotrophin

Heartburn A burning sensation in the midline of the chest caused by the regurgitation of acid stomach contents

Hepatic Relating to the liver

Hereditary Genetically transmitted from parents to offspring

Hernia The protrusion of an organ through a membrane such as the abdominal wall

Hindwaters Amniotic fluid situated behind the presenting part of the fetus

Histamine An enzyme released by cells which causes local vasodilation

Homeostasis The physiological process which maintains the body systems in constant balance

Hormone A chemical secreted by an endocrine cell or gland, which has its effect on another part of the body

Human chorionic gonadotrophin (hCG) A hormone produced by early chorionic villi

Human immunodeficiency virus (HIV) A virus that invades cells of the immune system, principally T-lymphocytes, and can lead to AIDS

Human placental lactogen A hormone released by the placenta that encourages breast development and the metabolism of carbohydrates

Humoral immunity An antibody response to an antigen

Hyaluronidase An enzyme released by spermatozoa to dissolve the zona pellucida and corona radiata surrounding an ovum

Hydrocephalus Excessive cerebrospinal fluid distending the ventricles of the brain

Hymen The membrane covering the vagina, which either perforates spontaneously before puberty, or ruptures on first sexual intercourse

Hyperemesis Excessive vomiting

Hyperglycaemia High blood glucose levels

Hyperplasia The increased production and growth of normal cells

Hypertension High blood pressure

Hypertonic Describes frequent strong contractions

Hypertrophy The enlargement of muscle fibres due to cells increasing in size, rather than dividing

Hypoglycaemia Low blood glucose levels

Hypotonic Describes deficient muscle tone during labour

Hypoxia Decreased level of oxygen in body tissues

Immune response The immune system's reaction to antigens

Immunity The body's resistance to infections

Immunoglobulin An antibody

Implantation The embedding of the fertilised ovum into the decidua of the uterus

Inborn error of metabolism A congenital disorder involving the absence of an enzyme

Incontinence The involuntary passage of urine

Induction of labour Initiating labour by amniotomy or the use of hormones

Infarct An area of dead tissue caused by inadequate blood supply

Infertility The inability of a woman to conceive, or of a man to induce conception

Infibulation A type of female circumcision

Inheritance The transmission of genetic information from parent to offspring

Innate immunity Non-specific immunity

Inner cell mass A collection of cells in the blastocyst

Inorganic Derived from neither animal nor vegetable matter

Instrumental delivery Delivery of the fetus with the use of forceps or ventouse

Insulin A hormone which initiates the storage of glucose as glycogen

Integumentary Relating to the skin

Interstitial Between cells

Intracellular Inside cells

Introitus The entrance into a cavity or space, e.g. the vaginal orifice

Involution The return of the uterus to its non-pregnant state

Ischaemia A deficiency of blood flowing to a particular part of the body, caused by a constriction or blockage of blood vessels

Isthmus A narrowed part of an organ or tissue

Jaundice The yellow discoloration of the skin or the whites of the eyes caused by an excess of fat-soluble bilirubin in the blood

Juxtaglomerular apparatus Specialised cells found in the kidney involved in the control of blood pressure

Kernicterus A condition in the newborn characterised by abnormal movements, caused by damage to the basal ganglia of the brain by high levels of bilirubin

Ketone bodies Acids released during the process of fat metabolism

Ketonuria The presence of ketones in the urine

Labour The process of childbirth

Lactation The production of colostrum then milk by the mammary glands of the breast

Lactiferous Relating to the movement or secretion of breast milk e.g. the lactiferous ducts

Lambda The posterior fontanelle

Lanugo Fine hair present on the fetus, shed at about 40 weeks

Leucocyte A white blood cell

Leucorrhoea Whitish or yellowish vaginal discharge, which may increase during pregnancy

Linea nigra Pigmented line running from the umbilicus to the mons pubis which women develop during pregnancy

Lipids A group of organic substances including fats that are insoluble in water, and provide a source of body fuel

Lipolysis The breakdown of fats and other lipids into fatty acid

Liquor amnii (also called Amniotic fluid) The fluid produced by the amniotic membrane in which the fetus is contained

Living ligatures The oblique muscle fibres of the uterus which ligate blood vessels after the delivery of the placenta

Lochia Discharges from the uterus during involution

Lumen The space within a tube, e.g. blood vessel, intestine

Luteinising hormone A hormone released by the pituitary gland that acts on the corpus luteum

Lymphocyte A type of white blood cell associated with the immune system

Lymphopoietin A hormone involved in the production of lymphocytes

Lysozyme An antibacterial enzyme found in tissue fluids such as tears

Macrophage A large phagocyte derived from a monocyte

Macrostructure Structure that can be viewed with the naked eye

Malaise A general feeling of being unwell

Malformation Incorrect formation of a body structure

Mammary gland The milk-producing gland, i.e. the breast

Mast cell A cell found in body tissue, involved in the inflammatory and allergic responses

Mastitis Inflammation of breast tissue

Maternal Relating to the mother

Meatus A passage or opening

Mechanism Description of the rotation and accommodation of the fetus to the pelvis and pelvic floor during labour and delivery

Meconium Waste material formed in the gut of the fetus in utero, excreted as the first stools of the newborn baby

Meiosis The type of cell division by which gametes are formed, with the haploid number of chromosomes in each cell

Menarche The start of menstruation at puberty

Mendelson's syndrome A condition in which acid is inhaled from the oesophagus into the lungs causing irritation and oedema

Meninges The membranes covering the brain and spinal cord

Menopause Cessation of egg cell production and menstruation

Menstrual cycle The cyclical physiological changes in the endometrium of the uterus, controlled by ovarian and pituitary hormones, which culminates in menstruation

Menstruation The shedding of the endometrium, along with blood, at intervals of about 1 month in non-pregnant women of child-bearing age

Mentum Chin

Mesoderm The middle germ layer of cells of the early embryo, which gives rise to e.g. connective tissue, bone, muscle, blood and kidneys

Metabolism The sum of all the biochemical reactions involved in the continued growth and functioning of the human body

Microcephaly Abnormal smallness of the head

Micturition The passage of urine

Milk ejection reflex The contraction of myoepithelial cells around the alveoli moving milk towards the nipple

Mitochondrion An organelle in the cytoplasm of every cell involved in the production of energy

Mitosis A type of cell division resulting in two genetically identical daughter cells, each containing a full complement of chromosomes

Mittelschmerz Lower abdominal pain felt by some women at ovulation

Monozygotic twins see Uniovular twins

Morbidity rate The number of cases of a disease present in a stated population

Morning sickness Nausea and vomiting related to early pregnancy

Mortality rate The number of deaths in a population in a defined period

Motility The ability to move

Moulding The overlapping of the fetal skull bones

Multigravidous A woman who is pregnant for the second or subsequent time

Multiple sclerosis A progressive disease involving the destruction of the myelin sheaths surrounding nerves in the brain and spinal cord

Mutation An alteration in the genetic code, not caused by normal genetic processes

Myoepithelial cells Contractile epithelial cells surrounding the alveoli of the breasts

Myometrium The muscle layer of the uterus

Narcotic A substance that produces insensibility and stupor and relieves pain, e.g. morphine

Nausea Sensation of being about to vomit

Necrosis The death of cells in tissue or an organ

Neonate A newborn, up to 4 weeks after birth

Neural tube defect A congenital abnormality of the spinal column

Neuroendocrine Involving the interaction of both the nervous and endocrine systems

Neuroglia Supporting cells of the nervous system consisting, in the central nervous system, of astrocytes, oligodendrocytes and microglia

Neurone A nerve cell, which transmits electrical nerve impulses

Neurotransmitter A chemical substance released by a synaptic end bulb to stimulate the adjacent neurone

Nidation The implantation of the embryo into the decidua of the uterus

Nocioceptor A nerve ending that detects painful stimuli

Nocturia The passage of urine during the night

Non-shivering thermogenesis The production of heat in the neonate by the metabolism of brown fat

Noxious Poisonous, harmful

Occiput The back part of the head

Oedema An excessive amount of interstitial fluid

Oestrogen A female sex hormone

Oligohydramnios A condition in which the volume of amniotic fluid is abnormally low

Oliguria A reduced output of urine

Oogenesis The development of ova in the ovaries

Ophthalmia neonatorum A form of conjunctivitis, characterised by a purulent discharge from the eyes of the neonate before the age of 21 days

Organelle A small structure within a cell, specialized for a specific function, e.g. the nucleus, mitochondrion

Organogenesis The formation of organs

Os An opening or a bone

Ossicles Small bones, such as the three auditory ossicles of the middle ear

Ossification The formation of bone

Ovarian cycle The cycle of development and release of an ovum

Ovary The main female gonad, or reproductive organ

Ovulation The release of an ovum by the ovary

Ovum A mature female gamete

Oxytocin A hormone released by the posterior pituitary gland which is involved in the contraction of the uterus and the myoepithelial cells around the alveoli of the breast

Palate The roof of the mouth, separating the mouth from the nasal cavity

Palpation Examination by touch

Partial pressure Pressure exerted by one gas in a mixture of gases

Paternal Relating to the father

Pathology The study of disease processes

Pelvimetry Measurement of the internal diameters of the pelvis

Pendulous abdomen Extreme laxity of abdominal muscles during pregnancy

Perimetrium The outermost layer of the uterus

Perinatal The period around the time of birth, defined as being from the 24th week of pregnancy until 1 week postpartum

Perinatal mortality rate The death rate during the perinatal period

Perineal body The area of muscle between the vaginal orifice and the rectum

Perineum The pelvic floor and associated structures

Peristalsis Spasmodic muscular contractions that create a wave-like movement along some hollow tubes of the body, e.g. the intestines

Phagocyte A cell which ingests particles or microorganisms

Pharmacology The study of use and effects of drugs

Phenylketonuria An inherited condition in which excessive phenylalanine accumulates in the blood, damaging the nervous system and leading to mental retardation

Physiology The study of the functioning of living organisms

Pituitary gland An endocrine gland situated beneath the hypothalamus

Placenta The structure in the uterus responsible for the developing fetus's respiration, excretion and nutrition

Plasma The straw-coloured fluid part of blood

Platelet (also called Thrombocyte) Small disc-shaped cells in the blood, involved in the formation of a clot

Plexus An intertwined collection of nerves or blood vessels

Polydipsia Excessive thirst

Polyphagia Excessive hunger

Polyuria The production of excessive amounts of urine

Postnatal After childbirth

Postpartum After delivery

Preeclampsia (also called Pregnancy-induced hypertension) A condition that can occur in pregnancy, characterised by hypertension, proteinuria and oedema

Precipitate delivery Rapid labour and delivery

Preconception Before conception

Pregnancy The period of time between conception and delivery

Pregnancy-induced hypertension see Preeclampsia

Prenatal Before delivery

Prepregnancy Before pregnancy

Presentation That part of the fetus entering the pelvis first

Primigravida A woman who is pregnant for the first time

Primordial follicle A follicle present in the ovary since its development

Progesterone A female sex hormone

Prognosis The probable outcome of a condition

Prolactin A hormone involved in milk production

Prolapse The downward displacement of an organ or part of an organ

Proliferate Multiply

Prostaglandin A hormone involved in the initiation of labour and in the inflammatory response

Proteinuria The presence of protein in the urine

Pruritus gravidarum Itching during pregnancy

Psychology The study of the mind and behaviour

Psychosis Severe mental illness, whose symptoms include loss of contact with reality

Puberty The period during which the reproductive organs become active

Puerperium The period of up to about 6 weeks after childbirth, when the reproductive organs return to their non-pregnant state

Pyelonephritis Inflammation of the kidneys and ureters

Pyloric sphincter The sphincter between the stomach and the duodenum

Pyrexia Fever

Referred pain Pain that is felt in an area remote from its origin

Regeneration The natural renewal of a structure such as lost tissue

Relaxin A hormone that loosens the joints of the pelvis during pregnancy

Renal Relating to the kidneys

Renal threshold The level at which substances in the blood begin to be excreted in urine

Reproduction The formation of new cells or organisms

Reproductive cycle The cycle encompassing all of the hormonal changes relating to the functioning of the female reproductive organs

Respiratory distress syndrome Difficulty in the establishment of respiration in the preterm infant due to lack of surfactant, needed for the initial inflation and normal expansion of the lungs

Retinopathy of prematurity (also called Retrolental fibroplasia) Damage to the retina caused by high levels of inhaled oxygen in the preterm infant, possibly leading to blindness

Retraction Shortening of muscle fibres

Retraction ring A muscular indentation felt between the upper and lower uterine segments

Retrolental fibroplasia see Retinopathy of prematurity

Retroperitoneal External to the peritoneal lining of the abdominal cavity

Retroplacental Behind the placenta

Rhesus factor A group of antigens found on the surface of red blood cells, forming the basis of the rhesus blood group system

Rheumatic fever An acute fever, caused by streptococcal infection, that may damage the valves of the heart

Ripening see Effacement

Rubella German measles

Rugae Large folds in the mucous membrane of an organ e.g. the vagina

Sacral Relating to the sacrum

Sacrococcygeal joint The hinge joint between the sacral vertebrae and coccyx

Sagittal suture A suture (immovable joint) situated between the two parietal bones on the fetal skull

Sclerosis Hardening of a tissue

Secondary sexual characteristics The physical characteristics which form or mature under the influence of the hormones of puberty

Secretory phase The phase of the menstrual cycle in which the glands of the endometrium increase production

Sedative A drug which calms the mood, relieving anxiety and tension

Semen The mixture of spermatozoa and seminal fluid discharged from the penis during ejaculation

Septum A wall dividing two cavities

Sinciput Forehead

Sinus A hollow in tissue

Somatic Relating to the body

Somite A group of specialised cells in the fetus that develop into vertebrae

Spasticity Hypertonic muscle tone with abnormal reflexes

Spermatogenesis The production of mature spermatozoa in the testis

Spermatozoon A male gamete

Spermicide A substance which kills spermatozoa

Sphincter The circular muscle surrounding an orifice e.g. anal sphincter

Spina bifida A congenital malformation of the vertebral column

Stasis A halt in the flow of fluids such as blood or lymph

Station The position of the presenting part of the fetus in relation to the ischial spines of the pelvis

Status asthmaticus A prolonged asthmatic attack

Stenosis The abnormal narrowing of a passage or opening e.g. a blood vessel or a heart valve

Stillbirth Delivery of a fetus which has shown no sign of life

Stratified In layers

Stress Any undue strain exerted on the mind or body

Stress incontinence The involuntary passage of urine on coughing and straining, common in women with weak pelvic floor muscles following childbirth

Stressor Any agent or stimulus that produces stress

Striae gravidarum Stretch marks that may appear on the abdomen, breasts and thighs during pregnancy, and seem to result from overstretching of the elastic fibres of the skin

Sulcus A groove or furrow, e.g. the groove between the cotyledons of the placenta

Supine hypotension Low blood pressure when lying on one's back caused by the pregnant uterus compressing the vena cava

Supplement A substance added to the diet to make up a deficiency

Surfactant A phospholipid present in the alveoli of the lungs which decreases surface tension, so preventing the alveoli from collapsing

Suture A fibrous joint between the bones of the skull

Symphysis pubis The cartilage between the pubic bones

Symptom Any evidence of disordered physiology perceived by the patient

Synergy Enhanced action resulting from the combined effect of two or more substances

Synthesis The production of more complex molecules from simple molecules/atoms

Syntocinon A synthetic form of oxytocin

Systemic lupus erythematosus An autoimmune disorder characterised by a widespread inflammatory response within tissues

Tentorium cerebelli The double layer of dura mater that separates the cerebrum from the cerebellum

Teratogen Any factor that causes a congenital defect

Testosterone The male sex hormone

Thermogenesis The production of heat

Thermoregulation The control of body temperature

Thrombocyte see Platelet

Thrombophlebitis Inflammation of the wall of a vein resulting in clot formation

Thrombosis The formation of a clot in a blood vessel

Thrombus A blood clot

Thyrotoxicosis Overactivity of the thyroid gland

Toxin A poison

Trauma A physical wound or injury; or a psychologically painful event

Trimester A 3-month period of pregnancy

Trophoblast The outer covering of the blastocyst from which the placenta develops

Tubal pregnancy A pregnancy in which the embryo embeds in the uterine tube

Ultrasound Sound waves which can be transmitted through tissue to indicate changes in density

Umbilical cord The temporary structure that carries blood from the placenta to the body of the fetus

Uniovular twins (also called Monozygotic twins) Identical twins, derived from the division of one fertilised ovum

Urinalysis Analysis of the constituents of urine

Uterine polarity The difference between the strength of contractions in the upper and lower uterine segments, resulting in cervical dilatation

Uterus (also called the Womb) The hollow muscular organ in the female in which the embryo embeds and is nourished

Vaginitis Inflammation of the vagina, leading to itching, increased vaginal discharge and pain on passing urine

Varicose vein Swollen vein resulting from structural changes in its walls

Vasectomy A surgical operation involving the ligation of the vas deferens to prevent the ejaculation of semen, leading to sterility if performed on both ducts, and therefore used as form of birth control

Vasoconstriction The narrowing of blood vessels

Vasodilation The dilation of blood vessels

Ventricular septal defect An abnormal opening in the septum between the ventricles

Vernix caseosa The greasy covering of the skin of the fetus

Vertex (of skull) That area of the fetal skull surrounding the posterior fontanelle that presents first in a fully flexed fetus

Vesical Relating to or affecting the bladder

Vestibule A cavity at the entrance to a hollow part of the body, e.g. the area enclosed by the labia minora

Villus Root-like structure of the placenta which lies in the maternal sinuses under the placenta

Viscosity Thickness

Vulva External genitalia of the female

Womb See Uterus

X chromosome The sex chromosome present in both sexes. The female has two X chromosomes

Xiphisternum The lowest portion of the sternum

Y chromosome The male chromosome

Zona pellucida The thick layer of cells surrounding the ovum, which is penetrated by at least one spermatozoon to permit fertilisation, and which remains until the blastocyst reaches the uterus

Zygote The cell formed from the fertilisation of an ovum by a spermatozoon

Index

Page numbers in **bold** type refer to illustrations and tables.